The Complete Body, Mind, and Spirit

Edited by
Nancy Allison, CMA

Keats Publishing

Chicago   New York   San Francisco   Lisbon   London   Madrid   Mexico City
Milan   New Delhi   San Juan   Seoul   Singapore   Sydney   Toronto

Library of Congress Cataloging-in-Publication Data

The complete body, mind, and spirit / edited by Nancy Allison.
       p.   cm.
      Rev. ed. of: The illustrated encyclopedia of body-mind disciplines. 1999.
      Includes bibliographical references and index.
      ISBN 0-658-00704-1
      1. Alternative medicine.   2. Mind and body therapies.   I. Allison, Nancy,
1954– .   II. Illustrated encyclopedia of body-mind disciplines.

R733.I46   2000
615.5—dc21   00-053477

Keats Publishing

A Division of The McGraw·Hill Companies

Originally published in 1999 by The Rosen Publishing Group, Inc.

1 2 3 4 5 6 7 8 9 0 VL/VL 0 9 8 7 6 5 4 3 2 1

ISBN 0-658-00704-1

This book was set in Palatino by Wendy Staroba Loreen
Printed and bound by Vicks Lithograph and Printing Corporation

Interior design by Wendy Staroba Loreen

McGraw-Hill books are available at special quantity discounts to use as premiums and sales promotions, or for use in corporate training programs. For more information, please write to the Director of Special Sales, Professional Publishing, McGraw-Hill, Two Penn Plaza, New York, NY 10121-2298. Or contact your local bookstore.

The purpose of this book is to educate. It is sold with the understanding that the publisher and author shall have neither liability nor responsibility for any injury caused or alleged to be caused directly or indirectly by the information contained in this book. While every effort has been made to ensure its accuracy, the book's contents should not be construed as medical advice. Each person's health needs are unique. To obtain recommendations appropriate to your particular situation, please consult a qualified health care provider.

About the Editor

Nancy Allison, CMA, has always been interested in the role of movement in human society, its inner impulses and outer forms. This interest led her to pursue a career in dance. During her childhood she performed with the National Ballet of Washington, D.C., and with Moscow's world-renowned Bolshoi Ballet during its 1963 American tour. She graduated with honors from Ohio University at Athens with a B.F.A. in dance. While at Ohio University she augmented her study of dance with courses in philosophy and psychology. As a young professional dancer she joined the Theater of the Open Eye in New York City, founded by choreographer Jean Erdman and the late Joseph Campbell. From the 1970s through the 1990s, Allison distinguished herself as the leading interpreter of Erdman's dance repertoire from the 1940s and 1950s, producing the three-volume video archive *Dance and Myth: The World of Jean Erdman.*

Inspired by both Erdman and Campbell, Allison expanded her exploration of movement to include the body-mind relationship. She has studied hatha yoga, t'ai chi ch'üan, the Pilates Method, bioenergetics, authentic movement, and Laban movement analysis, in which she earned a degree as a certified movement analyst. A much-sought-after educator, Allison has taught master classes and workshops throughout the United States. She resides in New York City, where she is a professor at the School of Education of New York University.

Contents

Acknowledgments xi

Introduction xiii

1. Alternative Health Models 1
   Ayurvedic Medicine   4
   Holistic Health   6
   Homeopathy   9
   Naturopathic Medicine   13
   Shamanism   16
   Traditional Chinese Medicine   20
   Wellness   25

2. Skeletal Manipulation Methods 29
   Chiropractic   33
   CranioSacral Therapy   35
   Network Chiropractic   38
   Osteopathy   40
   Zero Balancing®   44

3. Nutritional and Dietary Practices 47
   Herbal Medicine   52
   Orthomolecular Medicine   55

4. Mind/Body Medicine 59
   Biofeedback Training   63
   Guided Imagery   65
   Hypnotherapy   68
   Interactive Guided Imagery℠   71
   Psychoneuroimmunology   73

5. Sensory Therapies 77
   Aromatherapy   81
   Bates Method   83
   Behavioral Vision Therapy   85
   Eye Movement Desensitization and Reprocessing   88
   Flower Remedies   90

Hydrotherapy   92
Light Therapy   95
Sounding   100
Tomatis Method   102

6. Subtle Energy Practices 105
Do-In   108
Feng Shui   110
Magnet Therapy   113
Polarity Therapy   115
Qigong   118
Reiki   121
SHEN®   124
Therapeutic Touch   126

7. Massage 129
Bowen Technique   135
Connective Tissue Therapy℠   136
CORE Structural Integrative Therapy   138
Infant Massage   139
Muscular Therapy   142
Myofascial Release   143
Myofascial Trigger-Point Therapy   145
Reflexology   146
Rolfing®   149
Rosen Method   151
St. John Method of Neuromuscular Therapy   154
Swedish Massage   155

8. Acupuncture and Asian Bodywork 159
Acupressure   162
Acupuncture   164
Jin Shin Do® Bodymind Acupressure™   167
Jin Shin Jyutsu® Physio-Philosophy   169
Process Acupressure   171
Shiatsu   173
Tui Na   175

9. Movement Therapy Methods 179
Alexander Technique   183
Aston-Patterning®   185
Bartenieff Fundamentals℠   187
Body-Mind Centering®   190
Feldenkrais Method®   192
Hanna Somatic Education®   194
Hellerwork   197
Ideokinesis   199
Kinetic Awareness   201
Meir Schneider Self-Healing Method   203
Sensory Awareness   206

Soma Neuromuscular Integration   208
Somatorespiratory Integration   210
Trager Psychophysical Integration   211

10. Somatic Practices 215
Brain Gym®   218
Contact Improvisation   220
Continuum   222
Eurythmy   224
Gurdjieff Movements   226
Pilates Method of Body Conditioning®   229
ROM Dance   232
Skinner Releasing Technique   234
Spatial Dynamics℠   236
T'ai Chi Ch'üan   239

11. Martial Arts. 243
Aikido   247
Capoeira   248
Ju Jutsu   251
Judo   254
Karate   256
Kendo   259
Kung Fu Wu Su   262
Taekwondo   265

12. Yoga. 269
Integral Yoga   276
Iyengar Yoga   277
Kripalu Yoga   278

13. Meditation. 281
Relaxation Response   286
Transcendental Meditation   288

14. Psychophysical Evaluation Frameworks. 291
Enneagram   293
Kestenberg Movement Profile   296
Laban Movement Analysis   298
Movement Pattern Analysis   301

15. Expressive and Creative Arts Therapies 305
Art Therapy   311
Authentic Movement   313
Dance Therapy   315
Drama Therapy   318
Halprin Life/Art Process   321
Journal Therapy   323
Multimodal Expressive Arts Therapy   325
Music Therapy   328
Poetry Therapy   331
Sandplay Therapy   334

16. Body-Oriented Psychotherapies 337
    Bioenergetics   341
    Bodynamic Analysis   344
    Core Energetics   346
    coreSomatics®   350
    Emotional-Kinesthetic Psychotherapy   351
    Focusing   352
    Gestalt Therapy   355
    Hakomi Integrative Somatics   358
    Holotropic Breathwork™   360
    Medical Orgone Therapy   363
    Organismic Body Psychotherapy   366
    Pesso Boyden System Psychomotor   368
    Process-Oriented Psychology   371
    Psychodrama   372
    Psychosynthesis   375
    Radix   377
    Rebirthing   378
    Rubenfeld Synergy Method™   380
    Unergi   383

Contributors 385

Acknowledgments

So many people have helped create this volume that it is impossible to name them all, but given this opportunity, I would like to try. I am deeply indebted to Joseph Campbell, whose personal encouragement guided my early explorations into the world of body-mind and whose spirit and knowledge are a constant wellspring of inspiration to me. I also want to thank my husband, who believed in my ability to complete this project and nurtured both it and me with his constant love and support.

I am eternally grateful to all of the distinguished teachers, healers, and writers who contributed entries to this volume. Their dedication to their respective fields and their generous gifts of time and knowledge to this project have earned my undying respect and admiration. I believe each of them, in his or her own wonderfully unique way, is helping to make this world a better place.

Certain writers and consultants have been particularly influential in my own development, and I want to acknowledge their gifts to me: t'ai chi master Sophia Delza, who passed away during the course of our work, taught me to follow the flow of the life force in its endless cycle from full to empty and back to full again; Ed Groff, Janet Hamburg, Clio Pavlantos, and Jackie Hand, who taught me to recognize the endless permutations of that force through the language of Laban movement analysis; Nina Robinson, who introduced me to the thrill of liberating that force through bioenergetics; Lillo (Leela) Way, who taught me the true nature of a spiritual practice; Jane Magee and Jackie Hand, whose healing hands managed to untangle the knots into which I seem to endlessly entangle my body; and Dr. Domenick Masiello, whose healing artistry has restored me and so many of my loved ones to a vibrant state of health. I am also indebted to Dr. Masiello for the many fine contributing writers he recommended for this project. In that regard I am also deeply indebted to Thomas Claire and Ken Frey.

There are also those who, while not contributing writers, were important to my ability to realize this project: Clifford Schulman, Jeff McMahon, Anne Johnson, Joanna Kosartes Vergoth, and Cynthia Reynolds, all of whom recommended contributing writers; Romana Kryzanowska, who gave me my first teaching job in the body-mind arena at the Pilates Studio; Carol Walker and Steven Giordano, who encouraged me to expand and explore that skill and knowledge at SUNY, Purchase; Miriam Roskin Berger, who has supported so many of my creative endeavors and gave me the opportunity to develop my teaching at New York

University; and all of my students over the years who continually show me through their amazing transformations that my approach to this material is valuable and life-enhancing.

With such a huge task spanning so many years, I'm sure there are others I have missed. Please forgive me and know that you have my deepest respect and gratitude.

—*NANCY ALLISON, CMA*

Introduction

Body-mind is a term often seen in print and heard in conversation today. It is used frequently both in private discussions about disease and healing and in public forums on health care, where the value of alternative or complementary medicine continues to gain recognition. Today, many educators are developing new methods that use the body-mind connection to help children learn how to live productive and creative lives in today's complex technological society. The phrase *body-mind* resonates through the halls of gymnasiums, in physical conditioning studios, and in self-defense classes. It echoes in theaters, dance studios, and music practice rooms. What exactly is this concept that is exciting so many people and changing the way we heal, learn, work, and play?

Body-mind is a way of seeing and understanding the human organism. To see a human being in terms of body-mind is to see that person as a totality wherein his physical, psychological, and spiritual aspects are interrelated and reflective of one another. In other words, the body is not simply the material receptacle of the mind or spirit, but the medium through which we experience, each in a unique and individual way, the unfolding, transforming nature of spirit itself.

From this perspective, the functioning of the body influences the functioning of the mind and the emotions. In a like manner, thoughts and feelings have a profound and direct effect on the body. On a deeper level, many body-mind models believe that the physical, emotional, and mental aspects of human experience are a reflection of and are inextricably linked to an all-pervasive spiritual essence. In different cultures and in different times, this spiritual essence has had many names: Atman, the Tao, God, energy, the force.

A body-mind discipline is an organized program of activity that seeks to awaken and activate the links between body, mind, and spirit. The practice of a body-mind discipline may involve a variety of activities, all of which aim to incorporate the physical body with the sensing, feeling, thinking, and/or intuiting faculties of the mind. Through the practice of a body-mind discipline, one develops awareness of physical sensations and mental and emotional processes. This awareness can be the basis of healing and improved health, greater efficiency and expressiveness in one's activities, more rewarding relationships and interactions, and a deeper, clearer sense of purpose in one's life.

The practice of body-mind disciplines is ancient. We have evidence that some, such as yoga and various forms of touch therapy, were widespread well before written treatises were available. The ancient disciplines were based on one of the earliest and most steadfast of human desires: to live a long, meaningful, and healthy life. For most of human history this meant living in a state of balance and harmony, both within oneself and within one's environment. The body-mind disciplines that evolved in all cultures addressed, each in its own particular way, the many elements that create and maintain this balance and harmony.

Western culture, with its roots in the civilizations of the Fertile Crescent and ancient Greece, once shared this same value for balance and harmony. The Greek physician Hippocrates understood the importance of balance and believed his patients' health could be affected by many factors. He believed it was more important to know the kind of person he was treating than to know what kind of disease the person had. He was known to prescribe herbs, changes in diet, forms of hydrotherapy, skeletal manipulation, movement therapy, and creative arts therapies to help his patients regain a state of balance and harmony.

Over many centuries, however, there has been a gradual erosion of this holistic viewpoint as Western culture developed a highly technical and specialized perspective. By comparison, today most of us no longer have a single physician who knows us as a total human being and draws on any number of healing methods. Instead, we go to one specialist for a problem in our ears, nose, and throat, another for our gastrointestinal tract, and still another for troubling emotional situations. Although each specialist may have a wealth of information regarding her area of expertise, no one seems to be looking at the whole picture. Often, the pharmaceutical or surgical solutions each specialist recommends address only one aspect of our problem and sometimes create new ones.

This segmented, specialized perspective is evident not only in our approach to health care, but in our approach to education and the arts as well. Instead of encouraging each person to feel alive, whole, and connected to the rest of the world, this perspective seems to foster a lack of confidence in one's experience and judgment, a weakened sense of personal agency, and a feeling of spiritual isolation. For this reason more and more people today are seeking the holistic, centering experience of body-mind disciplines.

In this volume we have tried to include all of the major disciplines with which a reader may come into contact. With a subject of such scope, it was necessary to set certain limits in order to complete the task. We deliberately excluded any art or skill that is used primarily for performance or competition, although we recognize that any such art or skill may be practiced from a body-mind perspective. We also excluded any practice that is exclusively associated with a specific religious practice, although here again we do not intend to diminish the value of any religious practice in its ability to incorporate body and mind. What we have included is a cross-cultural sampling of techniques and methods that seek to develop the body-mind connection and that have evolved in the worlds of health care, education, physical conditioning, self-defense, spirituality, psychology, and the arts.

We have arranged the entries in sixteen sections that generally reflect the world in which the disciplines developed, highlight the multicultural approaches to a particular practice, or sometimes draw attention to historical connections. Each section is introduced by an essay that provides an overview of the histories, theoretical foundations, and methodologies of the disciplines included in that section. The introductory material also helps relate each individual section to other sections of the encyclopedia. It is possible to gain a broad perspective of the entire world of body-mind by simply reading the sixteen introductory essays.

Most of the entries are written by certified practitioners of these disciplines. The entries describe in detail the history, philosophy, and techniques of the specific disciplines. The entries also describe what it feels like to practice or experience the discipline. It is our hope that the reader not only will gain intellectual knowledge from reading an entry, but will be stimulated on a sensory level as well.

Within each of the sections, the reader will find disciplines that work along several different continuums. The broad spectrum of approaches reflects the belief of body-mind disciplines that each individual is unique and has specific strengths, weaknesses, and predilections. The first of these continuums may be best described as the percentage of physical work compared to the percentage of mental or emotional work required of the practitioner. For example, somato respiratory integration requires the practitioner to remain relatively still, focusing the mind on physical sensations and emotional memories, whereas the Feldenkrais Method® develops awareness of mental and emotional patterns by moving the body through prescribed spatial forms. This continuum, found within individual sections of the encyclopedia, is also apparent from section to section. All of the practices in the Meditation section approach the process of building the body-mind connection somewhat more from the use of the mind, whereas all of the disciplines in the Somatic Practices section come at the process somewhat more from the use of the body. A person may enter the world of body-mind at any point along this continuum that suits one's needs or temperament.

Another continuum along which the various practices can be viewed concerns the degree of spontaneous action compared to structured action used by the discipline. For example, contact improvisation and Skinner release technique work largely through improvisational forms created by the practitioner. The quality of one's conscious control of the movement patterns is loose and free-flowing. By contrast, the Pilates Method and t'ai chi ch'üan use intricately structured movement sequences that rarely vary. They require a different kind of control in order to achieve a free-flowing connection of body and mind.

Another of the continuums concerns the degree of involvement of the practitioner, or receiver, as a whole. In any of the forms of massage therapy, the receiver is relatively passive in contrast to the active participation required by any of the forms of martial arts. All body-mind disciplines, however, ultimately encourage the active participation of the practitioner on some level. As the practice awakens awareness of physical sensations and mental or emotional processes, the participant naturally becomes more capable of taking an active role in the practice, whether that means learning how to relax and experience physical sensations more deeply, or learning to follow complex thought, breath, and movement patterns more effortlessly and subtly. This active awareness and participation is a basic value of all body-mind disciplines.

Some of the disciplines in this volume have as their primary goal the relief of physical pain. It may not seem immediately clear how such practices develop the body-mind connection. In body-mind terms, the response to pain can be the first step toward awakening a deeper awareness of the body. The theoretical underpinnings of every discipline included here view pain as a message from the body to the mind that some vital link between the two is not functioning. Pain is the cry of the body when it has been ignored, when the body-mind connection has not been honored. When viewed this way, pain is transformed from a symptom to be eradicated into a call to undertake a journey of self-discovery.

We hope this volume offers you, the reader, useful information for your unique journey. We wish each of you a voyage filled with the excitement of discovery, the creativity of transformation, and the joys of fulfillment.

PART 1:

Alternative Health Models

Alternative health models consist of a variety of ways of viewing health and sickness and depicting the relationship between body and mind. Each model has developed a system of health care with associated practices and disciplines. These health models are categorized as alternative because they are different from the allopathic paradigm, the scientific framework of contemporary Western health care.

In the allopathic model the body is viewed as a self-contained machine or collection of systems that malfunction with age or injury, or when invaded by infectious microbes or germs. A battery of defensive techniques was developed to deal with these causes of malfunction. In contrast, alternative health models see the body as one aspect of a whole person, along with mind and spirit. They view illness as an imbalance between these three interdependent aspects, or between a human being and his environment. Since the 1960s, because of the high cost and sometimes ineffectiveness or damaging side effects of allopathic health care practices, more and more people have begun exploring the possibilities of alternative health models.

AYURVEDIC
MEDICINE

HOLISTIC HEALTH

HOMEOPATHY

NATUROPATHIC
MEDICINE

SHAMANISM

TRADITIONAL
CHINESE MEDICINE

WELLNESS

A Historical Survey of Health Models

The oldest and most widespread alternative health model is used in shamanism and contemporary shamanistic counseling. Shamanic healers believe that all things have a spirit, including rocks, rivers, the sky, and the earth. According to the shamanic model of health, spirits are responsible for the physical and psychological health or sickness of all individuals and communities. Ancient shamans developed methods of interacting with spirits to affect individual or communal health. Contemporary shamanic counselors continue to use these traditional healing techniques today.

Over time, more abstract metaphors evolved to describe the spirit world and its interactions with the material world. The concept of energy or energetic forces replaced the discussion of individualized spirits in human philosophical and medical thought. Practitioners of health models such as ayurveda in India and traditional Chinese medicine throughout the rest of Asia developed intricate theories and practices to work with the complex patterns of energies they perceived moving through the universe and all the people in it.

The ancient Greeks also conceived of the world as a complex of energies, and many of their healing practices reflected an integrated view of spirit and matter. The philosopher Aristotle (384–322 B.C.E.) articulated an important new tendency in Western thought. He believed that the workings of the natural world could be known through observation, experimentation, and classification. Whereas Aristotle himself believed that spiritual truth could be known through a study of the material world, his scientific method created the possibility of a split in Western thought between spirit and matter.

During the Renaissance important Greek texts were rediscovered. Many of the great thinkers of the day embraced the Aristotelian scientific method of the pursuit of knowledge. This method of inquiry met with tremendous opposition from the dominant religious and political institution of that time, the Church. The Church regarded science as a threat to its most basic theological doctrines. This opposition created in Western thought a deeper schism between the material and spiritual realms. Certain Western philosophers and scientists, however, continued to investigate health models that unify body, mind, and spirit. Health models such as Samuel Hahnemann's (1755–1843) homeopathy, which combines the science of chemistry and biology with the belief in an invisible vital life energy, developed in Europe toward the end of the Age of Reason. Later, healers such as Father Sebastian Kneipp (1821–1897) found other ways to integrate spiritual beliefs with scientific inquiry. His reexamination of ancient herbal cures and indigenous European health modalities eventually made its way to the United States in the form of naturopathy.

Spiritual and material models of health coexisted in Europe and the United States for many years. In the 1930s, however, the materialistic allopathic model of health became institutionalized in organizations such as the American Medical Association, which proceeded to discredit holistic methods of healing. The successful control of infectious disease with penicillin, along with other pharmaceuticals developed throughout the 1930s through the 1950s, appeared to substantiate the allopathic approach and helped it become the dominant health model.

In the 1960s dissatisfaction with social conventions and institutions, including allopathic health care, caused Westerners to investigate the ancient health models of Eastern and indigenous cultures, as well as older European-based models. Many people began to feel that allopathic strategies did not provide a complete approach to health care. Disciplines combining Western psychological insights with ancient concepts of harmony and balance, such as holistic health and wellness, became more popular.

In the 1970s and 1980s soaring health care costs and the appearance of many chronic health problems sparked even greater interest in alternative health models. Today, these disciplines are practiced individually and as a complement to allopathic care. The philosophical viewpoint on which these disciplines are based continues to exert an ever-growing and far-reaching influence on the practice of contemporary medicine.

Some Theoretical Considerations

All of the health models presented in this section believe that in addition to the physical body, human beings are composed of nonmaterial aspects. These include thoughts, emotions, and intuitions of the mind, along with a person's spiritual essence. In these holistic models, all three aspects—body, mind, and spirit—are interdependent and determine an individual's state of health. Many of the disciplines adhering to this viewpoint believe that each person's spiritual essence interacts with the spiritual essence of the universe in much the same way that her body interacts with the material environment. Health care modalities that developed from this philosophical viewpoint seek to maintain the balance between all aspects of human beings and their relationship with their environments.

One of the major differences between the practices based on these health models and those based on allopathic health care is the emphasis the former place on the maintenance of health, rather than the spectacular and dramatic treatment of illness. Maintaining health requires monitoring the subtle physical, mental, and emotional ways that the spirit manifests itself in the body. Symptoms are viewed as physical evidence of a spiritual imbalance. They are rarely suppressed. These health models generally believe that although the suppression of symptoms may offer temporary relief from physical pain, it blocks the natural healing process and will invariably result in more serious problems. Instead of suppression, a physician follows the sequence of symptoms to find the proper way to help the body, mind, and spirit regain their state of balance.

The models in this section hold that each individual has the potential for self-healing. While each model recognizes that there are many similarities in self-healing processes, each individual's process is respected as unique. Specialists in these modalities use various techniques to enhance a person's self-healing abilities. They help clients interpret and find patterns in their symptoms, develop greater sensitivity to their physical bodies, and create a broader awareness of the interrelationship among body, mind, and spirit. In this way, these methods encourage each person to participate in his own healing.

Adopting One of These Models

These models aim to help each individual live a happy, healthy, meaningful life. Adjusting to the methods and practices of a new health model may cause a healing crisis. Once a person no longer suppresses symptoms, old physical or emotional problems may temporarily reappear, causing a person to feel weaker or more vulnerable. Eventually these suppressed causes of illness are released, and physical and emotional trauma are diminished, laying the foundation for many years of continued good health and development.

—*NANCY ALLISON*, CMA

Further Reading

Manning, Clark A., and Louis J. Vanreen. *Bioenergetic Medicines East and West: Acupuncture and Homeopathy*. Berkeley, Calif.: North Atlantic Books, 1988.

Ayurvedic Medicine

 Ayurvedic medicine, the ancient Indian science of healthy living, places great emphasis on disease prevention. It encourages the maintenance of health by achieving a balance of one's body, mind, and spirit through proper lifestyle, diet, exercise, use of herbs, and meditation. Practitioners of ayurveda learn to identify the patient's personal "constitution," understood as a unique mixture of three distinct life energies, or doshas. A healthy person employs positive thinking, diet, and lifestyle to maintain a perfect proportion of life energies.

History

Ayurvedic medicine is considered by many scholars to be the world's oldest healing science. It dates back 5,000 years to the ancient Vedic culture of the Rishis, the philosophers and religious leaders of ancient India. *Ayurveda*, which means "the science of life" in the ancient Indian language of Sanskrit, was passed on in the oral tradition from master to disciple for thousands of years. Some of this knowledge was published a few thousand years ago, notably in the ancient holy texts of Hinduism, one of the world's oldest existing literatures. It is believed that much of the tradition has actually been lost.

Ayurveda has been practiced in daily life in India for more than 4,000 years. Western medicine has influenced (and been influenced by) ayurvedic medicine, but the traditional ayurvedic lifestyle management is, for many Indians, still the primary therapy for ailments. The principles of many natural healing methods now familiar in the West, such as homeopathy, wellness, and polarity therapy, have their roots in ayurveda.

Philosophy

According to ayurvedic philosophy, the entire cosmos is made up of the five great elements—space (also known as Ether), air, fire, water, and earth. These five elements combine to form three distinct types of energy, called doshas, that are present in all people and things. There are no words in English to describe these energies, so we use the original Sanskrit words *vata, pitta,* and *kapha.* In the physical body, vata, composed of air and ether, is the subtle energy associated with movement. It governs breathing, blinking, muscle and tissue movement, pulsation of the heart, and all movements in the cytoplasm and cell membranes. Pitta, made up of fire and water, is considered the body's metabolic energy. It governs digestion, absorption, assimilation, nutrition, metabolism, and body temperature. Formed from earth and water, kapha is the energy that creates the body's structure—bones, muscles, tendons—and provides the "glue" that holds the cells together. Kapha also supplies the water for all bodily parts and systems. It lubricates joints, moisturizes the skin, and maintains immunity.

All people have vata, pitta, and kapha; one is usually primary, one secondary, and the third least prominent. In ayurveda the cause of disease is viewed as the lack of proper cellular function because of an excess or deficiency of one of these three energies and/or the presence of toxins.

Just as everyone has an individual face or thumbprint, according to ayurveda each person has a particular pattern of energy—an individual combination of physical, mental, and emotional characteristics—that is her constitution. This constitution is determined at conception. Many factors, both internal and external, can disturb this balance, which is reflected as a change in one's constitution.

When all of the three doshas are properly proportioned, they nourish and build mental and physical health in a person. The proper amount of vata promotes creativity and flexibility; pitta engenders understanding and intelligence; kapha is expressed as love, calmness, and forgiveness.

Disease is viewed as improper body functioning caused by an excess or deficiency of vata, pitta, or kapha compared to the original balance of these doshas. This imbalance can be caused by any number of factors. Genetic or congenital traits may predispose a person to develop unhealthy habits such as overeating or smoking. Accidents or other upsetting events can cause physical, mental, or emotional trauma, further disrupting the individual's balance. Furthermore, all of us have certain personal sensitivities, such as to weather conditions, spicy food, and flower pollen, which can disrupt the body's functioning.

In all of these cases, an upset in mind and/or body creates an imbalance in the doshas. When this happens, the process of disease begins, as fear and anxiety can be caused by too much or too little vata. Similarly, pitta can stir anger, hate, and jealousy, and kapha can lead to greed, attachment, and envy.

Practice

In times of health, when there are no dominant outside traumas or toxins afflicting a person, practitioners of ayurveda pay strict attention to diet and lifestyle. Just as each person has a unique constitution, there exists for each person a specific "right" lifestyle, tailored to cultivate the perfect levels of the three doshas. This right lifestyle engages body, mind, and spirit—three distinct but interrelated aspects of each person—in a regimen of diet, breathing exercises, meditation, and physical activity.

In times of illness, an ayurvedic physician must first determine which of the three basic constitutional types the patient is. Then the symptoms must be understood as to whether they are of vata, pitta, or kapha. Vata heart pain is different from pitta or kapha heart pain. Accordingly, a battery of tests is performed, including taking the pulse, observing the tongue and eyes, and listening to the tone of the patient's voice. The results of these tests, coupled with a patient's physical attributes and family traits, are used to understand the cause of disease, the dosha(s) involved, and the stage of the disease process.

The assessment provides the doctor with a standard of the patient's normal functioning. Armed with this knowledge, the ayurvedic physician can suggest steps to help return the client's health to a balanced state. Typically this involves the implementation of a different lifestyle with a new diet, exercise, and meditation plan. In cases where disease can be attributed to toxins or other external stresses, the ayurvedic physician may prescribe additional herbal remedies, breathing exercises, and sun and massage therapies. In some cases, participation in an intensive cleansing program known as *panchakarma* is suggested to help the body rid itself of accumulated toxins.

Benefits and Risks

Ayurvedic medicine is and has been practiced throughout the world for thousands of years. Its patients claim increased longevity and better health. Proper ayurvedic practice demands adherence to a strict, carefully planned lifestyle. Furthermore, many in the ayurvedic field have integrated Western medicine into their practices, acknowledging that different systems can complement one another. Those interested in pursuing ayurveda, particularly patients with preexisting conditions, should consult an established clinic or ayurvedic physician.

—DR. VASANT LAD

Resources

American Institute of Vedic Studies
   1701 Sante Fe River Road
   Sante Fe, NM 87501
   Tel: (505) 983-9385
   Provides information on training programs
   and practitioners.

American School of Ayurvedic Sciences
   10025 N.E. 4th St.
   Bellevue, WA 98004
   Tel: (206) 453-8022
   Offers a program in ayurvedic medicine.

Ayurvedic Foundation
   P.O. Box 900413
   Sandy, UT 84090-0413
   Tel: (801) 943-1480
   e-mail: Dean@ayur.com
   Web site: www.ayur.com
   Conducts workshops and custom training.
   Also produces cassette tapes and provides
   ayurvedic counseling.

Ayurvedic Institute
   11311 Menaul N.E., Suite A
   Albuquerque, NM 87112
   Tel: (505) 291-9698
   Offers a two-year program in ayurveda, as
   well as panchakarma workshops and ayurvedic herbs, supplies, and products.

Further Reading

Chopra, Deepak. *Ageless Body, Timeless Mind.*
   New York: Harmony Books, 1993.
———. *Perfect Health.* New York: Harmony
   Books, 1991.
———. *Quantum Healing.* New York: Bantam
   Books, 1990.
Frawley, David. *Ayurvedic Healing.* Salt Lake City:
   Morson Publishing, 1990.
Lad, Vasant. *Ayurveda: The Science of Self-Healing.*
   Wilmot, Calif.: Lotus Light Press, 1984.
———. *Secrets of the Pulse: The Ancient Art of Pulse
   Diagnosis.* Albuquerque: The Ayurvedic Press,
   1996.

Holistic Health

 Holistic health is an approach to life. Rather than focusing on illness or specific parts of the body, this ancient approach to health considers the whole person and how she interacts with her environment. It emphasizes the connection of mind, body, and spirit. The goal is to achieve maximum well-being, in which everything is functioning at the highest level possible. With holistic health, people accept responsibility for their own level of well-being, and everyday choices are used to take charge of one's health.

History

As far back as 5,000 years ago, ancient healing traditions in India and China stressed living a healthy way of life in harmony with nature. Socrates (fourth century B.C.E.) warned against treating only one part of the body, "for the part can never be well unless the whole is well." Although the term *holism* was introduced by South African prime minister Jan Christiaan Smuts in 1926 as a way of viewing living things as "entities greater than and different from the sum of their parts," it wasn't until the 1970s that *holistic* became a common adjective in our modern vocabulary.

Holistic concepts fell temporarily out of favor in Western societies during the twentieth century. Scientific medical advances had created a dramatic shift in the concept of health. Germs were identified as outside sources causing disease. Gaining health became a process of killing microscopic invaders with synthesized drugs. People believed they could get away with unhealthy lifestyle choices, and modern medicine would "fix" them as problems developed.

For some conditions, however, medical cures have proven more harmful than the disease itself. In addition, many chronic conditions do not respond to scientific medical treatments. In looking for other options, people are turning back to the holistic approach to health and healing. The holistic health lifestyle is regaining popularity each year, as the holistic principles offer practical options to meet the growing desire for enjoying a high level of vitality and well-being.

Basic Principles

Holistic health is based on the law of nature that a whole is made up of interdependent parts. The earth is made up of systems, such as air, land, water, plants, and animals. If life is to be sustained, these systems cannot be separated, for what is happening to one is felt by the others. In the same way, an individual is a whole made up of physical, mental, emotional, and spiritual parts. When one part is not working at its best, it impacts all of the other parts. Furthermore, this whole person is constantly interacting with everything in the surrounding environment. For example, when an individual is anxious about a history exam or a job interview, his nervousness may result in a physical reaction such as acne or a stomachache. When a person suppresses anger at a parent or a boss over a long period of time, she can develop a serious illness such as migraine headaches, emphysema, or even arthritis.

The principles of holistic health state that health is more than just not being sick. A common explanation is to view wellness as a continuum along a line. The line represents all possible degrees of health. The far left end of the line represents premature death. On the far right end is the highest possible level of wellness, or maximum well-being. The center of the line represents a lack of apparent disease. This places all levels of illness on the left half of the wellness continuum. The right half shows that even when no illness seems to be present, there is still a lot of room for improvement.

Holistic health is an ongoing process. As a lifestyle, it involves a personal commitment to move toward the right end of the wellness continuum. No matter what their current status of health, people can improve their level of well-being. Even when there are temporary setbacks, movement is always headed toward wellness.

The U.S. Centers for Disease Control and Prevention reports that the key factors influencing an individual's state of health have not changed significantly over the past twenty years. Quality of medical care is only 10 percent, heredity accounts for 18 percent, and environment is 19 percent. Everyday lifestyle choices are 53 percent. The decisions people make about their lives and habits are, therefore, by far the largest factor in determining their state of wellness.

The most obvious choices people make each day are what they "consume"—both physically and mentally. The cells in a person's body are constantly being replaced. New cells are built from what is available. Harmful substances or lack of the necessary building blocks in the body can result in imperfect cells that are unable to do what is required to keep that person healthy. Similarly, on the nonphysical level, a person's mental attitudes are "built" from what he sees and hears.

The majority of illnesses and premature deaths can be traced back to lifestyle choices. There are the well-known dangers connected with drugs, alcohol, nicotine, and unprotected sexual activity. Less recognized is the impact of excesses in things like sugar, caffeine, and negative attitudes. Combined with deficiencies in exercise, nutritious foods, and self-esteem, these gradually cause the accumulation of harmful effects. With time they diminish the quality of the "environment" within that human being, and can set the stage for illness to take hold. Quality of life, now and in the future, is actually being determined by a multitude of seemingly unimportant choices made every day.

The conventional (or allopathic) medical model taught in most Western medical schools does not include the holistic principles. Complementary (or alternative) medical traditions such as acupuncture, chiropractic, homeopathy, massage therapy, and naturopathy incorporate many of the principles of holistic medicine. Yet some medical doctors are holistic in how they deal with their patients, and some practitioners using complementary therapies are not holistic. Patients are learning to look for both technical expertise and whether a practitioner uses holistic principles.

Those interested in a career as a holistic practitioner must first become qualified in one or more methods of delivering health care, such as chiropractic, massage therapy, medicine, naturopathy, or psychology. They can then apply holistic qualities and philosophy to their specialties.

Practice

Although preventing illness is important, holistic health focuses on reaching higher levels of wellness. The right half of the wellness continuum invites people to constantly explore which everyday actions work for them and discover what is appropriate to move them toward maximum well-being. People are motivated by how good it feels to have energy and enthusiasm for life, knowing that what they are doing that day will allow them to continue to feel this great for years to come.

When disease and chronic conditions do occur, the holistic health principles also can be applied. The term is usually changed to *holistic medicine,* and additional factors are added. Health care professionals using the holistic approach work in partnership with their patients. They recommend treatments that support the body's natural healing system and consider the whole person and the whole situation.

A holistic approach to healing goes beyond just eliminating symptoms. Taking an aspirin for a headache would be like disconnecting the oil light on the dashboard of a car when it flashes. The irritation is eliminated, but the real problem still exists. In holistic medicine, a symptom is considered a message that something needs attention. The symptom is used as a guide to look below the surface for the root cause and address what truly needs attention.

Benefits

Holistic health supports reaching higher levels of wellness as well as preventing illness. People enjoy the vitality and well-being that results from their positive lifestyle changes, and are motivated to continue this process throughout their lives.

—*SUZAN WALTER*

Resources

American Holistic Health Association
　　Dept. R
　　P.O. Box 17400
　　Anaheim, CA 92817-7400
　　Tel: (714) 779-6152
　　e-mail: ahha@healthy.net
　　Web site: www.ahha.org
　　This nonprofit educational organization has compiled lists of self-help resources available in the United States. These free materials and a booklet, *Wellness from Within: The First Step,* which introduces the holistic approach to creating wellness, are available on the Internet or by mail.

Graduate Certificate Program in
Holistic Health Care
　　Director: Molly B. Vass, Ed.D.
　　Western Michigan University
　　College of Health and Human Services
　　Kalamazoo, MI 49008-5174
　　Tel: (616) 387-3800

Fax: (616) 387-3348
e-mail: Brenda.Bell@wmich.edu
Unique opportunity to study holistic health care in an accredited academic program. Consists of eighteen semester hours of study in holistic health care and related topics. Can be taken as an independent certificate or used to supplement graduate training in related fields. Three main areas of holistic health care (promotion, prevention, and treatment) are addressed through a combination of education, research, promotion, training, administration, program planning, and program development efforts. Graduates are able to work within their chosen professional areas from a holistic perspective.

Further Reading

Collinge, William. *The American Holistic Health Association Complete Guide to Alternative Medicine.* New York: Warner Books, 1996.

Gordon, James S. *Holistic Medicine.* New York: Chelsea House Publishers, 1988.

Travis, John W., and Regina Sara Ryan. *The Wellness Workbook.* Berkeley, Calif.: Ten Speed Press, 1988.

Homeopathy

 Homeopathy is a holistic system that is used to treat chronic and acute illness and disease. Founded by Samuel Hahnemann in the late 1700s, homeopathy is based on the concept of "like cures like," which means that remedies are matched to symptom patterns in the patient. The physician analyzes a patient's symptoms, then finds a substance, usually from plants, minerals, and animals, that induces the same symptoms in a healthy person. By ingesting small, diluted doses of these substances, the body is stimulated to fight illness. In recent times, homeopathic practices have increased dramatically in popularity as people all over the world rediscover the inexpensive, natural remedies used to cure illnesses that do not respond to conventional treatment.

History

Samuel Hahnemann was born in Meissen, Germany, in 1755. Thin, delicate, and highly intelligent, with an interest in the natural sciences and languages, he established his first medical practice in 1780. Hahnemann was appalled by the prevalent practices of bloodletting, purging, vomiting, and the administration of large doses of harsh drugs.

It was not until 1789, when translating *A Treatise of Materia Medica* by Dr. William Cullen, that Hahnemann first conceived of his homeopathic method. He decided to experiment on himself with *cinchona* (Peruvian bark), one of the drugs mentioned in that work. He noticed that when a healthy person took cinchona, the substance from which quinine is derived, it produced many of the symptoms that it was intended to alleviate.

The official birth date of homeopathy is 1796, when Hahnemann published an article in the *Journal of Practical Medicine,* in which he delineates three methods of healing: preventative treatment, which is the removal of the causes of illness; palliative treatment through the principle of *contraria contraris,* which means healing by opposites; and the treatment of likes with likes, namely the prescribing of medicines that cause similar symptoms in healthy individuals. Hahnemann coined the term *homeopathy,* from the Greek words *homois,* "similar," and *pathos,* meaning "disease." The word *homeopathic* first appeared in print in an article he published in 1807.

Published in 1810, the *Organon of Rational Medicine* is Hahnemann's quintessential work, a complete exposition of his healing method. To this day it forms the foundation of homeopathy. The principle of *similia similibus,* first set forth in his essay of 1796, was now expanded to *similia similibus curentor*—let likes be treated by likes—the core principle of homeopathy. The reception of this work was lukewarm. Nevertheless, Hahnemann attempted to teach homeopathy through his newly formed Institute for the Postgraduate Study of Homeopathy. Not one person responded to his advertisement. In 1812 Napoleon was driven from Germany, and the war flooded the area with refugees, starvation, and no less than 80,000 dead and another 80,000 wounded. Hahnemann and other physicians were pressed into service, trying to help the many who suffered not only from the battle but also from an outbreak of typhus. Armed with twenty-six homeopathic remedies, Hahnemann achieved remarkable results. He would later report that only two of the 180 typhus patients he treated had died.

In 1819 a group of envious physicians and angry pharmacists filed a court action against Hahnemann to prevent him from dispensing his own medicines in Leipzig, where he was living at the time. Despite Hahnemann's growing reputation and successful treatment of royalty and famous people such as Johann Goethe, Hahnemann did not prevail. Although he subsequently won in the Appeals Court of Dresden, Hahnemann closed his practice and left Leipzig for the city of Kothen in 1821.

Shortly after his arrival, Hahnemann, through his political and social connections, procured permission from the Kathen authorities to practice homeopathy with total immunity. He wrote his last great work, *Chronic Diseases: Their Peculiar Nature and Their Homeopathic Treatment.* First published in Dresden in 1828, it ultimately ran to five volumes by 1839 and totaled in excess of 1,600 pages. This work set forth another deep insight: not only could patients be cured of acute conditions, but their patterns of acute conditions over the years allow for a classification of chronic tendencies toward types of disease. These chronic tendencies Hahnemann called *miasms,* the patient's inherited predisposition toward certain types of illness. By knowing the miasmatic type, a homeopathic physician could now treat pre-

ventively, and this tendency could be mitigated so that the next generation's health could be improved. Hahnemann had intuited the basis for treating genetic disorders.

In 1831 a cholera epidemic swept through Europe. The Hahnemannian protocol for treating cholera, which also included cleanliness, ventilation, and disinfection, resulted in a drastic reduction in mortality. Records at that time indicate that under homeopathic treatment, mortality was between 2 and 20 percent, while conventional treatment carried a mortality rate of over 50 percent.

Homeopathy began to spread to England and the United States. By 1844 the American Institute of Homeopathy was founded by homeopathic physicians from New York, Philadelphia, and Boston. The first national medical organization in the United States, it was established to promote standardization of the practice and teaching of homeopathy.

This period in American homeopathy was its golden age. Literally thousands of homeopathic books and journals were published. There were no less than twenty-two homeopathic medical schools and countless homeopathic hospitals and clinics throughout the United States. Estimates are that by the turn of the century about 15,000 homeopathic physicians were in practice in the United States.

Around the same time, the sciences of cellular and molecular biology, as well as physiology, began to replace the rudimentary medical knowledge of Hahnemann's time. Together these sciences produced medicines used by conventional physicians to quickly and effectively remove or modulate their patients' symptoms at relatively low cost. By the 1960s homeopathy in the United States was virtually dead, and medical historians predicted the complete demise of this "medical heresy" by 1980. Instead, by the late 1970s American homeopathy was well into a revival. By 1996, the bicentennial anniversary of Hahnemann's discovery, more books and articles were being written about homeopathy than at any time since the turn of the century. Sales of homeopathic medicines have increased by 30 percent per year in the United States since 1990.

Basic Principles

As laid down by Hahnemann, the eight fundamentals of homeopathy are as follows:

1. There is a natural and universal scientific law of cure; namely, that likes can be cured by likes. This means that small amounts of any substance that causes disease in a healthy person can be used to treat that same disease in a patient.
2. The knowledge of the action of remedies is harvested from single- or double-blind experiments in which small doses are given to healthy subjects who later record their detailed reactions to the test substance. This is called a homeopathic proving. The knowledge base for a particular substance or remedy is also determined from case histories of treatment with the substance, which has not undergone a proving but which has yielded a cure in clinical practice. Added to this is the information on symptoms produced by accidental poisonings with toxic substances. The proving, clinical, and toxicological data form the *materia medica* of the remedy.
3. The ability of an organism to feel, sense, act, or achieve homeostasis (or equilibrium) is maintained by a nonmaterial principle called the dynamis. This dynamis, or "spiritlike" vital force, is, according to Hahnemann, similar in nature to gravity or magnetism. It is a force that to date has eluded explanation or classification by the natural sciences. Diseases, therefore, are not actual material things, but descriptions or classifications of symptom patterns. Symptoms are not things to be removed or suppressed by drugs; rather, they are an expression of the vital force's attempt to heal. The properly prepared, selected, and administered homeopathic remedy somehow "resonates" with the vital force and stimulates the healing process.
4. A single remedy is given at a time. This allows a clear evaluation of its efficacy.
5. A minimum dose must be used. Small doses of a substance stimulate healing, medium doses paralyze the patient, and large doses kill.
6. Individualization of the treatment is essential. No two people are exactly alike in either sickness or health, and although homeopaths use classifications of disease types, finer, individual distinctions must always be made since, although the action of two remedies may often be similar, they are never exactly the same.
7. The mere removal of symptoms by suppressive means is a grave danger because it defeats the vital force's attempt at homeostasis and puts the patient at risk for a more serious disease.
8. There is a distinction between acute or epidemic diseases and chronic disease patterns of patients. Preventative homeopathic care requires an understanding of these chronic patterns.

Despite more than two hundred years of clinical efficacy, the way these remedies work remains a mystery. We do not yet possess the technology or methodology necessary to unlock homeopathy's secrets.

Philosophically, homeopathy is holistic (not merely alternative) because the essential task is to understand the patient as a whole person. As a method, homeopathy is a synthesis of the natural science approach and the phenomenological or descriptive approach. The physician must blend his natural science training in anatomy, physiology, pathology, biochemistry, physical diagnosis, and other areas with observation of the patient and understanding of the patient's self-description. The challenge of homeopathy, even in the treatment of apparently purely physical conditions, is to select a few probable remedies from the thousand or more possible remedies.

Women figured prominently in the history of American homeopathy. By 1900 an estimated 12 percent of homeopathic physicians were women. The Cleveland Homeopathic College was one of the first coeducational medical institutions in the country. Women's auxiliaries raised large amounts of money to open many of the homeopathic hospitals, and it was women, in their role of family caretaker, who were the lay prescribers introducing homeopathy to many communities. Some members of the early women's suffrage movement were either homeopathic physicians or their patients. Dr. Susan Edson, a graduate of the Cleveland Homeopathic College, was personal physician to President James Garfield.

Like a novel with many chapters and plot twists, so a patient's cure unfolds. The process is highly individual. The homeopathic physician will be guided by certain principles of cure: healing occurs from above downward, from the center to the periphery, from more vital organs to less vital organs, and in reverse order of the appearance of the original symptoms.

Practice

A typical session begins with the patient's history. The patient is allowed to tell her story without interruption. Only after the patient is finished will the physician ask specific questions to understand the symptoms, namely how they vary according to time of day or season, rest or activity, temperature, bathing, position, eating, thirst, sleep, social intercourse, perspiration, external stimuli, emotions, and so forth.

Most important, the physician attempts to understand the patient's personality. Inquiries are made into how the patient copes with stress, and about the patient's fears and worries. The patient describes herself. This process is often the most revealing. The physician uses these descriptions to generate an understanding of the patient. He also obtains a conventional medical and surgical history, and finally performs a physical examination.

The physician then attempts to rank various symptoms, modalities, and generalities by degree of intensity. A list of symptoms is generated and the symptoms are then repertorized, that is, cross-indexed with the remedies known to have caused or cured these same symptoms. This labor-intensive process was for centuries performed by hand but is now done by computer.

Having narrowed the field to several probable remedies, the homeopathic physician must then determine whether the patient's problem is an acute, chronic, or inherited illness, or perhaps an illness due to the suppressive effects of previous treatment.

The art of homeopathy is in the ability of the homeopathic physician to process all of this information into a synthesis, a "remedy portrait" or gestalt, which corresponds to the remedy likely to stimulate a healing response. Having given a dose of the indicated remedy, the patient and physician must now wait. Depending on the patient, the nature of the problem, and the potency of the remedy, a return visit is scheduled weeks or months after the initial dose. While there have been miraculous homeopathic cures after just one dose, most chronic cases take months or years to cure. The process is highly individual.

Benefits

Homeopathic treatment is appropriate and safe for all ages and is especially useful in childhood and during pregnancy, labor, and the postpartum period. Homeopathy has successfully treated patients with conditions such as otitis, bronchitis, pneumonia, migraines, hepatitis, pancreatitis, appendicitis, and cholecystitis. Historically, homeopathy has been used to treat potentially dangerous infections such as cholera, influenza, syphilis, gonorrhea, scarlet fever, polio, measles, and tuberculosis. Chronic conditions such as arthritis, asthma, eczema, psoriasis, and chronic fatigue syndrome have all been alleviated by homeopathic treatments. It is reported that devastating diseases such as multiple sclerosis can be brought to remission if treated early enough. Historical homeopathic literature contains many references to cures of various types of cancer, though admittedly these are some of the most difficult for any system of medicine to cure and are best dealt with on a preventive basis.

—DR. DOMENICK MASIELLO

Resources

American Institute of Homeopathy
    1585 Glencoc St., Suite 44
    Denver, CO 80220-1338
    Tel: (303) 321-4105
    Facilitates conferences, publishes a journal, and provides referrals.

The National Center for Homeopathy
    801 N. Fairfax, Suite 306
    Alexandria, VA 22314
    Tel: (703) 548-7790
    e-mail: nchinfo@igc.apc.org
    Nonprofit organization that promotes homeopathy in the United States. Publishes monthly magazine entitled *Homeopathy Today*.

Videotape

Winston, Julian. *The Faces of Homeopathy: A Pictorial History*. Alexandria, Va.: The National Center of Homeopathy, 1995.

Further Reading

Cook, Trevor M. *Samuel Hahnemann: His Life and Times*. Middlesex, U.K.: Homeopathic Studies Ltd., 1981.

Coulter, Harris. *Homeopathic Medicine*. St. Louis, Mo.: Formur, 1972.

Hahnemann, Samuel. *Organon of Medicine*. Translated by Jost Kunzli, Alain Nuadé, and Peter Pendleton. Los Angeles: J. P. Tarcher, 1982.

———. *The Chronic Diseases: Their Peculiar Nature and Their Homeopathic Cure*. New Delhi: B. Jain Publishers, 1985.

———. *Materia Medica Pura*. New Delhi: B. Jain Publishers, 1984.

Kent, James Tyler. *Lectures on Homeopathic Philosophy*. Richmond, Va.: North Atlantic Books, 1979.

Roberts, Herbert. *The Principles and Art of Cure by Homeopathy*. Santa Barbara, Calif.: Health Science Press, 1942.

Weiner, Michael, and Kathleen Gross. *The Complete Book of Homeopathy*. Garden City, N.Y.: Avery Publishing Group, 1989.

Wright-Hubbard, Elizabeth. *A Brief Study Course in Homeopathy*. St. Louis, Mo.: Formur, 1977.

Naturopathic Medicine

 Naturopathic medicine is a form of health care that utilizes and integrates different natural therapies such as clinical nutrition, homeopathy, hydrotherapy, botanical medicines, minor surgery, Oriental medicine, physical medicine, and lifestyle counseling with a knowledge of traditional diagnostic and medical therapies to treat a range of afflictions. A licensed doctor of naturopathy (ND) must complete a four-year program that specializes in not only naturopathic studies, but also basic medical science. Practitioners are then qualified to provide primary care, perform diagnostic testing, and prescribe a course of treatment that draws from a long list of natural remedies and techniques.

Origins

The development of naturopathic medicine began with Benedict Lust, a German who immigrated to the United States in 1892. A few years after arriving, Lust was struck down by tuberculosis. When American doctors couldn't help him, Lust returned to Europe and sought out Father Sebastian Kneipp, a priest living in Bavaria who was known for his "nature cure" treatments.

Kneipp did what Lust's doctor could not—he successfully treated Lust. This was a turning point in Lust's life. In 1896 Kneipp gave Lust permission to bring his treatments to America. Back in the United States, Lust researched other natural health philosophies and used them to reshape and mold Kneipp's ideas to appeal to the American people. By broadening the scope of his work, Lust and other Kneipp disciples developed what is now known as naturopathic medicine.

In 1902 Lust bought the word *naturopathy* from a New York physician who had coined the term seven years earlier. Seven years later California became the first state to recognize the new discipline by enacting regulatory laws regarding the practice of naturopathic medicine. Popularity of naturopathy rose significantly early in the century, but began to decline with the improvement and accessibility of pharmaceutical drugs. Alternative methods of health care, including naturopathic medicine, have enjoyed a resurgence of interest as people rediscover that natural remedies are also valuable.

Basic Principles

Today's brand of naturopathic medicine embodies five main principles. The first, *vis medicatrix naturae*, means "the healing power of nature." Naturopathic physicians use therapies that help the body to heal itself.

Primum non nocere, the second principle, means "first do no harm." This translates into safe, naturopathic treatments that have minimal side effects or none at all. Naturopathic physicians refer patients to other health care practitioners, such as medical doctors (M.D.s), when it is appropriate for the patient.

True health can be achieved only when your doctor practices *tolle causam*, or "finds the cause." Diagnosing the true cause of disease and illness is fundamental to naturopathic care. Sometimes it is as simple as poor diet or sleeping habits. These basic issues can significantly affect one's health. Other times, more complex factors are responsible.

A commitment to treating the whole person is an important principle of naturopathic healing. Illness is generally the result of many factors. Part of "whole person," or holistic, care is investigating not only physical symptoms, but emotional and mental ones, too. How and what you eat, lifestyle habits, genetic tendencies, and social interactions are important in assessing and treating health problems.

The final principle of naturopathic medicine is its emphasis on preventative medicine. Practitioners aim to lessen and even eliminate the chance of disease by encouraging patients to take a proactive role in their health care by implementing and maintaining a healthy lifestyle.

Practice

Naturopathic physicians are often primary caregivers. This means they can serve as family or general practitioners, differing only in their use of natural treatments. When you call an N.D.'s office, a receptionist will greet you and ask when you'd like to make an appointment, much as in a medical doctor's office.

On the day of your visit, you'll find that a naturopathic medical office is just that—a

Before applying to naturopathic medical school, one must complete a minimum of three years of college, including specific prerequisite courses. It takes four years of graduate-level study to earn the degree of Doctor of Naturopathic Medicine. Anatomy, pharmacology, gynecology, and radiology are just some of the medical sciences taught. Training in natural therapeutics is also included, as is time spent working in a clinical setting seeing patients.

Although an N.D. degree specifically prepares you for naturopathic medical practice, there are other career opportunities. N.D.s also teach, do research, work within the natural health industry, write, lecture, and serve as consultants. As natural medicine expands and grows, so does the potential for naturopathic medicine.

medical office. You might fill out some forms and then be invited to see the doctor. Your naturopathic physician will ask what's wrong, and will then spend about an hour to discover the cause of your ailment.

Your N.D. will take a lengthy medical history and perform a thorough physical examination. Laboratory tests will be ordered as needed. An N.D. relies on both standard medical lab tests and specialized tests more fitting to a natural medical practice.

Your N.D. then recommends treatment based on his or her investigation. Diet is discussed, and perhaps vitamins or other nutrient supplements suggested. Herbs are common medicines used by N.D.s as well as homeopathic remedies, which are specially prepared substances used to boost healing. Various techniques like hydrotherapy, exercise, or ultrasound, just as physical therapists use, might be employed. And where appropriate, stress management or counseling is suggested.

N.D.s are trained to perform minor surgery such as repairing superficial wounds, but will refer you to surgeons and other doctors for major operations. Some states allow qualified N.D.s to prescribe some drugs like antibiotics.

It's perfectly appropriate, and sometimes desirable, to mix and match naturopathic therapies with allopathic treatment. This should be done only under professional guidance to prevent potential problems. While all naturopathic doctors are trained in the basics of Oriental medicine, there are some who specialize in acupuncture, herbal medicine, and related therapies. Some N.D.s offer natural childbirth, including pre- and postnatal care, for pregnant women.

Benefits

Naturopathic medical care is suitable for all age groups and most acute and chronic conditions. Its whole-person, natural care approach allows patients to attain the best health possible in an effective and safe manner. Because naturopathic physicians are concerned with solving, not masking, symptoms, healing can take longer than with conventional treatment. Naturopathic medicine also requires that patients take an active role in their health care. N.D.s take their role as teacher very seriously as they instruct their patients in how to stay healthy.

As primary caregivers, N.D.s cooperate with other medical and health professionals. An N.D., like any general practitioner, is the gatekeeper for your health care. When you're sick, see your N.D. first. She will consult with or refer you to other physicians and specialists when appropriate.

—LAURI M. AESOPH, ND

Resources

American Association of Naturopathic
Physicians
  601 Valley St., Suite 105
  Seattle, WA 98109
  Tel: (206) 298-0125
  Web site: www.infinite.org/naturopathic.
  physician
  e-mail: 74602.3715@compuserve.com
  This professional organization provides re-
  ferrals to naturopathic physicians in the
  United States. A myriad of information on
  naturopathic medicine is also available.

Bastyr University
  14500 Juanita Dr. N.E.
  Bothell, WA 98011
  Tel: (206) 823-1300
  Web site: www.bastyr.edu
  Four-year postgraduate university that offers
  degrees in naturopathic medicine and related
  health care disciplines.

Canadian Naturopathic Association
  4174 Dundas St. W., Suite 304
  Etobicoke, ON M8X 1X3
  Canada
  Tel: (416) 233-1043
  Fax: (416) 233-2924
  This professional group offers referrals to
  naturopathic doctors throughout Canada.

National College of Naturopathic Medicine
  049 S.W. Porter
  Portland, OR 97201
  Tel: (503) 499-4343
  Web site: www.ncnm.edu
  A postgraduate, four-year institution that
  provides classes in naturopathic medicine.

Southwest College of Naturopathic Medicine &
Health Sciences
  2140 E. Broadway
  Tempe, AZ 85282
  Tel: (602) 858-9100
  Fax: (602) 858-0222
  Web site: www.healthworld.com/pan/pa/
  naturopathic/aanp/SW/SW.college. home.
  html

Four-year postgraduate college that offers
degrees in naturopathic medicine and related
health care disciplines.

Further Reading

Aesoph, Lauri. *How to Eat Away Arthritis.* Para-
mus, N.J.: Prentice Hall, 1996.

Brown, Donald. *Herbal Prescriptions for Better
Health.* Rocklin, Calif.: Prima Publishing,
1996.

Kirchfeld, Friedhelm, and Wade Boyle. *Nature
Doctors: Pioneers in Naturopathic Medicine.* East
Palestine, Ohio: Buckeye Naturopathic Press,
1994 (distributed by Medicina Biologica, Portland, Ore.).

Murray, Michael, and Joseph Pizzorno. *Encyclopedia of Natural Medicine.* Rocklin, Calif.:
Prima Publishing, 1991.

Murray, Michael. *The Healing Powers of Foods.*
New York: Ballantine Fawcett, 1993.

Ullman, Robert, and Judith Reichenberg-Ullman.
The Patient's Guide to Homeopathic Medicine.
Kent, Wash.: Pacific Pipeline, 1995.

Shamanism

 Shamanism is an ancient healing
method that allows a person to
enter and interact with an unseen world of spirits. Contemporary shamanism encompasses a wide
range of spiritual practices originating in
civilizations in North and South America,
Siberia, Indonesia, Australia, Southeast Asia,
Japan, and Tibet. Throughout history, shamanic healers have been known by many
names, including medicine man or medicine
woman, witch, warlock, or, in African-based
vodoun religions, priest or priestess. The
word *shaman* was derived from the Asian
word *saman* by nineteenth-century European scholars intrigued by the cultures and
practices of ancient shamanism. Currently

many Western medical researchers and psychologists are exploring shamanism not as a curiosity, but as a creative and constructive way of viewing the world.

History and Philosophy

In ancient times, shamans served many roles in their societies. They performed rituals to mark the migrations of the animals that their societies hunted. Hunters consulted shamans to learn where animals could be found. The shamans also designed and performed rituals to mark the changing of seasons, the migration of their people to different locations, and individual rites of passage such as birth, the transition from adolescence to adulthood, marriage, and death.

Early shamans were also teachers. In many early societies, storytelling was an important part of the shaman's skills. Often, the stories he told taught lessons about the society's beliefs, fears, and traditions.

Shamans were also healers. Since many societies believed that all illnesses had a spiritual source, the shamans were often chosen for their ability to communicate with the spirit world. Healing rituals designed to remove harmful spirits from individuals or communities often took place in sacred spaces such as caves or mountains, and included wearing ceremonial clothing; using herbs; playing drums, rattles, and flutes; and dancing.

Shamans believe there are two realities: the "seen" world, which is the world we perceive through our five senses, and the "unseen" or "invisible" world, which our five senses cannot detect. The unseen world can be compared to the world of dreams, emotions, instincts, and intuition. Emotions such as fear, joy, love, grief, and human sexual drives cannot be seen but are real forces in human life. Ancient shamanic cultures honored the forces of the unseen world in the form of gods, goddesses, and monsters in the narratives of their mythologies.

Shamanism is founded on a belief that most diseases and grievances between individuals or nations are caused by an imbalance in the natural order of the seen and unseen worlds. A shaman interacts with the invisible world of forces and energies and restores the balance. Her stories, rituals, and dances are used to subdue or stimulate feelings that may bring new hope, motivate a person to act, or simply increase energy for healing and change.

It is unlikely that you will find the services of a shaman advertised at your family health clinic, but many clinics do refer patients to therapists who use techniques borrowed from the shamanic tradition. For example, psychologists and hypnotherapists use hypnosis and mental visualization (a traditional shamanic technique) to help people stop smoking, control appetite, reduce anxiety, manage chronic pain, or recover from an addiction. Mental visualization is a process in which a person sets a goal by imagining himself accomplishing it. For example, a person who wants to calm his anxiety before delivering a speech may imagine stepping up to the podium, confidently delivering a successful talk, and receiving a standing ovation. For many people these images can replace the old memories that caused the fear. While shamans helped their communities by telling stories or performing rituals, today's practitioners sometimes use "guided imagery" to achieve a similar goal.

There are also an increasing number of organizations teaching traditional shamanic practices throughout the world. Courses are taught by anthropologists, psychologists, and shamans from Native American, African, Hawaiian, South American, Australian, or other traditions. Typical workshops might include lectures about basic principles of shamanism, drumming workshops, and experiences in the basic shamanistic technique of "journeying" into the unseen world.

Other shamanic techniques are described below:

Vision Quests: In this practice a person spends a day or more alone in the wilderness. There he is able to fast and meditate without distractions. This can be used to help people contemplate their own inner worlds, fears, dreams, strengths, and gifts. It can also be used to experience a oneness with nature.

Sun Dances: The sun dance was originally used to help warriors get in touch with their inner strengths and to draw strength from the spirits of nature such as those found in trees, rocks, clouds, and sky. Usually over a period of several days, the young warrior was prepared through fasting, meditation, and counsel with an elder. Then small hooks or barbs were placed in the fleshy portions of his chest. Cords fastened these hooks to a tree or post, and the dancer leaned back, naturally causing some pain. The dancers stood in this way from dawn to dusk, usually in the hot sun. It was a test of one's endurance and one's ability to deal with his own fears and discomforts. People who experienced the sun dance claimed to have gained dramatic self-knowledge. Even today there are those who repeat the sun dance every year.

Drumming Circles: This practice uses drums for therapeutic purposes. Usually there is a lead, or "mother," drum with a deep voice that sets a simple rhythm based on the heartbeat. People participate in these circles to help focus their energies, rather than to perform or make music. In a

Practice

Shamanic counseling is available today in many parts of the United States. It is used to aid a person's physical, emotional, or spiritual health. A typical session may begin with a "smudging" ceremony. This consists of burning a small amount of dried sage, often mixed with other herbs such as sweet grass and cedar. Smoke from the smudge pot might be wafted with a feathered fan over the person's body, sometimes from head to toe. Shamans believe that the person is "cleansed" as the smoke lifts away dark or negative influences and energies.

The smudging ceremony may be followed by a "journey" in which the shaman enters the unseen world in order to consult guiding spiritual forces. A person may also journey to the unseen world for herself. In this practice, the shamanic counselor may begin by discussing the person's problem. The person may then be told to close her eyes, relax, and imagine the journey that she is about to make. With the image clearly in the person's mind, the shaman or shamanic counselor begins a steady rhythm with a hand drum, a rattle, or recorded music. She may use a rhythm similar to the human heartbeat—between fifty-five and seventy beats per minute. This rhythm puts the person into a light trance, allowing her to relax and enter a dreamlike state.

Upon entering the trance state, the person might meet and work with an inner guide or adviser. During the journey, the person might ask her guide questions, listen for answers, and possibly carry on a dialogue for several minutes or more. Eventually, the shamanic counselor will change the rhythm of the drum to indicate that the person should return to the "seen" world. After returning, there might be further discussion with the shamanic counselor to help the person interpret the meaning of the journey.

drumming circle, there are many conversations with the drums, which are used to teach participants how to listen and communicate with one another. Some people look upon drumming circles as times of communion, in which people are brought together at a deep spiritual level.

Medicine Wheel: The medicine wheel is an important practice in most shamanic traditions. Evidence of its use can be found in every part of the world. People form a wheel by gathering in a circle to discuss a problem or to bring about a change that affects them all. At the wheel, all people have equal status and an equal chance to speak. The wheel is used to allow a joining of their "spirits," that is, the inner worlds of each participant. It is understood that no single person at the wheel ever has the ultimate answer; rather, the solution is to be found as a community.

Sweat Lodge: A dome-shaped structure is constructed with willow branch poles and covered with hides or blankets. Prayers are offered and each participant is blessed upon entering the lodge. Rocks, which have been heated at a fire outside the lodge, are brought inside and placed in the center. Water is poured over the rocks and the heat inside the lodge rises. In this steamy, hot environment, the participants meditate and contemplate their own lives or the lives of their community. The ceremonies and rituals that are performed vary with each lodge. Some create a medicine wheel. Others may sing. Still others may eat ritual herbs or peyote, a drug that produces hallucinations. The purpose of the sweat lodge, as with most shamanic practices, is to get in touch with the forces and energies of the invisible world in order to improve the quality of life.

Benefits

Although many people still view the practices of shamanism more as fiction than as fact, a growing number of people value the emphasis these practices place on the unseen world of emotions, dreams, and spiritual forces to help heal illnesses and provide guidance in living a healthy and fulfilling life. While shamanism rarely offers a quick fix for acute illnesses, many people have reported profound physical and emotional relief through contemporary shamanic practices. With a history as long and enduring as humankind itself, it is hard to find a more time-tested method for bringing harmony and comfort to body and mind.

—*HAL ZINA BENNETT*

Resources

Conference on the Study of Shamanism and Alternative Modes of Healing
    Ruth-Inge Heinze, Ph.D.
    2321 Russell St., Suite 3A
    Berkeley, CA 94705
    Promotes shamanism as a healing practice.

The Foundation for Shamanic Studies
    P.O. Box 1939
    Mill Valley, CA 94942
    Tel: (415) 380-8282
    Sponsors workshops on shamanic training. Call or write for a catalog.

Further Reading

Books
Andrews, Lynn. *Medicine Woman.* San Francisco: HarperCollins, 1981.

Beck, P. V., Anna Lee Walters, and Nia Francisco, eds. *The Sacred Ways of Knowledge, Sources of Life.* Flagstaff, Ariz.: Northland Publishing, 1990.

Bennett, Hal Zina. *Spirit Guides.* Ukiah, Calif.: Tenacity Press, 1997.

———. *Zuni Fetishes: Using Native American Objects for Meditation, Reflection, and Personal Insight.* San Francisco: HarperCollins, 1995.

Campbell, Joseph. *Primitive Mythology.* New York: McGraw-Hill, 1978.

Castaneda, Carlos. *The Teachings of Don Juan: A Yaqui Way of Knowledge.* New York: Ballantine, 1968.

Harner, Michael J. *The Way of the Shaman: A Guide to Power and Healing.* San Francisco: Harper-Collins, 1980.

Morgan, Marlo. *Mutant Message Down Under.* New York: HarperCollins, 1994.

Journals

Shaman's Drum: A Journal of Contemporary Shamanism.

Traditional Chinese Medicine

 Traditional Chinese medicine (TCM) is an ancient approach to health care. Still practiced today in one form or another by almost one-quarter of the world's population, TCM traces its mixture of herbal medicine, acupuncture, and massage therapy back to the origins of Taoism and Confucianism. With a heavy emphasis on understanding the patient and his needs, as opposed to focusing on the illness and its symptoms, TCM offers a counterpoint and complement to the bioscience of Western medicine.

TCM was studied and practiced in many Asian countries such as Japan as long ago as 600 C.E. Some countries such as Korea and Japan have developed their own modifications to TCM. For this reason, the term *Oriental medicine* is sometimes used instead of Chinese medicine. However, all forms of traditional Oriental medicine are considered to have originated from the work done in China during the Han dynasty.

Because of the sociopolitical climate in modern China, a wide gap exists between current TCM theory and traditional TCM. Unfortunately, English translations of TCM have been available for only the past fifteen years, and even then they are usually a modern, officially sanctioned version of TCM. Different translations often contain confusing variations. For example, an important word like *qi* may be spelled *chi* (using an older translation system) or *ki* (in Japanese). All three versions have the same meaning. In this section the modern Pinyin form of Chinese is used when possible. Understanding these translation principles can help you to read and understand other books and articles on the subject of TCM.

History

In China an extremely organized system of healing developed during the period known as the Han dynasty (approximately 213 B.C.E.–240 C.E.). At this time in Chinese history the country was finally reunited into one empire after hundreds of years of fighting in the Warring States period (476–221 B.C.E.). Both Confucian and Taoist philosophies emerged from this period, and each had an important impact on TCM. During the Han dynasty there were many different kinds of healers and teachers in China. Confucianism was the main political power in court. When Ssu-ma Chien became Grand Historian of the Court, great importance was placed on organizing and recording written records.

From this period emerged three books that are still considered the cornerstones of TCM. The first was *The Yellow Emperor's Classic of Internal Medicine (Huang di-nei Jing,* or simply *Nei Jing). The Nei Jing* refers to both Taoist and Confucian concepts. The Taoist perspective of health emphasizes living in harmony with nature and achieving longevity. The Confucian ideals describe an integrated system within the human body that reflected the orderly social structure finally made possible by the reunification of China into one unified state. This organized structure was eventually mapped into the specific lines and pathways we see on acupuncture charts. The lines or pathways are usually called meridians. Places where the *qi* comes right up to the surface are called acupoints. The *qi* is believed to circulate through this system, connecting the deepest internal organs to places on the skin where the energy can be influenced and treated. The points can be treated with needles (acupuncture), heat (moxibustion), or manipulation (acupressure).

The *qi* system was described in more detail in the second book, the *Classic of Difficult Issues (Nan Jing)*. The *Nan Jing* is believed to have been written at least one hundred years after the *Nei Jing*. The *Nan Jing* refers to information in the *Nei Jing* and expands on those ideas. The *Nan Jing* goes so far as to say that a person's health can be directly analyzed just from carefully feeling the *qi* and blood as it moves through the radial artery in the wrist. This is called the radial pulse. Modern practitioners of TCM still use this map of the *qi* system to diagnose and treat their clients.

The third book is believed to have been written around 220 C.E. by a famous physician and scholar named Zhang Zhong-Jing. Called the *Treatise on Harm Caused by Cold (Shang Han Lun)*, it deals with how outside influences such as colds, flu viruses, and plagues can attack people and make them sick, and describes how to treat these problems with Chinese herbal medicine. Zhang Zhong-Jing described six specific layers of the body's defense system and matched these with already recognized meridian pathways. He described the qualities of illness as they invaded each layer and gave specific herbal formulas that could be used for treatment. Using a wide variety of herbs given in specific dosages, he created formulas that could match detailed patterns of diagnosis. Zhang's use of herbal medicine introduced a whole new level of sophistication within the possibilities of TCM. Although he cannot be credited with inventing Chinese herbal formulas, his ability to understand and match patterns of illness with the herbs that will cure them established his place as one of the founding fathers of Chinese herbal medicine.

Over the next fifteen hundred years, China continued to develop and perfect the ideas that originated in the Han dynasty. Many physicians and scholars practiced and wrote about their ideas and results. Ideas that were originally used by particular authors and schools of thought were eventually homogenized into guiding principles for one predominant system of medicine.

By the end of the Ming dynasty (1643 C.E.) another idea, now described as the eight principles, began to emerge. This model included all of the dynamics that impact health. These are internal and external factors, hot and cold, yin and yang, and excess versus deficiency. This model was used to integrate many of the previous models in TCM. The Ming was the last dynasty in which traditional Chinese medicine continued to evolve and flourish without being influenced by Western thought and medicine.

The introduction of Western culture in China began a period of slow decline for TCM. The obvious realities revealed through anatomical study made many Chinese physicians and scholars feel less confident about some of TCM's less tangible theories. The Chinese government also applied political pressure that affected the publication of certain literature. Eventually there began a trend to weed out the more esoteric ideas from Chinese medical literature. While ideas as fundamental as the *qi* and blood remained intact, references to the spiritual components became more and more simplified. Under the Communist regime, many ideas came to be viewed as superstitious and unscientific. These ideas were disregarded and systematically eliminated from revised texts.

To this day little of the original TCM literature has been translated into Western languages. Subsequently, TCM is often described in terms of the clinical approach presently being used in hospitals in mainland China. While this system offers effective clinical applications for the treatment of disease, much of the broader perspective and theories remain buried in literary Chinese characters.

Basic Principles

Influenced by its Taoist origins, TCM views the human body as an image of the natural world. This is reflected in the terminology of TCM. Energy is said to flow through the body in "rivers," often to a bodily "reservoir" or "sea." A diagnosis might describe an ailment as "liver fire," or an entire organ system as part of the water element. These terms do not reflect a lack of sophistication, but rather a conscious decision to accept that the human body is a participating, not an isolated, part of the surrounding world. The language of TCM reflects how the ancients tried to reconcile their observations of the human body with what they observed in nature.

Continuous, dynamic movement is something the ancient Chinese observed both in the human body and in all nature. They viewed this movement as an interaction between two opposite but complementary energies called yin and yang. In Chinese philosophy these forces complement and help nourish each other. Neither can exist without the other. Examples of dynamic interaction between pairs of opposites can be seen in the constant interplay of day and night, male and female, hot and cold. All the organs and actions of the body may be categorized as either yin or yang.

TCM identifies five essential substances at work in the human body:

1. Spirit *(shen)*, which determines how people direct and conduct themselves in life.

2. Energy, or electromagnetic force *(qi)*, a Chinese concept that cannot be translated into one English word. *Qi* is how the spirit moves and becomes materialized in the body. It describes both activity and a material substance. The concept of *qi* bridges the line of distinction that the English language makes between energy and matter.

3. Blood, the same blood we refer to from a Western anatomical view. In TCM, however, blood is imbued with the nutritional and energetic qualities TCM attributes to *qi*. This aspect of blood is called the *ying qi,* and it circulates with and in the blood as it moves through the vessels and performs its various functions.

4. Body fluids *(jin ye)*, which include sweat, tears, cerebral spinal fluid, and other fluids of the body.

5. Essence *(jing)*, which in English may be understood as potential. This includes our genetic potential as well as the potential of any person or thing to take an action.

These essential substances are understood to exist as a continuum of one another. None can be considered as entirely separate, just as no one part of the body can be treated as entirely separate from the whole.

TCM uses the term *resonance* to describe the relationship among the five essential substances and their role in our health. Resonance is the idea that certain qualities may be identified as similar within different spheres of existence. For example, morning has a quality of energy that is similar to or resonates with springtime. This quality of rising energy identifies both as a particular stage in a cycle of change. Such stages of change are referred to as elements or transformations. The spring and morning are categorized as belonging to the wood-element stage of what is known as the five-element cycle. This cycle is used to explain how energy is constantly changing. It can be applied to the day, the year, the human body, or anything else we want to understand.

In TCM the five-element cycle has proven to be an exceptionally versatile frame of reference for explaining the patterns of dynamic change in our physical bodies. Each of our ten primary organs is correlated with one of the five elements of nature: fire, soil, metal, water, and wood. Doctors of Chinese medicine then correlate the ways in which these elements interact in nature at large with the way these organs and the dynamic qualities of yin and yang work together in the physical body. An inflamed liver might be seen as having too much fire. The solution to the problem is best deduced from the way nature cools fire with water. In the case of "liver fire," a yang excess condition, the patient will naturally be very thirsty and want to drink large quantities of cold water. The practitioner treating such a condition knows that the excess "fire" needs to be dispersed or drained and more "water" quality added to the meridian in order to keep the fire in check. Using needles, acupressure, magnets, or other techniques, a skilled practitioner will choose to use a dispersing technique on the fire point of the liver meridian and will tonify the water point. Understanding that the entire kidney organ system reflects the water element, a practitioner may also choose to bring in more water, or yin quality, using specific kidney meridian points.

Just as the five essential substances are all seen as part of one living whole, the dynamic interplay of yin and yang energies and the five elements are understood as having a complex interactive relationship with one another. Extensive study of Chinese medicine is needed to truly understand and effectively direct these complex interactions.

Traditional Chinese Herbal Medicine

Over the last two decades, the ancient arts of acupuncture, Chinese herbology, and Oriental bodywork therapy have emerged from the privacy of Asian American communities and into the greater American consciousness.

Unlike acupuncture and Oriental bodywork therapy, which use physical pressure and manipulation to effect changes in the way a patient's body functions, Chinese herbal medicine counts on the properties of different plants and foods to stimulate or calm different parts of the body. In many ways this is similar to the drugs of Western medicine, but because Chinese herbal medicine employs "whole," naturally occurring food substances, the risk of causing harmful side effects is greatly reduced.

Chinese herbal medicine must be studied as a distinct skill. Its practitioners must learn the *pharmacopiae*, a term for the knowledge of the names, characteristics, and actions in the body of all the individual herbs. Dosage formulas must be memorized along with various modifications for each. Knowledge of contraindications and hidden effects for specific herbs is important. This information can take years to assimilate. Nevertheless, all of it is necessary for the experienced clinician to create formulas that match the patient's condition.

Chinese herbal medicine stores can usually be found in any major American city where there is a significant Asian population. Often these herb shops are owned or run by practitioners or "doctors" of Chinese herbal medicine. "Customers" have the option of becoming "patients" when they enter the store. Often a number of practitioners in one area will refer all their patients to one local store to have their herbal prescriptions filled. In this way Chinese herbal medicine stores act as pharmacies.

Practice

TCM practitioners use a system called the four examinations to diagnose a patient and determine a proper course of treatment. The examinations include the following steps:

1. *Questioning:* Starting with information about a specific complaint or condition,

the experienced practitioner asks about other symptoms and signs that can help point toward a specific pattern. In the Ming dynasty Zhang Jie-Bin developed a set of ten specific questions, and modified versions of these are still used today.

2. *Looking:* The practitioner carefully observes the patient's appearance. This usually includes looking at the person's tongue, face, and body structure.

3. *Touching:* The practitioner carefully feels the radial pulse in the patient's wrist for a very specific assessment of the patient's *qi*, blood, and other essences. Some practitioners can get most of their information from this one source. If the person's complaint is a pain or injury, then the practitioner must examine the afflicted area. A number of other sets of points and microsystems (the hand, foot, ear) may also be palpated.

4. *Listening and smelling:* This aspect of the four examinations involves listening to the patient's voice, noticing any strange odors (which could, for example, indicate infection), and otherwise gleaning information that a patient does not actually report to the practitioner.

Once the assessment is clear, the doctor writes out a prescription to be filled with exact dosages of each herb. Some prescriptions call for bags or batches of herbs, which are often packed in wrapped paper. For such prescriptions, dosage is determined by the number of bags to be cooked and used within a specified time frame. Patients who are unfamiliar with their formulas need to be instructed on how to cook their prescription into a tea or soup. Some herbs may need to be added separately to either reduce or increase their cooking time. For less serious problems, experienced customers are able to use the herbal store as a pharmacy, buying familiar, simple remedies without a prescription.

Benefits and Risks

The three disciplines of TCM have evolved over thousands of years and are considered safe for almost anyone who wishes to try them. Many schools for TCM have adjusted their programs to incorporate more training in modern Western science. Some schools, such as Harvard Medical School, are including courses to help Western physicians refer to and work with alternative medicine. For this reason, anyone thinking about choosing a full program of TCM should consult with both TCM and Western doctors to understand the strengths and shortcomings of each.

As with all health programs, choosing a therapist is a crucial decision. To decide whether an herbalist or therapist is properly qualified, a prospective patient should carefully ask the doctor where and how he learned this discipline. For Chinese herbal medicine, national certification through the National Commission for Certification of Acupuncture and Oriental Medicine (NCCAOM) is one clear way to be sure that a practitioner is at least competent. It is quite possible, however, to find master-level practitioners who have not chosen to acquire such a credential.

—CINDY BANKER

Resources

American Association of Acupuncture and Oriental Medicine
    4101 Lake Boone Trail, Suite 201
    Raleigh, NC 27607
    Tel: (919) 787-5181
    Offers information on TCM.

National Certification Commission for Acupuncture and Oriental Medicine
    1424 16th St. N.W., Suite 501
    Washington, DC 20026
    Provides certification for practitioners of acupuncture, Chinese herbal medicine, and Oriental bodywork therapy.

The New Center for Wholistic Health,
Education and Research
   6801 Jericho Turnpike
   Syosset, NY 11791
   Promotes the study and practice of TCM.
   Web site: www.acupuncture.com
   Provides information and referrals on tradi-
   tional Chinese medicine and acupuncture.

Further Reading

Cheng, Xinnong, ed. *Chinese Acupuncture and Moxibustion*. Beijing: Foreign Language Press, 1987.

Enqing, Dr. Zhang, ed. *Practical English-Chinese Library of Traditional Chinese Medicine*. Shanghai: Publishing House of Shanghai College, 1990.

Kaptchuk, Ted J. *The Web That Has No Weaver*. New York: Congdon & Weed, 1983.

Unschuld, Paul, ed. *Introductory Readings in Classical Chinese Medicine*. Dordrecht, Netherlands: Kluwar Academic Publishers, 1988.

Yubin, L. and L. Chengcai. *Advanced Traditional Chinese Medicine Series*. Amsterdam: IOS Press, 1996.

Wellness

 Wellness programs are based on holism, sometimes called holistic wellness, a philosophy of health that believes well-being is not just a condition of physical health or the absence of disease and illness. Rather, health is a balance of elements that include the mental, emotional, spiritual, and physical aspects of the human condition. In other words, wellness is the integration, balance, and harmony of mind, body, spirit, and emotions, where the whole is thought to be greater than the sum of the parts. Wellness professionals believe that the lines separating the mental, physical, emotional, and spiritual aspects exist in theory but not actu-

ality. Research in the field of psychoneuroimmunology (the relationship between emotions and the body) reveals that there is no division between these aspects, and they should be regarded as one.

History

Although the concept of wellness is thousands of years old, the word *wellness* was introduced into the American vernacular in the 1960s. Thought by many to be an expansion of the fitness movement of the late 1970s and early 1980s, wellness is considered to be a more comprehensive approach to optimal health than standard health education programs that treated specific symptoms or were used to prevent disease. Addressing more than physical ailments, wellness programs integrate, balance, and harmonize the physical, mental, emotional, and spiritual aspects of the wellness paradigm. Today programs are offered in corporate, community, hospital, and fitness club settings.

Basic Principles

It may seem as though mind, body, spirit, and emotions are separate aspects—indeed, a premise proposed by the French philosopher René Descartes (1596–1650) stated that the mind and body are separate entities. Descartes's premise, known as the Cartesian principle, inspired the mechanistic paradigm, which eventually led to the belief that the human body acts like a machine and the way to treat disease and illness (the opposite of health) was through medications and surgery.

The wellness paradigm holds that there is no separation among mind, body, spirit, and emotions. All aspects of the human condition are so tightly connected that it is impossible to distinguish one from the other. An ancient theory that is supported by many experts in several disciplines suggests that each aspect of the human condition is composed of energy, with the densest energy being the most obvious and tangible: the physical body. Here then are definitions for each aspect of the wellness paradigm:

- Emotional well-being is best defined as the ability to feel and express the entire range of human emotions from anger to love, and to control them, not be controlled by them.
- Physical well-being is defined as the optimal condition of each of the body's physiological systems. These include the pulmonary, cardiovascular, nervous, immune, reproductive, urinary, endocrine, musculoskeletal, and digestive systems.

- Mental well-being is understood as the ability to gather, process, recall, and communicate information. Like a computer, the mind can gather and store mass quantities of information.
- Spiritual well-being is defined as the maturation of higher consciousness as developed through the dynamic integration of three facets: relationships (internal—how you relate to yourself and a higher power, however you conceive this to be; and external—how you relate to and interact with all the people in your life), a personal value system, and a meaningful purpose in life.

When evaluating the dynamics of wellness applications, many programs and services need to be considered. Below is a partial list of services, organized according to their respective holistic components. Keep in mind that a service listed in one area has a crossover effect in all the other areas.

Physical Well-Being:
Aerobic Fitness
Cholesterol Screenings
Blood Pressure Screenings
Blood Sugar Screenings
Weight Training
Nutritional Assessments
Biofeedback
Massage Therapy
Hatha Yoga
T'ai Chi

Mental Well-Being:
Meditation
Mental Imagery
Stress Management
Time Management
Creativity and Creative Problem Solving
Communication Skills
Dream Analysis

Spiritual Well-Being:
Values Clarification and Assessment
Journal Writing
Dance Therapy
Meditation
Communing with Nature
Inner Resource Development
Human Potential Development
Community Service Projects
Social Support Groups

Emotional Well-Being:
Humor Therapy
Music and Art Therapy
Aromatherapy
Codependency Therapy
Grieving Therapy
Communication Skills
Creative Anger Management
Stress Management

An important figure in the wellness area, Dr. Elisabeth Kübler-Ross, outlines a theory that suggests that although all four components are always present in the human condition, each component dominates in our lives as we journey through the life cycle. The first component is the emotional, in which we experience the array of human emotions. During this time we may be conditioned by parents, guardians, or even society to suppress our feelings, which could likely result in emotional dysfunction later in life. The influence of physical development begins to dominate at puberty and continues throughout the teen years. The mental or intellectual aspect kicks in during the college years and endures into midlife, as we exercise our mental capabilities through the thinking processes of the right and left brain and the conscious and unconscious mind. The last section of the wellness paradigm, the spiritual, emerges during the midlife years. As Kübler-Ross and others note, many people never move into this phase of development out of laziness, mistrust, or fear.

Practice

With the help of a thorough personal history and open discussions between patient and practitioner, the practitioner can recognize an imbalance or problem in one of the four areas. She will then be able to guide the patient toward programs or services that address the patient's needs. The wellness professional has a whole range of programs to choose from and is aware of how these services and programs will interact and affect the patient. Wellness professionals work in partnership with their patients and recommend treatments that support the body's natural healing system.

Benefits

Wellness programs focus on reaching higher levels of wellness as well as preventing illness. Many patients are motivated by the energy and vitality that result from a holistic approach to life, especially when they realize that the benefits could continue and allow them to feel good for many years.

—BRIAN LUKE SEAWARD, PH.D.

Resources

National Wellness Association
   1045 Clark St., Suite 210
   Stevens Point, WI 54481-0827
   Tel: (715) 342-2969
   Fax: (715) 342-2979
   e-mail: nwa@wellnesswi.org
   Web site: www.wellnesswi.org/nwa.html
   A nonprofit professional membership organization that disseminates information and provides services to professionals working in wellness areas.

National Wellness Institute
   1045 Clark St., Suite 210
   Stevens Point, WI 54481-0827
   Tel: 1-800-243-8694
   Fax: (715) 342-2979
   Founded in 1977, this is a full resource center for wellness practitioners and those interested in wellness programs.

Further Reading

Edlin, Gordon, Eric Golanty, and Kelli McCormack Brown. *Health and Wellness.* Sudbury, Mass.: Jones and Bartlett, 1996.

Travis, John, and Regina S. Ryan. *The Wellness Workbook,* 2nd ed. Berkeley, Calif.: Ten Speed Press, 1988.

PART 2:

Skeletal Manipulation Methods

Skeletal manipulation methods are a group of healing practices that focus on the form of the skeleton to improve the functioning of the whole person. They are part of a larger group of practices that have come to be known collectively as bodywork. *Bodywork* is a general term describing a wide variety of methods that use touch to enhance awareness of feelings and sensations in the body and improve physical functioning. Bodywork methods are also used to relieve pain and encourage relaxation. Many of the disciplines in this book are considered part of the bodywork category: see under Acupuncture and Asian Bodywork, Body-Oriented Psychotherapies, Massage, Movement Therapy Methods, Somatic Practices, and Subtle Energy Practices.

The oldest methods in this section, chiropractic and osteopathy, were developed in response to the conventional medical practices prevalent in America in the mid– to late nineteenth century. The other methods evolved from these seminal practices. In addition to their historical roots, these methods also share a theoretical framework. They view the human being as an integrated whole of body, mind, and spirit, possessing its own innate healing and balancing mechanisms that guide communication among the interrelated systems of the body. The goal of all of these drugless methods is to remove any structural alterations to the natural skeletal alignment that may impede the operation of these innate healing and balancing mechanisms. Osteopathy and chiropractic are used by millions as primary health care modalities for treating a wide variety of health problems. The remaining methods derived from them are generally used to treat specific problems or to enhance general physical health and emotional well-being.

CHIROPRACTIC

CRANIOSACRAL
THERAPY

NETWORK
CHIROPRACTIC

OSTEOPATHY

ZERO BALANCING®

History

The practice of manipulating the skeleton for optimal health is ancient and widespread. Some medical historians report that the Egyptians used such techniques. The earliest written record of skeletal manipulation comes from China, where methods of bodywork were developed several thousand years ago as part of a complete health care system. The Asian bodywork methods practiced today that are derived from these ancient practices are similar to the skeletal manipulation methods described in this section, in that both manipulate the physical body with the goal of influencing a vital life force. There is no evidence that these Eastern practices directly influenced the development of the earliest skeletal manipulation methods. It is likely, however, that the philosophy on which these Eastern practices are based, which was introduced into American cultural discourse in the late nineteenth century, indirectly influenced the founders of chiropractic and osteopathy.

Hippocrates (c. 430–377 B.C.E.), the father of modern Western medicine, is reputed to have said that dislocations of the spine are the origin of many ailments, but it is unclear how this belief affected his medical practice. The recorded history of manipulating the skeleton as a means of treating disease and creating optimum health began in the West with the work of Andrew Taylor Still, M.D. (1828–1917). A controversial figure in American medical history, Still rebelled against the medical practices of his day, which included heavy use of drugs, purging, and bloodletting. He formulated the gentle, drugless, noninvasive principles and techniques of osteopathy and established its first school in Kirksville, Missouri, in 1892.

Unlike Still, Daniel David Palmer (1845–1913), the founder of chiropractic, had no formal medical training but practiced various forms of energy healing popular at the end of the nineteenth century. Chiropractic was formally introduced as a healing modality in 1895. Some medical historians report that Palmer was treated by Still in Kirksville in 1893. Whether or not this particular treatment occurred, given Palmer's lifelong interest in unconventional healing techniques, it is certainly probable that he was familiar with Still's groundbreaking work.

Both osteopathy and chiropractic have had long, arduous struggles for acceptance within the conventional medical establishment. Today doctors of osteopathy (D.O.s) and doctors of chiropractic (D.C.s) are licensed to practice throughout the United States and Canada. In recent years a number of D.O.s and D.C.s have added their own insights to these century-old healing modalities to create more personalized approaches to healing the whole person through manipulation of the skeleton. These new methods include CranioSacral therapy, which focuses primarily on manipulating the bones of the skull; network chiropractic, which blends Western psychotherapeutic theory with gentle chiropractic techniques; and Zero Balancing®, which integrates Eastern concepts of energy with skeletal manipulation.

Using the Body's Inborn Healing Potential

All the methods described in this section are built on the theory that the body has an inborn healing potential. This potential goes by many names, such as "energy," "spirit," or "innate intelligence." Andrew Taylor Still believed this energy was transmitted primarily through the blood, whereas Daniel David Palmer postulated that it moved primarily through the nervous system. In either event, both methods, and all the methods derived from them, when practiced in their most pure form, are drugless, concentrating on releasing structural misalignments in the skeleton and thereby allowing the body's own internal healing and balancing systems to work freely.

Practitioners of skeletal manipulation methods see the relationship between structure and function in the body as interdependent. Just as the steel frame of a building supports its heating, plumbing, and electrical systems, practitioners of skeletal manipulation methods see our bones as the supporting framework of all other systems of our bodies. If the framework is faulty or has collapsed at any point, it is likely to cause damage to the interior systems. Likewise, if there is a problem in an interior system, such as a leaky pipe, which in our bodies might correspond to a diseased organ such as the kidney, liver, or heart, that malfunction will eventually cause a structural defect in the building, such as a bulge in a wall with peeling paint. In the body this would correspond to misalignments in the skeleton and to pain caused by muscles responding to skeletal changes.

Furthermore, skeletal manipulation methods view the systems of the body as interrelated. A common everyday activity such as reaching high for something on a closet shelf or vigorously swinging a baseball bat could initiate a series of systemic changes that begin as a small change in the alignment of the upper spine. If left unchecked, this dislocation could cause localized muscular pain in the shoulder or upper back area, followed by shortness of breath as the muscles between the ribs in the upper torso contract in response to the structural change. Restricted breath may in turn lead to any number of complicated health problems, including bronchitis, asthma, heart conditions, and even depression.

In a like manner, emotional problems such as a traumatic experience, phobias, and even addictions, which can cause chemical toxicity, are seen as possible causes of structural changes in the body. These changes initiate a chain reaction in the interdependent systems of the body, which stimulates further emotional or physical cravings. Many practitioners of skeletal manipulation methods extend this holistic view to every aspect of a person's life, including genetic inheritance, diet, exercise, daily activities, and stress from work and personal relationships.

Experiencing Skeletal Manipulation

Practitioners of skeletal manipulation methods rely predominantly on the use of the hands, physical contact, and knowledge of anatomy to diagnose patients. Touching and physically moving the patient in various ways allows the practitioner to feel the alignment of the skeleton and the state of the muscular system. In this way they are able to treat a spectrum of chronic and acute health problems.

Each of these disciplines has its standard techniques for manipulating the skeleton. Chiropractors focus on the manipulation of the spine itself. They see the flow of information from the central nervous system housed inside the spine as the primary self-regulating system of the body. CranioSacral therapists focus on the relationship of the bones of the skull to each other to monitor the wavelike flow of cerebrospinal fluid, which they believe to be a barometer of healthy functioning throughout all the systems of the body. Zero Balancers focus on special joints, called foundation joints, which they believe are the primary regulators of energy throughout the body. Osteopaths may manipulate the spine, including the skull, or any other joint of the skeleton where they feel skeletal misalignment is negatively affecting the whole person. Although in their original and most pure forms osteopathy and chiropractic used only manipulation techniques, today many

D.O.s and D.C.s augment their treatment plans by recommending specific exercises, dietary or lifestyle changes, and in some cases herbal or pharmaceutical remedies.

Providing Relief for Millions of People Each Year

Skeletal manipulation methods reportedly help more than 15 million people each year who are suffering from a variety of physical and emotional problems. They have been found to help with problems that have not responded to conventional Western medical practices. Whether you are looking for a comprehensive health modality or relief from a specific pain or condition, these methods may offer unique, drug-free, holistic approaches to healing and maintaining optimum health of body and mind.

—*NANCY ALLISON, CMA*

Resources

American Chiropractic Association
    1701 Clarendon Blvd.
    Arlington, VA 22209
    Tel: (703) 276-8800
    Provides information about chiropractic, including monthly publications, newsletters, and clinical councils.

American Association of Colleges of Osteopathic Medicine
    5550 Friendship Blvd., Suite 310
    Chevy Chase, MD 20815-7231
    Tel: (301) 968-4100
    Web site: www.aacom.org
    Offers educational and professional support to osteopathic physicians.

Further Reading

Montagu, Ashley. *Touching: The Human Significance of Skin*. New York: Columbia University Press, 1986.

Chiropractic

 Chiropractic is a mode of body-work that promotes self-healing by manipulating the spine to remove blocks in the transmission of nerve impulses from the brain through the spinal nerves and out to all parts of the body. It postulates that malfunction in any aspect of the individual can be attributed to subluxations, misalignments of the vertebrae that disturb the spinal nerves in their mediation of mind and body. Further, chiropractic subscribes to the basic principle that the immune system will function perfectly and maintain robust, good health as long as misalignments of the spine do not constrict the nervous system. Other therapeutic methods such as nutritional counseling may be included, but treatment always focuses on detection and adjustment of vertebral misalignments. Chiropractic is the second largest primary health care field in the world. Proponents credit it with a wide range of benefits, from relief of chronic back pain to successful treatment of asthma and depression.

History

There is strong evidence that adjustment of the spine has been used as a form of medical treatment since civilization first began. A Chinese manuscript from 2700 B.C.E. records details of soft tissue manipulation, and the Greeks are known to have developed similar practices around 1500 B.C.E. In a treatise dating from the fifth century B.C.E., Hippocrates encouraged his patients to "get knowledge of the spine, for many diseases have their origin in dislocations of the vertebral column."

Daniel David Palmer is responsible for developing the form of spinal adjustment used today. Born in 1845, Palmer was an American who worked as a healer most of his life but had no formal medical training. While its Greek name, *chiropractic*, meaning "done by hand," evokes ancient Hippocratic teachings, virtually all of chiropractic's principles and techniques are late nineteenth century in derivation. Manual "bone-setting" was accepted practice, and irregularities in the nervous system were commonly viewed as the cause of illness. The third major component in chiropractic, the use of the hands to harmonize the circulation of nervous energy, came from Palmer's experience as a magnetic healer, or Mesmerist. In Mesmerism the hands are passed over the person's field of electromagnetic energy with the aim of correcting imbalances regarded as the cause of illness.

Palmer advanced beyond Mesmerist concepts as his work progressed, but he never relinquished its vision of a treatment that bypasses drugs and surgery in favor of direct contact between the hands of the healer and the life force of the person. By 1895 he had put together the basic principles of chiropractic and was winning renown throughout the Midwest for "miracle cures" of apparently irreversible problems. His son, Bartlett Joshua Palmer (1881–1961), transformed chiropractic into a profession with a following that was devoted but rocked by persistent controversy. Doctors of Western medicine were generally opposed to the growth of a competing system of health care and led efforts to make chiropractic illegal. Attacks on its lack of scientific rigor intensified debate about the interpretation of Palmer's legacy within the chiropractic community. "Straights" argued that chiropractic should consist solely of hands-on vertebral adjustment and condemned as traitors those who mixed spinal adjustment with other forms of therapy or used mechanical devices in lieu of their hands.

Present-day chiropractors continue to identify themselves as either "straights" or "mixers," but the struggle to win public respect and authority is largely over. During the 1930s John J. Nugent started a movement that gradually raised the standards at chiropractic schools and set up chiropractic licensing laws in all the states. More recently, chiropractic has benefited from a swing toward natural medicine that stimulated broad interest in its history and potential as an alternative mode of health care. Because of the experiments of "mixers," chiropractic is rapidly becoming more diversified and offers nutritional counseling, massage, and an increasing use of mechanical devices.

Theory

Palmer believed a human being is born with an ever-vigilant "innate intelligence" or "innate mind" that superintends all the body's functions and seeks to achieve homeostasis, a state of balance that extends "to every individual cell in the living organism." In chiropractic, much as in therapeutic touch or osteopathy, virtually unlimited powers of self-healing are imputed to the person, and drugs are seen as detrimental to the workings of the body's own defense mechanisms. Palmer also taught that diagnosis of disease through the study of symptoms generally overlooks the true cause. Ninety-five percent of all disease, he contended, is attributable to vertebral misalignment that interferes with the transmission of information from the innate intelligence to the spinal nerves.

Contemporary chiropractors are more apt to speak of an inborn switchboard than of innate intelligence, but they adhere to Palmer's belief that illnesses are often caused by subluxated vertebrae and in numerous instances are misdiagnosed because the symptoms do not point directly to back trouble. For example, chronic bladder infection may be the result of a misalignment of the lower vertebrae that irritates the nerves leading to the bladder. Palmer performed his most famous cure—restoring the hearing of a man deaf for seventeen years—by correcting a subluxation of the upper spine.

Diagnosis and treatment in chiropractic are therefore organized not around disease, but around signs of systemic malfunction likely to originate in vertebral misalignment: aberration of musculoskeletal development, or kinesiopathology; abnormality in the muscles proper, or myopathology; irritation of the nerves, or neuropathology; inflammation indicative of abnormality in the blood cells, or histiopathology; and deterioration of the sense of mental and physical well-being, or pathophysiology. The misalignments themselves are attributed to any of several causes, such as injury, mental or physical stress, and genetic defect or predisposition.

Chiropractic education consists of a four-year, postgraduate program similar in overall structure to medical school. Graduates receive the degree Doctor of Chiropractic (D.C.) and are required to take courses basic to Western health care during the first two years of training. Study in the third and fourth years is devoted to the diagnostic and therapeutic tools specific to chiropractic. Work with patients at clinics affiliated with the chiropractic school is a standard part of advanced training.

Practice

Chiropractic treatment begins with the taking of a thorough case history and a physical examination that includes analysis and touching of the spine to determine imbalances and subluxations. X rays of the spine are sometimes taken to get additional information. Recommendations for rest, physical therapy, or diet may be made as part of a therapy plan that generally entails spinal adjustments carried out over a series of sessions. The adjustments are done through hands-on contact that varies from gentle touch to firm pressure, depending on the needs of the patient and the orientation of the chiropractor. Some advocate a maneuver in which the joint is stretched to just beyond its normal range of motion and makes an audible click. Others rely on a repertory of "nonforce" techniques to manipulate the vertebrae. The adjustments are not painful and are often described as relaxing, relieving, liberating, or energizing. Length and frequency of the sessions are established by the chiropractor and patient and depend on the nature of the problem.

Benefits

A wide variety of health problems respond favorably to chiropractic treatment. It is beneficial for musculoskeletal disorders, particularly whiplash injuries, neck and back pain, scoliosis, sciatica, arthritis, and bursitis. It can be effective in alleviating migraine headaches and other organic conditions, sinusitis, gastrointestinal disorders, bronchial asthma, high blood pressure, and heart trouble. Spinal adjustment is also regarded as a drug-free means of releasing nervous tension that contributes to the formation of mental and physical disability. Extensive research today is also testing the efficiency of chiropractic in the treatment of addictions.

—DR. TRINA MARX

Resources

American Chiropractic Association
1701 Clarendon Blvd.
Arlington, VA 22209
Tel: (703) 276-8800
Provides a myriad of information about chiropractic, including monthly publications, newsletters, and clinical councils.

International Chiropractors Association
1110 North Glebe Road, Suite 1000
Arlington, VA 22201
Tel: (703) 528-5000

A professional organization dedicated to chiropractic.

World Chiropractic Alliance
2950 N. Dobson Road, Suite 1
Chandler, AZ 85224
Tel: 1-800-347-1011
Fax: (602) 732-9313
Web site: www.worldchiropracticalliance.org
A professional support group that provides referrals for chiropractors nationwide.

Further Reading

Coplan-Griffiths, Michael. *Dynamic Chiropractic Today: The Complete and Major Guide to This Major Therapy.* San Francisco: HarperCollins, 1991.
Gevitz, Norman. *Other Healers: Unorthodox Medicine in America.* Baltimore: The Johns Hopkins University Press, 1988.
Martin, Raquel. *Today's Health Alternative.* Tehachapi, Calif.: American West Publishers, 1992.
Moore, J. Stuart. *Chiropractic in America: The History of a Medical Alternative.* Baltimore: The Johns Hopkins University Press, 1993.
Palmer, Daniel D. *The Chiropractor's Adjuster.* Davenport, Iowa: Palmer College Press, 1992 (first published 1910).

CranioSacral Therapy

CranioSacral therapy is a gentle form of bodywork based on releasing restrictions in the craniosacral system to help one achieve one's highest levels of physical, mental, and emotional well-being. It was developed over a twenty-year period by Dr. William Sutherland, an osteopathic physician intrigued by the movement of different bones in the skull. He discovered that by exerting gentle pressure on selected areas of the skull or the rest of the body, a craniosacral therapist could effectively treat chronic pain, lowered vitality, recurring infections, and dysfunctions affecting the head, spine, and whole body.

History

CranioSacral therapy developed from cranial osteopathy, the origin of which dates back to the 1890s, when Andrew Taylor Still, M.D., founded osteopathy. Distraught over the death of his wife and two children from meningitis and not knowing whether the disease or the mercury used to treat them was responsible, Still began an intensive study of anatomy and nonpharmaceutical methods of healing. He realized that everything in nature was ordered: that the body functions as a unified whole, that structure and function are interrelated, that the body has an inherent self-corrective mechanism, and that drugs can be harmful. Based on these principles, Still founded the first osteopathic college. Still's star student was William Sutherland, who was intrigued by the idea that the bones of the skull were structured to allow for movement. For more than twenty years he explored this concept, eventually developing a system of treatment known as cranial osteopathy.

In 1970 osteopathic physician John E. Upledger observed the rhythmic movement of the craniosacral system during surgery. Upledger and his colleagues could not find an explanation for this mysterious movement. After studying the work of Sutherland, Upledger worked to scientifically confirm the mobility of the cranial bones and the subsequent existence of the craniosacral system. From 1975 to 1983 he served as clinical researcher and a professor of biomechanics at Michigan State University. There he supervised a high-level team of anatomists, physiologists, biophysicists, and bioengineers to test and document the influence of therapy on the craniosacral system. This team developed the theoretical PressureStat Model to describe how the craniosacral system functions. Upledger's continued work in the field resulted in the further development of CranioSacral therapy, including a ten-step protocol used to alleviate a range of conditions.

Basic Principles

The craniosacral system consists of the central nervous system, brain, and spinal cord, as well as the membranes and cerebrospinal fluid that surrounds and protects the cord. The central nervous system interconnects with the tissue that surrounds it, which in turn interconnects with all other bodily structures. As a result, there is one uninterrupted tissue sheath, called fascia, from the top of your head to the tips of your toes. CranioSacral therapists are highly trained in sensing through touch a restriction in your system and determining how it affects other areas in your body. For instance, practitioners believe a restriction in your leg might have a profound effect on your lower back, shoulder, neck, or even head. They use touch to track, identify, and release root restrictions affecting the person.

How does CranioSacral therapy work? First, as cerebrospinal fluid filters into the craniosacral system, pressure builds. As the amount of fluid increases, the increased pressure forces the fluid to travel down the spinal cord. As the fluid moves, the membranes surrounding the fluid and the interconnected fascial tissue of the entire body pulse in a rhythmic fashion, normally at a rate of six to twelve cycles per minute. It is this rhythm that the therapist monitors.

One unique feature of CranioSacral therapy is its emphasis on very delicate palpation. Therapists are taught to use, appreciate, and develop profound insights through applying a light, gentle touch—generally the pressure is equal to the weight of a nickel. It is believed that this light touch allows the therapist to receive as much information as possible from the patient's body, and to interact with it in a respectful, highly therapeutic manner.

Another distinction relates to its facilitation of the body's self-corrective ability. Therapists believe engaging body restrictions with a gentle touch can break down tissue, emotional, and energetic blocks to self-release. CranioSacral therapy is not a manipulative therapeutic modality in which therapists impose what they think should happen on their patients. Rather, therapists are trained to allow their patients' bodies to facilitate their own healing processes.

CranioSacral therapy aims to be very direct toward yet highly respectful of the patient. A gentle touch directed toward a patient's primary restrictions is believed to provide profound access to the fabric of an individual's being. This respect for the patient's own healing abilities reflected through touch creates a safe environment for people to frequently access deep, nonconscious parts of themselves they may have blocked or simply could not access by themselves. Training in CranioSacral therapy is recognized as a profound foundation for advancement in manual therapies, massage, and therapeutic bodywork.

Practice

A typical session of CranioSacral therapy lasts forty-five minutes to an hour. The client is fully clothed and lies on a comfortable, padded table. In a very gentle manner, the therapist evaluates the patient by testing for craniosacral motion in various parts of the body. Experienced practitioners are able to feel the craniosacral rhythm anywhere on the body. They can quickly gain valuable information by palpating the craniosacral motion for rate, amplitude, symmetry, and quality.

Lack of craniosacral rhythm or an asymmetrical craniosacral rhythm is used to locate problems throughout the body. The problem may be anything that causes loss of natural physiological responses, pain, trauma, adhesions, neurological and orthopedic disorders, systemic disease processes,

John E. Upledger is credited with introducing CranioSacral therapy to a broad spectrum of the world's health care professionals representing diverse specialties. In 1985 he founded the Upledger Institute to educate the public and health care practitioners about the benefits of CranioSacral therapy. To date, this health care resource center and clinic, based in Palm Beach Gardens, Florida, has trained more than 25,000 health care practitioners worldwide. Alumni include osteopaths, medical doctors, psychiatrists, psychologists, dentists, physical therapists, occupational therapists, acupuncturists, doctors of chiropractic, nurse practitioners, massage therapists, and bodyworkers.

and other conditions. The therapist's job is to restore the symmetrical craniosacral motion to problem areas. As the asymmetry is eliminated and normal physiological motion is restored, the problem is being or has been alleviated.

Benefits

CranioSacral therapy has been used to improve the functioning of the brain and spinal cord, to alleviate pain and the effects of stress, and to enhance general health as well as resistance to illness and disease. It has been especially effective for conditions such as migraines, hyperactivity, chronic neck and back pain, temporomandibular joint pain and dysfunction, chronic fatigue, eye difficulties, stress and tension-related problems, scoliosis, emotional difficulties, motor-coordination impairments, central nervous system disorders, learning disabilities, and childhood developmental disabilities.

—KENNETH I. FREY, PT, DIPLOMATE CST

Resources

Kenneth I. Frey, PT, Diplomate CST
Director, Institute of Physical Therapy
30 W. 60th St., Suite 1BC
New York, NY 10023
Tel: (212) 245-1700
World renowned for its clinical services and as an educational resource center in New York City dedicated to the application and development of advanced holistic physical therapies. Treatment integrates whole-body evaluation and advanced manual therapies, clinical sciences, and therapeutic exercise.

The Upledger Institute, Inc.
11211 Prosperity Farms Road, D-325
Palm Beach Gardens, FL 33410-3487
Tel: 1-800-233-5880 ext. 9283
An educational and clinical resource center that integrates the best of conventional health care with advanced complementary techniques. Dedicated to the natural enhancement of health, it is recognized worldwide for its continuing education programs, clinical research, and therapeutic services.

Further Reading

Claire, Thomas. *Bodywork*. New York: William Morrow, 1995.

Sutherland, William. *Teachings in the Science of Osteopathy*. Portland, Ore.: Rudra Press, 1990.

Upledger, John E. *Your Inner Physician and You*. Berkeley, Calif.: North Atlantic Books, 1991.

Upledger, John E., and Jon D. Vredevoogd. *CranioSacral Therapy*. Chicago: Eastland Press, 1983.

Network Chiropractic

 Network chiropractic is a branch of chiropractic, a health care method that views all health as a result of the body's inability to express, relay, and distribute energy and information through the nervous system. Chiropractors aim to enable the brain and the body to better communicate through the elimination of disruptions in the central nervous system, which is housed in the protective bones of the spinal column. To do this, they use gentle manual pressure and adjustment to reduce muscular tension, skeletal torsion or twisting, and compression of the spinal cord or the nerves branching from it, which may result in a disruption of the body's essential energy and information highway.

Network chiropractic is a form of chiropractic that seeks to develop the body's self-corrective mechanism. It is believed that this improvement will enhance a person's health, wellness, and quality of life.

History

Donald Epstein, D.CA., a 1977 graduate of New York Chiropractic College, developed this method of chiropractic, which has been researched through the Department of Anatomy and Neurobiology and Sociology at the College of Medicine at the University of California–Irvine, and at the University of Southern California, Department of Engineering. Epstein's method resulted from his efforts to incorporate many different approaches and theories into a single "network" of established chiropractic techniques. Also known as network spinal analysis, the system has been evolving since 1982 and is currently practiced by chiropractors under the trade name network chiropractic.

Philosophy

Adjustment is a central technique of chiropractic doctors. Adjustment means using the hands to apply leverage and thrust to a joint to restore function to the joint or muscles, nerves, and tissue around the joint. This therapy relies on the body's ability to recover without surgery or drugs.

Network shares the historical philosophy of chiropractic, which is based on the concept that the information the body needs to function is conveyed through oscillation, or vibration. The nervous system coordinates all vibration through the body, relaying energy and information to all body parts and influencing all body functions. Tension on the spinal cord or the nerves exiting from the spinal cord causes an energy disturbance. Network chiropractic seeks to enhance communication between the brain and the body through the correction (adjustment) of vertebral subluxations.

Network practitioners believe that subluxations are caused by physical, emotional, mental, or chemical stresses. In network care it is common for the body to express the energy unavailable to the body as spontaneous muscular movement, stretching, or the outward expression of emotion such as laughter or crying. This liberates the spine from the interference caused by the inability to effectively "move the energy" and circulates the body's information.

The largest study of health and wellness benefits of a chiropractic method was performed at the University of California–Irvine. Patients evaluated their own improvements through a wide range of health and wellness indicators. The study showed evidence of significant improvement in the areas of physical symptoms, emotional and mental state, stress evaluation, life enjoyment, and overall quality of life.

Practice

Before the start of a session, the chiropractor will request that individuals complete a questionnaire on the individual's physical, emotional, mental, and chemical stresses and history. The spine is then evaluated for posture, muscle tension patterns, tension in the extremities that may be related to spinal cord tension, range of motion, and the involvement of spinal motion with respiration. Some practitioners utilize various types of noninvasive instrumentation to further assess the functioning of the nervous system. Spinal X rays are not routine, however, and are taken as indicated on an individual basis.

A chiropractor's office usually contains a special device called an adjusting table, which allows patients to sit or lie in the optimal position for receiving care, whether that be faceup, facedown, seated, or on the side. Patients spend about ten minutes or so on the adjusting table—not an extended period.

Rather than addressing the structural misalignment as a primary distortion, the network practitioner views it as protection for a spinal cord under tension. The doctor begins with light pressure applied to the tissue around the spine. Precise touches and touch adjustments are used to release tension in the spinal cord and to assist the body in recognizing the distortion and generating self-correction.

As tension is relieved from the spine, a spontaneous release of emotional tension occurs. The practitioner will reassess the patient regularly, perhaps every two months, until the desired improvement has been made.

Benefits and Risks

Network chiropractic is one of the most nonaggressive types of adjustment. Adjustments are not given in the areas of maximum tension, fixation, swelling, or pain. Most adjustments are very gentle. The practitioner is not seeking to inhibit the body or alter pain; instead, the objective is to enhance the body's own self-corrective, self-healing mechanism. For these reasons, network is considered a safe application of chiropractic.

—*Donald Epstein, D.CA.*

Resources

Association for Network Chiropractors
444 N. Maine St.
Longmont, CO 80501
Tel: (303) 678-8101
Professional organization of network chiropractors.

International Chiropractors Association
1110 N. Glebe Road, Suite 1000
Arlington, VA 22201
Tel: (703) 528-5000
Provides information on practitioners.

World Chiropractic Alliance
2950 N. Dobson Road, Suite 1
Chandler, AZ 85224
Tel: 1-800-347-1011
Promotes the practice of network chiropractic.

Further Reading

Books

Epstein, Donald, and Nathaniel Altman. *The Twelve Stages of Healing: A Network Approach to Wholeness*. San Rafael, Calif.: Amber-Allen Publishing, 1994.

Maynard, Joseph E. *Healing Hands: The Story of the Palmer Family, Discoverers and Developers of Chiropractic*. 4th ed. Woodstock, Ga.: Jonorm Publishers, 1992.

Woodham, Anne, and David Peters. *Encyclopedia of Healing Therapies*. New York: DK Publishers, 1997.

Journals

Journal of Vertebral Subluxation Research, vol. 1, no. 1 (1996).

Osteopathy

 Osteopathy is a holistic and drugless approach to health and disease. It is based on the idea that a human being is not merely a collection of parts but a totality imbued with spirit. The human body functions as a unit and possesses self-healing and self-regulating mechanisms. Osteopathy maintains there is a reciprocal relationship between structure and function, meaning that an alteration in structure (the musculoskeletal system) through injury will result in a change in function (in internal organs), namely disease. Conversely, a diseased internal organ will result in an alteration in the musculoskeletal system. The osteopathic physician, through his intimate knowledge of human anatomy, can recognize even subtle deviations from normal bodily functioning and by the application of various techniques can restore the proper structure and function and assist the inherent self-healing powers of the body.

History

The practice of osteopathy was developed by Andrew Taylor Still, M.D. (1828–1917), the son of an itinerant Methodist preacher who supported his family by farming and by practicing medicine. While helping his father tend to the medical needs of Native Americans, Still decided to take up medicine himself, under the guidance of his father. He studied the standard medical texts of the time, including those on anatomy, physiology, pathology, surgery, and other topics.

Early on, Still became aware of the limitations of the medical practice of his day, particularly the almost total preoccupation of conventional, or allopathic, medicine with identifying and suppressing symptoms. To him, this understanding of disease was crude at best and based on vague notions of "physiological tension" that needed to be relieved by such devices as purging, bloodletting, and the administering of large doses of morphine, opium, alcohol, and mercury. Still believed that rather than treating only the symptoms of a disease with such agents, a doctor should attempt to discover the cause of the disease itself. He originated the concept of wellness and developed principles of proper exercise and diet to prevent disease. He also created a system of manipulating various joints and tissues to realign the bones and muscles and thereby increase blood circulation and nerve functioning.

In America in the 1870s, such a holistic perspective was heresy. Still's early life provided many unfortunate opportunities to witness the shortcomings of conventional medicine. He lost his first wife and six children to infectious diseases of one kind or another. He witnessed the impotency of medical care during his service as an Army field surgeon and when he cared for Native Americans during epidemics. He was stricken with pneumonia for three months and took three years to recover from typhoid. In many ways osteopathy was Still's unique synthesis of his personal experience and several major intellectual and philosophical movements making their way across America during his lifetime.

Over the years Still continued to practice conventional medicine—including service as a surgeon in the Union army during the Civil War—and to develop his unique healing methods. He devised a system of manipulation and spinal reflexes with which he treated all types of conditions. Despite his therapeutic successes he was viewed as a medical heretic, a grave robber, and a "crazy crank" because of his unorthodox views, study of corpses, long hours of solitary study, and casual dress. Because his methods obtained results that were seemingly inexplicable, some viewed his practice as the work of the devil. In 1873, while living in Kirksville, Missouri, Still saved many lives during an epidemic of infectious diarrhea without the use of any drugs. In spite of this success, his reputation as an eccentric followed him and he was shunned until he cured the crippled daughter of a prominent Presbyterian minister.

In 1874 Still severed his ties to conventional medicine and announced the founding of a new medical science, which he named osteopathy. This new school of medical thought was conceived as a reformation or improvement of conventional medicine, not an alternative system. Throughout the 1880s he continued to refine his science and made several attempts to train others. He also hoped to establish an osteopathic school. Patients flocked to Kirksville from all over America for his treatment. Hotels were built in the town to house the many patients arriving daily, and several railroad companies began advertising train service to Kirksville.

On November 1, 1892, Still opened the American School of Osteopathy. The first class of eleven students consisted of former patients, family friends, and five of Still's children. Five women were among the members of this first class, and Still was later reported to have said that he thought women made better osteopaths than men. Still was assisted in his teaching by William Smith, M.D., an 1889 graduate of the University of Edinburgh. After one year Still determined that for the most part his attempt to teach osteopathy was a failure. He issued certificates but beseeched the graduates to return for another year of instruction. Some did not return. In 1893, however, Still did receive some confirmation that his method could be successfully learned when two of his sons saved many lives during a black diphtheria epidemic in Minnesota. Graduation for those members of the first class who had returned was held on March 4, 1894. Slowly, the curriculum improved, more and better students graduated, and an infirmary was built in 1895. That year Still and his students performed 30,000 osteopathic treatments. By the late 1890s his school, infirmary, and new surgical hospital were increasingly successful both academically and financially.

In its struggle for acceptance, organized osteopathy had to battle the powerful American Medical Association, which sought to maintain its control of the practice of medicine in America. Denied the right to serve as physicians in the military and other government jobs, osteopathic professionals lobbied hard for inclusion. It wasn't until the Vietnam War that osteopaths were allowed to serve their country as physicians. Today there are seventeen osteopathic colleges. Some are state-supported schools where faculty and facilities are shared with students of allopathic medicine. Osteopathic physicians can now practice in all medical and surgical specialties and serve in all branches of the military and government health service organizations.

The curriculum at osteopathic schools is identical to its allopathic counterpart, with the exception that D.O.s learn osteopathic philosophy and manipulation. However, with equality comes paradox. As the osteopathic curriculum improved over the years, it became more like conventional medicine. Today there are approximately 35,000 osteopathic physicians in practice in the United States. Only about 3 to 5 percent of osteopaths practice the original healing art as envisioned by Still. Yet the original osteopathic concept is powerful and has made a lasting impression on medicine throughout the world. Chiropractic, Rolfing, and CranioSacral therapy borrow heavily from much of Still's pioneering work.

The osteopathic concept has also spread worldwide, giving rise to colleges in England, Canada, and Europe. To date, thirty-two countries have granted osteopathic physicians unlimited practice privileges, with an additional nine countries granting privileges limited to manipulation.

Philosophy

Osteopathy was Still's unique synthesis of his personal experience and several major intellectual and philosophical movements that were making their way across America at the time. He viewed disease as an effect of derangement from the anatomical perfection intended by God, the divine architect.

Still was most influenced by Herbert Spencer, a nineteenth-century British philosopher who coined the term *evolution* and influenced the thinking of Charles Darwin. In Still's philosophy of osteopathy one can find many of Spencer's ideas—the concepts of cause and effect, the relationship between structure and function, the holistic nature of humans, and the interrelatedness of parts.

These systems theorized the existence of the flow of certain healing and self-regulating electromagnetic and spiritlike fluids in the body, and Still incorporated these concepts into his notion of the healing effects of an unimpeded flow of blood. According to Still, osteopathic manipulation could relieve restrictions to the free flow of blood and nerve power by removing bony dislocations and easing muscle contractions. Toward the end of his life, Still revealed to one of his students that he was actually able to see the human aura, the human energy field.

There are currently around 35,000 osteopathic physicians in the United States, yet only about 500 osteopaths practice the original healing art, as many use manipulation techniques merely as an adjunct to their conventional practices. Nevertheless, the original osteopathic concept has made a lasting impression on medicine throughout the world. Osteopathic and conventional forms of research have validated and confirmed many of Still's original ideas. Today even the conventional medical world has many manual-medicine societies, and the specialties of psychiatry and rehabilitation medicine have benefited from Still's pioneering work.

Modern doctors of osteopathy take a holistic approach to the human body and mind and, accordingly, take the emotional and mental states into consideration, as well as physical condition. Osteopaths emphasize the interaction among the brain and nervous system and the musculoskeletal system, paying particular attention to the latter, which they believe influences all other organs and systems. They contend that physical and emotional disease is brought about by interrupted nerve flow caused by muscle spasms, injury, or improper alignment of the spine and other bones. By applying hands-on manipulation, palpation, and other physical therapies to the spine, bones, muscles, and connective tissues, D.O.s treat a variety of disorders.

Practice

A typical session begins with the taking of a history of the patient's current problem, including all medications or other therapies being used. This is augmented to include all past medical and surgical treatments and especially any physical or emotional traumas. Family and occupational histories are also obtained. In the case of an infant or child, the medical history includes the details of the pregnancy, labor, delivery, and perinatal period for that individual, and questions about developmental milestones are asked. Next comes a physical exam based on the patient's history, and laboratory and imaging studies (X rays, CT scans) may be ordered if appropriate.

In addition, the osteopathic physician performs either a regional (focusing just on the problem area) or a complete body examination, searching for areas of somatic (body) dysfunction, that is, impaired or altered functioning of parts of the musculoskeletal system. The dysfunction may lie in bone, joint, fascia, or muscle, or in related vascular, lymphatic, cerebrospinal, or neural elements. Once a diagnosis is made, treatment can begin. The entire body may be treated with a wide variety of natural techniques, using varying degrees of force according to the nature of the problem and the patient. Any point on or within the body that can be reached with the hands can be treated osteopathically.

The treatments are given on a padded table to a patient wearing comfortable, loose-fitting clothing (although the patient may have to undress partially for the initial screening examination). If it is performed properly, there is no contraindication for osteopathic manipulative treatment.

In osteopathic hospitals, treatments are given to patients in intensive care units, emergency rooms, labor and delivery rooms, and newborn nurseries, as well as in general medical and surgical units. After the first session, the patient's condition and treatment plan are discussed. Return visits are scheduled based on the individual's response to the first treatment and not on a fixed or routine basis.

—*Dr. Domenick Masiello*

Resources

American Association of Colleges of
Osteopathic Medicine
    5550 Friendship Blvd., Suite 310
    Chevy Chase, MD 20815-7231
    Tel: (301) 968-4100
    Web site: http://www.aacom.org
    Promotes the study of osteopathic medicine. Provides information on the seventeen osteopathic schools in the United States.

American Osteopathic Association
    142 E. Ontario St.
    Chicago, IL 60611
    Tel: 1-800-621-1773
    Fax: (312) 280-3860
    Web site: www.am-osteo-assn.org
    Offers educational and professional support to osteopathic physicians.

Further Reading

Gevitz, Norman. *The D.O.s: Osteopathic Medicine in America.* Baltimore: The Johns Hopkins University Press, 1982.

Hildreth, Arthur Grant. *The Lengthening Shadow of Dr. A. T. Still.* 3rd ed. Kirksville, Mo.: Osteopathic Enterprise, 1988.

Magoun, Harold Ives, Sr. *Osteopathy in the Cranial Field.* 3rd ed. Kirksville, Mo.: Journal Printing Company, 1976.

Still, A. T. *Autobiography.* Kirksville, Mo.: privately printed, 1897.

———. *Philosophy of Osteopathy.* Kirksville, Mo.: privately printed, 1899.

———. *Philosophy and Mechanical Principles of Osteopathy.* Kirksville, Mo.: privately printed, 1902.

———. *Osteopathy: Research and Practice.* Kirksville, Mo.: privately printed, 1910.

Still, Charles F., Jr. *Frontier Doctor, Medical Pioneer: The Life and Times of A. T. Still and His Family.* Kirksville, Mo.: The Thomas Jefferson University Press, 1991.

Sutherland, William Garner, and Ann L. Wales, eds. *Teachings in the Science of Osteopathy.* Fort Worth, Tex.: Sutherland Cranial Teaching Foundation, Inc., 1990.

Trowbridge, Carol. *Andrew Taylor Still: 1828–1917.* Kirksville, Mo.: The Thomas Jefferson University Press, 1991.

Ward, Robert C., ed. *Foundations for Osteopathic Medicine.* Baltimore: Williams & Wilkins, 1997.

Zero Balancing®

 Zero Balancing® (ZB) is a hands-on body-balancing and integrating approach that aligns body energy fields with body structure. ZB is based on the Western understanding of anatomy and physiology but includes Eastern concepts of energy as working tools as well as guiding principles for the integration of the whole person. Alignment through ZB balances body energy and structure; creates clearer fields of vibration throughout the body; releases tension patterns from the body tissue, the mind, and the emotions; and allows the vibration of stress to pass more freely through the person.

History

Fritz Frederick Smith, M.D., developed the system of Zero Balancing over several years. The son of a prominent chiropractor, Smith trained as an osteopath and medical doctor in the 1950s, and later as a five-element acupuncturist with Professor J. R. Worsley. He was also a student of shakti yoga as taught by Swami Muktananda, a massage therapist and certified Rolfer (while he was studying with Ida Rolf he was her model for seven of the ten-hour sessions). Out of these various experiences he formulated his own distinct set of ideas and techniques that later became known as Zero Balancing.

Basic Principles

According to Smith, Zero Balancing draws from Eastern concepts of energy and yet is fully consistent with contemporary quantum physics and the viewpoint that matter is composed of both particle and wave. In ZB the practitioner considers both of these components as they are found in the body—particle is represented by structure or matter, and wave by energy or vibration. If we compared the body to a sailboat, the sail would represent the structure and the wind the energy. ZB focuses on the interface and relationship of where the wind meets the sail—where the energy meets structure within the body and mind—with the knowledge on another level that all these aspects are forms of energy.

Smith postulates that the strongest fields of energy are in the bones of the skeletal system. This is the densest tissue in the body and therefore entraps the densest energy of the body. Whereas ZB also addresses soft tissue, its main focus is on the skeletal system. Within the skeletal system its main focus is on the foundation and semifoundation joints of the body—those joints that have more to do with the transmission, absorption, and equalization of energy than with locomotion or movement. Examples of these joints are the sacroiliac joints, the tarsal and carpal joints of the feet and hands, and the inter- and costovertebral articulations of the spine.

In addition to being intimately involved with energy forces in the body, these joints have several other characteristics that make them especially important in energy medicine. They have small ranges of motion, and when they become compromised in function the body tends to compensate around the dysfunction rather than resolve it directly. The compensatory patterns that result impact not only the physical body but the mind, emotions, and spirit as well. This means that these joints (and other tissues that hold vibration) can lock imbalances within the whole person. Many of these imbalances are at first subtle and do not come to the level of a person's awareness until symptoms (such as muscle pulls, increasing irritability, stress burnout) have manifested and magnified the problem. The structural/energetic work of ZB can release these patterns while they are still hidden from awareness and before they create symptoms. ZB can also improve the fundamental imbalance after a person develops symptoms and create a climate in which nature can improve or heal the person's complaint.

ZB is taught as a postgraduate studies program for the health care practitioner. It is not designed as a start-up program for the beginning health care student. A program of training has been established; the graduate of the program receives in-house recognition as a certified Zero Balancer and is given permission to use the registered trademark of ZB. It is not designed or intended to give the student any specific legal recognition or per-

mission to work in the health care field. ZB is practiced under the umbrella of other health care studies.

Practice

The Zero Balancer assesses the body by testing and evaluating the currents and/or stagnation of energy within bone, within the foundation joints of the skeleton, and within certain soft tissues. In places where the energy and structure are not well balanced, the ZBer uses touch to create a fulcrum, or balance point, in the tissue. When this balancing field of tension is held stationary for a few seconds, it allows the two variables—energy and structure—to reorganize. Improved function, movement of energy, and feelings of well-being ensue. By repeated use of fulcra, placed properly and where necessary, the skilled practitioner can balance a person in terms of the person's own energy and structure.

A typical ZB session requires about thirty to forty minutes and is done with the patient fully clothed. It is performed in two positions, with a person first sitting and then lying comfortably on his back on a massage table. Everything in ZB should either feel good to the client or "hurt good." If any of the procedures is ever uncomfortable or "hurts bad," the client should notify the ZBer.

Why Practice ZB?

Zero Balancing's major strength arises from the ability to balance and integrate a person in terms of her own body energy and body structure. This ability comes from integrating Eastern concepts of energy as working principles and tools into the practice of body handling. ZB is extremely effective in relieving stress and assisting a person as she is going through stressful periods in life. When a person is well balanced between energy and structure, the vibration of stress passes through the body more easily and has less tendency to become stuck, to cause tension patterns, and to progress toward physical or emotional dysfunction. ZB also has a particularly important place in relieving pain and suffering if they are the result of blocked energy.

Like any system of balancing or healing, ZB is not always the appropriate therapy for a given situation. The ZBer is schooled to know when ZB is of particular value, specific risks for the use of ZB, and situations in which a medical opinion is mandatory. ZB is not meant to delay or replace standard medical care; rather, it is an adjunct to high-level functioning and feelings of well-being.

—*FRITZ SMITH, M.D.*

Resources

Zero Balancing® Association
   P.O. Box 1727
   Capitola, CA 95010
   Tel/fax: (831) 476-0665
   e-mail: info@zerobalancing.com
   Web site: www.zerobalancing.com
   Conducts training programs throughout North America. Continuing education credit is granted for most programs by the Board of Nurses (California), Acupuncture Committee (California), and the National Certification Board for Therapeutic Massage and Bodywork (NCBTMB).

Further Reading

Smith, Fritz Frederick, M.D. *Inner Bridges: A Guide to Energy Movement and Body.* Atlanta: Humanics New Age, 1990.

PART 3:

Nutritional and Dietary Practices

Nutritional and dietary practices are body-mind disciplines that adhere to the popular adage "You are what you eat." Advocates of these practices believe that everything you ingest becomes a part of you, affecting your physical health, mental abilities, and emotional outlook. Nutritional and dietary practices are some of the oldest body-mind disciplines known to humankind. Although many specific practices are popular today, this section examines one ancient and one modern practice currently used to maintain wellness, prevent disease, and treat specific conditions, both chronic and acute.

HERBAL MEDICINE

ORTHOMOLECULAR MEDICINE

The Development of Nutritional and Dietary Practices

The roots of nutritional and dietary practices are firmly planted in the deepest biological and psychological instincts of the human race. When ill, humans and many other animals instinctively fast, which cleanses and rests the digestive system. In addition, animals have been observed in their natural environments searching out and eating specific plants for medicinal purposes.

Indigenous peoples also use plants from their surrounding environment for medicinal purposes. Much of our knowledge of herbal medicine comes from anthropologists who have lived with these peoples and learned their age-old wisdom. The diets of these peoples invariably include a variety of fruits, vegetables, grains, and sometimes animal products native to the area. These locally produced diets create a chemical balance within each person's body and between the people and their environment.

Nutritional practices and herbal medicine form an integral part of all classical healing systems. Doctors in both ayurvedic and traditional Chinese medicine diagnose patients in part through knowledge of their dietary preferences and cravings. Both systems prescribe dietary changes and herbal medicines to balance the body-mind disharmonies they perceive through their diagnostic methods. Like those of indigenous peoples, both of these highly developed healing systems are based on a belief that disharmony of body and mind, or of the body-mind complex and the surrounding environment, is the root cause of disease.

In classical Greece, where the modern Western healing system originated, the physician Hippocrates (c. 460–377 B.C.E.) also believed in health as a balance between the individual and the environment. Discussing the prescription of food as medicine, Hippocrates is believed to have said, "Food or drink which is in itself slightly inferior, but more pleasant should be preferred to that which is better in itself, but less pleasant." Hippocrates seems to affirm a belief not only that food could be used as medicine, but also that the human organism has the innate ability to direct its own healing, in part at least, through the sense of taste.

Throughout European history people continued to rely on their sense of taste to develop a varied, balanced, moderate diet that made use of local fruits, grains, and animal products. They also used various herbs and foods to heal specific conditions. Garlic has been used by people in many European countries for centuries to heal infections. Chamomile tea has long been recommended to calm the nerves.

In the mid–nineteenth century, Western medicine discovered the role of bacteria in the spread of disease. This momentous discovery led to many innovations in Western health care, including sterilization of surgical instruments, hygienic standards of cleanliness in hospitals, and the process known as pasteurization of milk and other liquids. It also led to the development of the germ theory of disease in which all disease was believed to be caused by outside organisms invading the human body. To fight these invaders, biochemists developed an arsenal of antibiotics and other pharmaceutical germ killers. These medicines appeared to work more quickly and to be more effective than the traditional dietary and herbal cures. Doctors began to pay less and less attention to the diets of their patients, and relied more and more on the growing stockpile of synthesized drugs to relieve painful and uncomfortable symptoms.

Throughout the nineteenth and early twentieth centuries, many voices of dissent arose against this shift away from natural whole-food diets and toward the dependence on pharmaceutical drugs. Some of those voices, such as that of American doctor Sylvester Graham (1794–1851), were dismissed as alarmist by allopathic, or conventional, Western doctors. Other individuals, such as Japanese physician Michio Kushi, a leading proponent of macrobiotics, were dismissed as exotic and extremist.

In the mid–twentieth century, scientists such as two-time Nobel Prize winner Linus Pauling (1901–1994) began using Western biochemical methods to study the effects of the individual vitamins found in foods on various physical, mental, and emotional conditions. The discoveries made by Pauling and other scientists form the basis of orthomolecular medicine, a contemporary scientific nutritional practice that recommends individualized whole-food diets and high doses of vitamins instead of drugs to heal disease and create optimum health.

A growing number of people in the 1960s became increasingly disillusioned with the use of pharmaceutical drugs. Some felt, as many feel today, that the drugs were costly, increasingly ineffective, and often produced as many side effects and complications as they appeared to cure. For these reasons many individuals, and eventually the U.S. government through the National Institutes of

Health, began to reconsider nutritional and dietary practices as a safe and effective means of disease prevention and health care.

Maintaining the Body's Natural Chemical Balance

The basic theoretical foundation of all dietary and nutritional practices is the belief that whatever we take into our bodies will affect our bodies. If we eat a diet that maintains the natural chemical balance of our cells and provides for extra vitamins and minerals in times of stress or high demand, we will remain healthy. If we don't eat a balanced diet, we may create an imbalance in our cellular chemistry. This may cause our organs and systems to malfunction and eventually may lead to disease and illness.

Scientific studies conducted by the National Institutes of Health and private foundations such as the National Cancer Institute have pointed to a strong connection linking diets high in fats, especially saturated fats, and low in fiber to diseases and conditions such as coronary artery disease, stroke, diabetes, high blood pressure, and breast and colon cancer. Conversely, changes in diet or eating specific herbs and nutrients seem to activate the body's natural defenses, enabling it to heal itself. Today scientists are looking at whole foods, specific vitamins, and herbs to discover, in scientific terms, how diet can prevent and cure illnesses. They have learned that orange and dark green vegetables like carrots, sweet potatoes, pumpkins, spinach, broccoli, and kale, which all contain high levels of beta carotene, seem to help prevent certain kinds of cancer. High doses of vitamin B_3 (niacin) have been used with positive results to help people suffering from a variety of mental and emotional symptoms often diagnosed as schizophrenia. And *Hypericum perforatum*, more commonly known as St. John's wort, seems to be a safe and effective remedy for mild to moderate depression.

Nutritional and Dietary Methods in Practice

Many different nutritional and dietary practices are in use today. Naturopaths, traditional Chinese medicine doctors, ayurvedic physicians, osteopaths, chiropractors, and bodyworkers may prescribe or suggest nutritional or dietary practices during a course of treatment. Herbalists and orthomolecular physicians are two types of practitioners who focus specifically on dietary or herbal practices as a means of maintaining health and curing disease.

A visit to one of these practitioners can be like a visit to a general practitioner. Both will want to know about the nature of your problems and information about your diet. The orthomolecular physician may make use of tests, whereas the herbalist may rely more on her physical observations and questioning of you to arrive at a diagnosis.

Once diagnosed, both will probably recommend changes in your diet and prescribe specific supplements. An herbalist may recommend that you buy a specific herb or combination of herbs that can be prepared and eaten in various ways, whereas the orthomolecular physician may recommend various doses of vitamins. Whichever practice you follow, these practitioners work with you and your other health care professionals to help you attain your maximum state of health.

Learning About Your Body

Like other body-mind disciplines, nutritional and dietary practices require that you take responsibility for your own health and healing. After all, an herbalist or orthomolecular physician can prescribe a course of treatment, but no one can make you prepare the prescription or take it!

Some people enjoy the heightened awareness of the body-mind connection that develops over time as they participate in a particular dietary or nutritional practice. Others find the process cumbersome, time consuming, or too restrictive. In addition, some people find the scents and tastes of various herbal cures unpleasant, whereas others enjoy the experience of preparing their own remedies and tonics.

Nutritional and dietary practices are designed to balance your body chemistry in order to develop its natural resilience and resistance to disease. After working with a dietary or nutrition professional, balancing your body chemistry, and becoming more knowledgeable about your nutritional needs, you may formulate a delicious and enjoyable diet that will help you heal minor ailments, prevent disease, and create optimum health of both body and mind.

—*Nancy Allison, CMA*

Resources

American Botanical Council
P.O. Box 201660
Austin, TX 78720-1660
Tel: 1-800-373-7105
Fax: (512) 331-1924
e-mail: custserv@herbalgram.org
Web site: www.herbalgram.org
Nonprofit research and educational organization. Offers a quarterly magazine called *HerbalGram*, which publishes the latest herbal research, legal and regulatory issues regarding herbal medicine, detailed profiles of herbs, conference reports, and book reviews.

The International Society for Orthomolecular Medicine
16 Florence Ave.
Toronto, ON M2N 1E9
Canada
e-mail: centre@orthomed.org
Web site: www.orthomed.org
Founded in 1994, this organization lists and recommends orthomolecular practitioners in Canada. Also publishes the *Journal of Orthomolecular Medicine*.

Further Reading

Books
Gladstar, Rosemary. *Herbal Healing for Women.* New York: Simon & Schuster, 1993.

Kowalchik, Claire, and Hylton Williams, eds. *Rodale's Illustrated Encyclopedia of Herbs.* Emmaus, Pa.: Rodale Press, 1987.

Santillo, Humbert. *Natural Healing with Herbs.* Prescott Valley, Ariz.: Hohm Press, 1984.

Journals
Willoughby, John. "Primal Prescription." *Eating Well*™ *Inc.,* May–June 1991.

Herbal Medicine

 Herbal medicine is one of the most popular forms of alternative medicine in the United States today. People use herbal remedies for a variety of reasons: to aid digestion; to relax; to alleviate minor aches, pains, and headaches; to stave off disease; and to diminish the symptoms of the common cold or flu. Besides addressing specific symptoms or needs, some herbalists believe these remedies bring the body and mind into balance and can therefore cure chronic or long-term illnesses.

History

Over the centuries herbal remedies have been utilized in many cultures to alleviate pain and cure disease. The ways herbs are used in diverse geographical areas reflect the philosophy and values of each particular culture as well as what herbs are available in each region. In traditional Chinese medicine, herbs are used to restore balance in the body and are part of a long-term treatment that seeks to maintain the health of both mind and body. In Western medicine, herbal medications have been developed to treat particular physical symptoms immediately. This pharmacologically based system has been especially successful in the treatment of acute illness.

Herbs form the basis of many modern pharmaceutical drugs. Today about 25 percent of all prescription medicines are derived from medicinal plants. Pharmaceutical companies are doing research on herbs from the Brazilian rain forests. In fact, the word *drug* derives from the old Dutch word *droge*, which means "to dry." During the Middle Ages, Dutch pharmacists dried plants for use as medicines.

In 1994 an estimated 17 percent of all Americans used herbs for some medicinal or health reason. The herbal industry is estimated to have earned $2 billion in sales in the United States in 1996, and sales are increasing at the rate of about 25 percent per year. A poll conducted in early 1997 indicated that one-third of adult Americans are using herbal medicines, spending an average of $54 per person annually, thus creating a total estimated retail market of $3.24 billion. Once found only in health food stores, mail-order catalogs, and marketing organizations, herbal medicines are now sold in drugstores and supermarkets, and by mass-market retailers, where herbal preparations constitute one of the fastest-growing areas.

Increased popular interest in herbs has been fueled in part by the passage of the Dietary Supplement Health and Education Act of 1994. In 1993 and 1994, when the act was being considered, Congress received more mail from American voters concerning this new law than they had concerning any other single issue since the Vietnam War. This overwhelming response suggests that consumers are interested in using herbs and other dietary supplements for their health.

In addition, the heightened interest in herbal medicine reflects consumer concern about the high cost of Western medicine in general and pharmaceutical drugs in particular. Further, there is a growing perception among consumers that many conventional medicines are toxic and produce adverse side effects, despite the fact that they have been approved by the Food and Drug Administration. These concerns have revived interest in many traditional herbs and medicinal plants, as well as other forms of alternative medicine. Many Americans have also become interested in this area because of the increased media coverage in alternative medicine and the creation of the Office of Alternative Medicine at the National Institutes of Health to study herbs and other alternative modalities.

Basic Principles

Herbs are popular all over the world. The World Health Organization estimates that about 80 percent of people in developing countries still rely on some form of traditional medicine for primary health care. In every type of traditional medicine, that is, medicine based on historical uses and used by indigenous cultures, herbs and medicinal plants constitute the major basis of the remedies used.

In a real sense, herbs are not alternative medicine; they are integral to the development of all medicinal systems, both modern and traditional. Despite the fact that many modern drugs are derived from plants, there is a major distinction between a plant-derived drug (e.g., quinine) and an herbal medicine. Plant-derived drugs are single chemical compounds that are extracted and purified from plants. Herbal medicines can be defined as a whole plant or plant part that is used for its medicinal properties. Thus, an herbal remedy contains small amounts of many naturally occurring chemicals from the plant.

Most herbal medicines are used for minor, self-limiting conditions or illnesses. Herbal medicines can be as simple as a cup of chamomile tea (*Matricaria recutita*) to help digestion after a big meal, to ease an upset stomach, or to serve as a relaxing beverage before bed. Other simple herbal medicines include an extract of the roots or leaves of echinacea (*Echinacea* spp.) to help reduce the severity or duration of a cold or flu, especially when taken at the onset of symptoms; the use of feverfew leaf (*Tanacetum parthenium*) to allay migraine headaches; and valerian root (*Valeriana officinalis*) to help assure a good night's sleep, especially for those with insomnia or other sleep disorders.

Today many people are also using herbs to help prevent long-term illness. Cardiovascular disease is the biggest killer of all Americans. Millions of Americans are turning to such simple remedies as garlic (*Allium sativum*) to help reduce cardiovascular risk factors. In fact, the German government has already approved garlic for such use, including the lowering of LDL cholesterol, known as "bad" cholesterol—a property of garlic that has been documented in more than two dozen clinical studies. Because the German government allows such claims on garlic tablets, garlic is the biggest-selling over-the-counter medicine sold in German pharmacies.

Herbs are being increasingly used as alternatives to modern synthetic prescription drugs. Millions of American men are using the extract of the fruits of the native American saw palmetto plant (*Serenoa repens*) as a safe and clinically documented remedy for benign prostatic hyperplasia, a nonmalignant enlargement of the prostate that affects about half of men over fifty years of age. Gaining popularity is the standardized extract of St. John's wort (*Hypericum perforatum*), which is considered a safe and effective remedy for mild to moderate depression. The efficacy of this herb, called a phytomedicine in Europe, has been established in numerous clinical studies.

Standardized extract of ginkgo leaf (*Ginkgo biloba*) has been shown in many clinical studies to be safe and effective in stimulating peripheral circulation, especially in the brain. This herb is especially useful in geriatric care to help treat senile dementia and short-term memory loss in elderly patients. Another useful phytomedicine is the standardized extract of milk thistle fruits (*Silybum marianum*). This preparation is a safe and effective tonic for the liver, especially for those who suffer from alcohol-induced cirrhosis of the liver, those who have been exposed to toxic industrial chemicals, or those who suffer from certain types of hepatitis.

Practice

Herbal medicines can be steeped or boiled in water (known as *infusion* and *decoction*, respectively), and taken as a tea. They can be

Following are types of herbs and their uses:

Adaptogenic: Helps to reduce and resist stress.
Alterative: Improves health and increases energy.
Antihelminthic: Kills or expels intestinal worms.
Anti-inflammatory: Soothes and reduces inflammation.
Antimicrobial: Strengthens resistance to dangerous microorganisms.
Antispasmodic: Reduces cramps and tension in skeletal muscles.
Astringent: Produces a barrier against infection.
Bitter: Functions as a general aid to disease prevention.
Carminative: Improves the operation of the digestive system.
Demulcent: Reduces inflammation.
Diuretic: Stimulates production of and increases the elimination of urine.
Emmenagogue: Aids in the functioning of the female reproductive system.
Expectorant: Helps to remove mucus from the lungs.
Hepatic: Strengthens the liver.
Hypotensive: Lowers blood pressure.
Laxative: Stimulates bowel movements.
Nervine: Promotes the healthy functioning of the nervous system.
Stimulating: Increases the metabolic activity of the body.
Tonic: Invigorates, supports, and calms the body.

ingested as powdered herbs in capsules and tablets, or as liquid extracts made with water and alcohol or just alcohol. They can also be taken as standardized extracts. In these extracts, the level of one naturally occurring chemical compound or group of compounds is chemically guaranteed from one batch to another in order to ensure reliable content.

Herbs can also be used topically. Fresh aloe gel (Aloe vera) can be applied directly to the skin to help reduce the pain of a minor burn or sunburn. Aloe is used as an ingredient in sunburn creams, skin lotions, and even shaving creams—all of which attest to the popularity and widespread acceptance of the healing dermatological properties of this plant recognized since ancient times. In Germany many skin care products rely on extracts of chamomile for their scientifically proven skin-healing properties. Also in Ger-

many, manufacturers sell echinacea products for external use on slow-healing wounds.

Benefits and Risks

A qualified herbalist or a well-respected herbal guide or specialist should be consulted for the most effective herbal treatment. Herbs have certain qualities and must be used with care. Like conventional drugs, they are not recommended in every instance. For example, the herb ephedra (Ephedra sinia, commonly called by its Chinese name, ma huang), functions as a stimulant and is not recommended for those with high blood pressure, diabetes, glaucoma, and related conditions in which hypertensives are contraindicated.

The world of plants is rich and diversified and produces numerous herbal remedies that have been used for thousands of years. Modern scientific research continues to document and validate the historical uses of many herbs as well as new uses of some traditional medicines. The safe and responsible use of herbal medicines offers an important way to lower health care costs and increase the wellness of the American public. More scientific research will continue to place herbs in a position to offer many benefits in the new medicine of the twenty-first century.

—MARK BLUMENTHAL

Resources

American Botanical Council
    P.O. Box 201660
    Austin, TX 78720-1660
    Tel: 1-800-373-7105
    Fax: (512) 331-1924
    e-mail: custserv@herbalgram.org
    Web site: www.herbalgram.org
    Leading nonprofit research and educational organization. Offers a quarterly magazine called *HerbalGram*, which publishes the latest herbal research, legal and regulatory issues regarding herbal medicine, detailed profiles of herbs, conference reports, and book reviews.

American Herbalists Guild
    P.O. Box 1683
    Sequel, CA 95073
    Provides a directory of schools and teachers of herbal medicine.

Further Reading

Castleman, Michael. *The Healing Herbs.* Emmaus, Pa.: Rodale Press, 1991.

Foster, Steven. *50 Herbs for Your Health.* Loveland, Colo.: Interweave Press, 1996.

Hoffmann, David. *The New Holistic Herbal.* Rockport, Mass.: Element Books, 1992.

Tierra, Leslie. *The Herbs of Life.* Freedom, Calif.: Crossing Press, 1992.

Orthomolecular Medicine

 Orthomolecular medicine strives to achieve the optimum health of its patients, as well as treat and prevent disease, by creating the uniquely individual levels of nutrients needed in each person's body through diet, vitamin supplementation, and lifestyle changes. Practitioners employ what is more commonly known as megavitamin therapy, which is the use of large doses of certain vitamins—based on thorough biochemical analysis—to correct ineffective or destructive chemical balances in the body. Orthomolecular medicine also addresses a variety of psychiatric disorders, such as schizophrenia and severe depression.

History

It was Linus Pauling, two-time Nobel Prize winner (for chemistry and for peace), who in 1968 first coined the term *orthomolecular medicine* to describe more accurately what had been popularly known as megavitamin therapy. Pauling's concept was to create an optimum nutritional microenvironment for every cell in the body by giving it the "right amounts of the right molecules"—vitamins, minerals, amino acids, enzymes, and other substances used by the body. This not only would correct the deficiencies or imbalances that make us more susceptible to disease and degeneration, but it also would promote the highest level of health, enabling us to reach our physical, mental, and spiritual potential and enjoy a maximum life span. The path to this goal is accomplished through dietary changes and supplementation.

For many years prior to his death in 1994 at the age of ninety-three, Pauling was an outspoken champion of nontoxic therapies and nutritional supplementation. He attracted considerable attention—and controversy—with his books on the beneficial effects of vitamin C supplementation against the common cold and cancer.

Pauling formulated a modern nutritional paradigm, an approach emphasizing optimum intake of nutrients for achieving powerful prevention and healing benefits. Orthomolecular physicians have used this approach to successfully treat schizophrenia, depression, alcoholism, drug abuse, and individuals with gastrointestinal disorders, arthritis, cardiovascular disease, and even cancer.

The first half of the twentieth century held much excitement and interest in vitamins because people believed they were a quick way to good health. From 1925 to 1940 many vitamins were isolated from food, then identified and synthesized. Nutritional pioneers began exploring the clinical uses of these newly available substances and using amounts that were above the levels considered necessary to prevent deficiency-state diseases such as scurvy, beri-beri, and pellagra.

In North Carolina, a country doctor named Fred Klenner used large doses of vitamin C effectively against viral illness. The infants delivered by mothers on his supplement program were so robust and healthy that the local hospital staff nicknamed them the "vitamin C babies." In Canada, two physician brothers, Evan and Wilfrid Shute, found that vitamin E offered a valuable treatment against heart disease. In the early 1950s, two other Canadian physicians, Abram Hoffer and Humphrey Osmond, began to use high doses of niacin (vitamin B$_3$) and other nutrients to help schizophrenic patients. The nutritional treatments they pioneered for a variety of mental conditions were later formalized into orthomolecular psychiatry. Over the years, the orthomolecular arsenal has expanded dynamically. Today it includes a broad spectrum of vitamins, minerals, amino acids, enzymes, hormones, and plant-derived supplements.

Many commentators believe that allopathic, or more conventional, medicine has shown little respect for nutritional therapy in an age of pharmaceutical, surgical, and high-tech methods. In the past vitamins and minerals were considered necessary only in tiny amounts in order to prevent certain diseases; furthermore, conventional Western medical practitioners maintained that if people ate right, they would obtain enough nutrients from food. As a result, conventional medical schools have not thoroughly educated their students about the role of nutrition in causing and healing disease.

Times may finally be changing. There is a growing interest in alternative treatments because of the cost and side effects of pharmaceuticals and the failings of modern conventional medicine to impact the crisis of chronic disease and runaway medical costs. A growing number of medical schools are offering programs in nontoxic treatments and clinical nutrition. In addition, quite a bit of research has proven that vitamin supplementation, at doses higher than those usually present in the diet, has a significant preventive and therapeutic effect and represents a potent, safe, and inexpensive medical option.

In 1992 the New York Academy of Science convened a landmark conference, "Beyond Deficiency: New Views on the Function and Health Effects of Vitamins." At this meeting researchers presented new findings on the positive effects of vitamins and minerals against cancer, heart disease, and other illnesses. A joint conference of the United Nations and the World Health Organization in 1996 on healthy aging reflected the growing recognition of nutrition in the fight against disease.

Basic Principles

"Let food be thy medicine and thy medicine be thy food," said Hippocrates to his students. More than 2,500 years later, this ad-

Is orthomolecular therapy dangerous?

Some people have argued that high doses of certain vitamins can be dangerous, even toxic, to those who take them. Studies have shown that the dangers are minor compared to the dangers of taking high doses of pharmaceutical medications.

If symptoms occur, or if you feel you are taking too much of a certain vitamin, ask your orthomolecular practitioner. He will be aware of the dangers and can tell you all you need to know about your treatment. If you are taking too much of a certain nutrient, the practitioner will lower your dosage immediately, and the level of that nutrient in your body will adjust within a short time. The most important issue is to keep your doctor aware of any changes or symptoms you might experience during the therapy.

vice from the father of medicine has been overlooked but not altogether ignored, by modern doctors using pharmaceutical drugs and sophisticated technology. Practitioners of alternative medicine, among them orthomolecular physicians, regard food and nutrition as the bedrock of their profession.

Orthos is a Greek word meaning "straight." Just as orthopedic medicine refers to the straightening of deformed or broken bones, and orthodontics to the straightening of crooked teeth, orthomolecular medicine literally means to straighten or correct the body's molecules.

Orthomolecular practitioners base their treatments on the concept of biochemical individuality, an idea put forward by Roger Williams, Ph.D., the University of Texas scientist who discovered vitamin B_5. This concept holds that each of us is uniquely different. We look different, react to stress and chemicals differently, live and work in different environments, have different genetic makeup, drink different water and eat different food, and have different requirements for various nutrients. Although the number of necessary nutrients is the same for each of us, the optimum amounts we need individually are very different. For this fundamental reason, orthomolecular physicians regard the government-promoted RDAs (recommended daily allowances) and MDRs (minimum daily requirements) as irrelevant. "Even if 90 percent of any population required only the minimal daily requirement of vitamins, it would leave huge numbers of people needing 10, 100, or 1,000 times as much," contends orthomolecular physician Abram Hoffer. "With sick people the range of need is many times greater."

The perspective of pioneers like Hoffer and other orthomolecular specialists is that their form of medicine is not a cure-all or a replacement for conventional treatment. Rather, explains Hoffer, "a proportion of patients will require orthodox treatment, a proportion will do better on orthomolecular treatment, and the rest will need a skillful blend of both."

Practice

Orthomolecular physicians practice throughout the world. They are primarily medical doctors (M.D.s), but also osteopaths (D.O.s), naturopaths (N.D.s), and chiropractors (D.C.s).

Orthomolecular practitioners zero in on the individuality of patients through laboratory tests and comprehensive medical reviews that consider diet, stress, exercise, levels of sensitivity to foods or chemicals, and the use of alcohol, drugs, or pharmaceuticals. These tests are performed in a physician's office.

Recommendations typically involve not just nutritional supplements but also the elimination or reduction of drugs, contaminants, and allergens, and the replacement of junk food and nutrient-poor diets with complete, fresh, and nourishing diets.

Benefits and Risks

Orthomolecular medicine is beneficial for a wide range of physical and mental conditions, and its concepts are widely practiced by health-conscious individuals concerned about preventative care.

To get comprehensive and effective treatment, one should see an orthomolecular specialist first rather than trying to attempt self-treatment.

—*Martin Zucker*

Resources

International Academy of Nutrition & Preventive Medicine
P.O. Box 18433
Asheville, NC 28814
Tel: (704) 258-3243
Offers a list of practitioners by state. Publishes the *Journal of Applied Nutrition*, a quarterly journal that covers nutritional issues.

The International Society for Orthomolecular Medicine
16 Florence Ave.
Toronto, ON M2N 1E9
Canada
e-mail: centre@orthomed.org
Web site: www.orthomed.org
Founded in 1994, this organization lists and recommends orthomolecular practitioners in Canada. Also publishes the *Journal of Orthomolecular Medicine.*

The Society for Orthomolecular Medicine of America
2698 Pacific Ave.
San Francisco, CA 94115
Tel: (415) 922-6462
Provides information on orthomolecular practitioners in the United States.

Further Reading

Hoffer, Abram. *Orthomolecular Medicine for Physicians—A Survey/Introduction Textbook.* New Canaan, Conn.: Keats Publishing, 1989.

Hoffer, Abram, and Morton Walker. *Putting It All Together: The New Orthomolecular Nutrition.* New Canaan, Conn.: Keats Publishing, 1996.

Janson, Michael. *The Vitamin Revolution in Health Care.* Greenville, N.H.: Arcadia Press, 1996.

Pauling, Linus. *Vitamin C and the Common Cold.* San Francisco: W. H. Freeman, 1970.

Pauling, Linus, with Ewan Cameron. *Cancer and Vitamin C.* New York: Linus Pauling Institute of Science and Medicine, 1979.

PART 4:

Mind/Body Medicine

Mind/body medicine is a contemporary term used to describe a number of disciplines that study or approach the healing of the physical body, or the transformation of human behavior, by engaging the conscious or unconscious powers of the mind. Whereas *mind/body medicine* is used in this book to describe a growing field of study and practice in contemporary Western medicine, it is used by others to describe ancient Eastern disciplines, such as yoga, meditation, traditional Chinese medicine, and subtle energy therapies. The disciplines that comprise mind/body medicine in this book combine a theory of the relationship between body and mind—which has much in common with these ancient Eastern disciplines—with Western scientific models of biology and chemistry. These disciplines are also characterized by an emphasis on individual motivation in the healing process and a more personal relationship between caregiver and receiver. Mind/body medicine has been used to treat stress-related conditions, such as chronic pain, allergies, chemical and emotional dependencies, and performance anxiety.

BIOFEEDBACK
TRAINING

GUIDED IMAGERY

HYPNOTHERAPY

INTERACTIVE
GUIDED IMAGERY^SM

PSYCHONEURO-
IMMUNOLOGY

Mind/Body Medicine— Ancient and Modern

Although the disciplines discussed in this section emerged from a context of contemporary Western science, the theories and techniques they use have much in common with approaches to healing developed by ancient cultures and still practiced worldwide. Both ancient and modern approaches to mind/body medicine believe that the cause of disease is not restricted to the physical body. In the ancient approach, the nonphysical causes of disease may include spirits, emotions, or the mind, which bridges spirit and body. From the modern perspective, the cause of disease is determined by investigating the effect of thoughts or emotions on behavior and the physical workings of the body.

Shamanism, an ancient method of healing, is based on the belief that all illness is a result of disharmony between the spirit world and the material world. Traditional shamanic practices include trance states and mental focusing techniques similar to those used by hypnotherapy and guided imagery today.

The highly disciplined Indian practice of hatha yoga is driven by the belief that all matter is a materialized form of the one great spirit motivating the universe. It includes numerous health-enhancing physical exercises, internal cleansing techniques, and breathing practices to help people refine the physical body and experience its spiritual nature. Hatha yoga practitioners develop a control of the body similar to that developed through biofeedback today.

In China healers practiced within the framework of the ancient Chinese religion of Taoism, which seeks a balanced, harmonious existence between humankind and nature. Over thousands of years Chinese herbal treatments evolved by correlating observations of the interaction of elements in nature with the physical, emotional, and mental characteristics associated with human illnesses. The relationships Chinese healers noted among elemental balances, emotional states, and physical health are similar to those recognized by psychoneuroimmunology today.

The Development of Mind/Body Medicine in the West

While ancient Greek medical practices were originally holistic, ways of viewing the body began to change with the influence of the philosophical pragmatism of Aristotle (c. 384–322 B.C.E.) and his desire to know and categorize all aspects of the material world. Ancient Greeks began to separate the observation and treatment of matter, or body, from the observation and treatment of spirit, or mind. This trend in Western thinking and healing was later reinforced by the medieval Christian Church, which glorified the devoted mind of humankind as the true channel to the spirit of God while denigrating the physical body as an instrument of the devil. In the seventeenth century, the French philosopher René Descartes (1596–1650) helped establish the philosophical foundation of the Enlightenment by proclaiming the mind a nonmaterial, transcendent aspect of human beings, separate and infinitely more valuable than the physical body.

Split off from philosophical or spiritual inquiry, Western medical science developed by studying the physical body and treating it as a purely mechanical instrument that could be broken down into smaller and more knowable components. Although this approach yielded many amazing, lifesaving achievements over the last three hundred years, it investigated only the physical treatment of ailments. The relationship of the mind and body was not fully investigated by Western medicine until the beginning of this century, gaining ever more momentum in the last thirty-five years. The neurologist Sigmund Freud's (1856–1939) theory of the unconscious mind introduced new ways of considering the mind's effect on behavior and physical health. The research that inspired Freud's theories employed many of the techniques that are a part of hypnotherapy and guided imagery practices.

Throughout the twentieth century, data pointing to a relationship between our thoughts, emotions, and health began to emerge from many branches of science, including sociology, anthropology, and psychology. For example, in 1956 Hans Selye, a Canadian physiologist, revealed the devastating effects of traumatic experiences, which he termed *stress,* on an organism's health. Then, in the 1960s, a more specific clue to the connections between mind and body appeared. Drs. Elmer and Alyce Green, pioneering researchers in biofeedback, documented the profound abilities of advanced yoga practitioners to consciously control their heart rate, temperature, and brain wave patterns. As the century wore on, scientists in the newly developing field of psychoneuroimmunology presented evidence linking particular chemical substances, such as endorphins, to specific human emotions, such as pleasure. They showed how certain levels of endorphins in the body may act as a chemical shield against invading viruses or germs.

Today mind/body medicine practices are a respected part of treatment in many major hospitals and clinics throughout the United States. They may be used for relief of pain before or during surgery and to aid in the postoperative process. In addition, individuals seeking help for a variety of chronic physical conditions, including cancer and AIDS, as well as those seeking to change painful and destructive behavior patterns, such as chemical addictions or eating disorders, are enhancing traditional Western methods of treatment with mind/body medicine practices.

Some Basic Mind/Body Medicine Beliefs

The disciplines discussed in this section represent an expansion of traditional Western approaches to medicine. While research in each discipline has yielded different theories and techniques, together these fields share certain basic principles. First, approaches to mind/body medicine are unified by their belief that real and useful connections exist between our bodies and our minds. Whether the discipline uses the powers of the conscious mind to interact with and affect the systems of the body, as in biofeedback, or employs the powers of the unconscious mind to effect changes in behavior, as in hypnotherapy, the pathways between body and mind are at the heart of these healing modalities.

Mind/body medicine holds that a person's emotions and attitudes will influence his or her body's innate ability to heal. In clinical studies in the 1940s and 1950s, patients were given a placebo, or neutral substance such as sugared water, and told it would relieve their chronic pain. The patients' emotional attitudes toward their pain, as well as their physical progress, were closely monitored. Researchers found that patients who believe they will recover are much more likely to do so than those who believe they won't or those who believe they will get worse. These results strongly suggest that emotions and mental attitudes play an important role in the body's ability to heal.

Finally, all mind/body medicine practices believe in the importance of personal motivation in the healing process. Clinical research has shown that cancer patients who become actively involved in their treatment are more likely to recover than those who passively accept their diagnosis and fail to examine their treatment options. Taking charge of one's life fends off feelings of hopelessness and lack of control, both of which have been shown through psychoneuroimmunology studies to reduce the number of disease-fighting cells in the body. By emphasizing personal responsibility, mind/body medicine practitioners aim to empower patients to make a successful healing journey.

Because practitioners emphasize the individual's participation in the healing process, special attention is given to the relationship between caregiver and receiver. In guided imagery the caregiver is often referred to as a guide or knowledgeable aide. The guide's role is viewed as helping the receiver access his own inner sources of physical, mental, and emotional health and offering positive reinforcement as he learns to navigate the channels between body and mind.

The Future of Mind/Body Medicine

Mind/body medicine practices have helped millions of people find relief from a multitude of physical and emotional problems. People suffering from migraine headaches, insomnia, hypertension, asthma and other respiratory conditions, ulcers and other gastrointestinal disorders, incontinence, cardiac and vascular irregularities, muscular problems caused by stroke or accidents, arthritis, anxiety, attention and learning disorders, depression, chemical and emotional addictions, and phobias and other stress-related disorders have all been helped. The field is still young, but with continued research, creative and caring practitioners, and courageous health care consumers willing to view illness as a message from the body to begin an active healing journey, mind/body medicine may provide new solutions for health care in the twenty-first century.

—NANCY ALLISON, CMA

Further Reading

Borysenko, Joan. *Minding the Body, Mending the Mind*. New York: Bantam Books, 1988.
Chopra, Deepak. *Quantum Healing*. New York: Bantam Books, 1989.

Biofeedback Training

Biofeedback training is a means of enhancing mental awareness of body changes. It is a process that offers techniques for regulating the body's vital functions and fostering overall health. Electronic biofeedback instruments supply information about the body not usually available to the consciousness. Heart rate, muscle tension, blood circulation, brain wave activity, and other body functions are made perceptible as visual and auditory signals that enable an individual to monitor her physiological reaction to various stimuli or situations. With the help of the biofeedback instrument, new, healthier patterns of response can be developed throughout the body's systems, even those patterns previously regarded as involuntary and outside the reach of the conscious mind. Biofeedback training has a vast range of diagnostic, therapeutic, and preventive applications, particularly in cases where stress and related psychological factors play a role.

History

The use of biofeedback devices to modify behavior originated in 1938, when Hobart G. Mowrer introduced an alarm triggered by urine to stop children from wetting their beds. Beginning in the 1940s muscle-tension biofeedback was successfully used in the field of neuromuscular rehabilitation. Biofeedback developed rapidly in America during the 1950s and 1960s because of a coincidence of two factors: the increasing awareness that stress was a principal cause of disease, and the growing interest in expanding the mind's ability to respond to stress more positively and nurture all parts of one's self. At the same time, the invention of the electroencephalograph machine (EEG) and similar electronic equipment gave scientists new tools for monitoring the internal workings of the body-mind connection. Alyce and Elmer Green used the EEG to study the techniques that enable masters of yoga meditation to alter the rhythms and responses of their bodies so extensively that they become impervious to extremes of temperature and pain. Under the direction of Joe Kamiya, volunteers in another study learned to use feedback from the EEG to recognize and achieve the alpha state, an alert sense of effortless well-being normally associated with advanced stages of meditation.

During the late 1960s the excitement generated by the initial findings of biofeedback research led to overly optimistic claims about "miracle cures" of the future. Nonetheless, it was clear that a fundamental concept in the human sciences, the distinction between voluntary and involuntary nervous activity, had been discredited. Vital functions like blood pressure were now seen as subject to the control of the individual. Behavioral modification accordingly became an ever more accepted mode of health care. The first professional meeting of feedback researchers was held in 1968. In 1969 researchers founded a professional support group, the Biofeedback Research Society, later renamed the Association for Applied Psychophysiology and Biofeedback (AAPB). The voluminous scholarly literature on various aspects of biofeedback attests to the interest it has attracted in the scientific community.

Theory

Biofeedback training sees the brain as a control center that sends impulses through the nervous system to program the body's vital functions: heart rate, blood pressure, circulation, digestion, breath, perspiration, and so forth. By automatically signaling the different systems when to turn on or off, people live safely and comfortably in their surroundings without deliberating over the body's basic activities. But stress, illness, or an accident can disrupt the natural process and cause it to send signals that produce common health problems like insomnia, muscular or vascular pain, and irritable bowel syndrome, to name just a few. While these stress-aggravated processes make the body seem unpredictable and beyond control, biofeedback training can help reverse overreactions.

The use of electronic instruments to measure and reflect the status of body functions is only one element of biofeedback training. The discipline also uses relaxation techniques derived from ancient meditation practice and requires participants to be open to the idea of attentional flexibility. Contrary to popular belief, the machines do not intervene in the information traveling between the body and mind. Instead, the instruments act as a mirror of one's internal reactions, allowing an individual to observe this behavior and to be aware of harmful reactions. This information helps uncover hidden patterns of physiological reactions to stress, for example, tensing of muscles and a fall in body temperature, that the person may never have noticed. Furthermore, the machines serve as a precise, objective gauge of the physiological effects accomplished by using a relaxation technique such as visualizing a pleasant scene or a soothing color. The true source of the self-healing promoted and reflected by biofeedback training are techniques that normalize physiological functioning. These techniques enable the person to stabilize erratic or unhealthy physical responses and to take responsibility for her own well-being.

Practice

In its most frequent application, biofeedback training is used to teach people how to cope with health problems that have already been diagnosed by a medical doctor or psychologist. The role of the certified practitioners who administer biofeedback training is to show the client how to interpret and control the electronic biofeedback. The client sits, remaining fully clothed, and sensors are placed on the skin over the region to be monitored. The sensors do not cause pain or discomfort. Body information from the biofeedback instrument is presented in any of several forms: flashing lights, beeping sounds, patterns on a computer screen, or tactile sensations. Currently available instruments have the capacity to monitor skin temperature, electrical conductivity in the skin, muscle tension, heart rate, brain wave activity, and other body processes.

The nature of the work varies according to the needs of the client. In the case of compulsive teeth grinding and temporomandibular joint (TMJ) disorder, training focuses on regulation of muscular tension in the jaw. Attention deficit disorder can be addressed by means of a computer game controlled by brain wave activity. The client watches the game but cannot play unless he produces brain waves of an appropriate pattern. In this way the client becomes minutely attuned to different levels of concentration and learns how to heighten, expand, and focus his attention.

As a biofeedback training session unfolds, the practitioner recommends techniques for attaining the desired result and provides positive reinforcement. Learning and achieving the body-mind benefits of a training program generally requires several sessions with a practitioner, who may advise additional work with home biofeedback instruments or audiotapes. Success in biofeedback training generally depends on the effort expended by the client. Over time and with consistent practice, one progresses to the point where one can monitor and adjust body processes without the aid of electronic instruments.

Benefits

Most practitioners still limit their practice of biofeedback to EEG and blood flow biofeedback. There is a growing movement, however, toward using other techniques, especially neurofeedback, to treat a variety of disorders. The most common applications are for headaches, pain management or pain dissolution, and general stress reduction. Stress reduction is therapeutic for a variety of symptoms such as irritable bowel syndrome, migraine headaches, hypertension, breathing difficulties, cardiac and vascular irregularities, anxiety, depression, insomnia, and symptoms related to addiction, as well as attention disorders and other learning disabilities. The AAPB can provide a list of clinical symptoms that have responded favorably to biofeedback treatment as well as a referral to a certified biofeedback provider in your area.

—LES FEHMI, PH.D.

Resources

Association for Applied Psychophysiology and Biofeedback
   10200 W. 44th Ave., Suite 304
   Wheat Ridge, CO 80033
   Tel: (303) 422-8436
   Provides a nationwide referral service. To receive a free copy of their brochure, "What Is Biofeedback?" send a self-addressed stamped envelope to the address above.

Biofeedback Certification Institute of America
   10200 W. 44th Ave., Suite 304
   Wheat Ridge, CO 80033
   Tel: (303) 420-2902
   A professional organization that determines minimum standards for certification in biofeedback training. BCIA also certifies organizations that provide training for biofeedback practitioners.

Further Reading

Crow, Mark, and David Danskin. *Biofeedback: An Introduction.* Palo Alto, Calif.: Mayfield Publishing Co., 1981.

Guided Imagery

Guided imagery is a therapeutic technique in which a person withdraws into one's mind, focusing on scenes and symbols pertaining to an illness, accident, or personal issue. Within that person's imagination, problems are replaced with a make-believe story of recovered health and happiness. Guided imagery is based on the principle that the imagination has the capacity to relieve pain and promote healing when it is optimistic and confident and, inversely, can help trigger a breakdown when it is consumed by worry. Individuals are taught how to use their powers of imagination to steer themselves away from negative thoughts and toward models of well-being. Guided imagery generally serves as an adjunct to medical treatment and has been incorporated in sports training programs and methods of self-care.

History

What is now called guided imagery can be traced back to practices found in early civilizations around the world. Symbols and spirits were summoned to promote healing, and envisioning one's health was a key element in rituals performed by shamans. When medicine was first separated from religion in classical Greek culture, imagery continued to be regarded as a valuable tool in the maintenance of physical and mental well-being. According to the Greek philosopher Hippocrates (c. 460–377 B.C.E.), inner pictures produce a "spirit" that arouses the heart and other parts of the body. These pictures need to be controlled if the person is to be healthy. Renaissance doctors took a similar view of the role of the imagination. Paracelsus, for example, wrote that "the power of the imagination is a great factor in medicine. It may produce diseases . . . and it may cure them."

After the Renaissance, interest in therapeutic imagery declined because of radical changes in the interpretation of the links between mind and body. Following the precepts of René Descartes, the body was considered a mechanical structure, and the imagination's role in either the body or the operations of the intellect was severely restricted. Sigmund Freud's study of hysteria, a psychosomatic disorder, marks the beginning of a revolution in medicine that can be viewed as a revival of ancient and Renaissance teachings about the power of the imagination. By explaining hysteria as a physical manifestation of emotional trauma, Freud challenged Descartes's notion that illnesses may have only a physical cause. He believed that an effective treatment must also address the patient's inner experiences.

The current American approach to guided imagery is based on Carl Simonton's work with cancer patients during the 1970s. By instructing patients to imagine white cells as warriors defeating the cancer cells, he discovered that these patients lived twice as long as those relying on medical treatment alone. After Bernie Siegel conducted an equally successful pilot program at Yale University, there was a rapid expansion in medical research into the benefits and workings of systems of internal visualization, from daydreaming to self-hypnosis to doodling and drawing. By 1990 guided imagery had emerged as an established mode of treatment, acclaimed by advocates of both traditional and alternative medicine.

Theory

Recent research has suggested that mental imagery can modify the functioning of the body. The brain responds to an image much as if it were the real thing, recalling past experiences and triggering a set of responses that lead from the cerebral cortex to the hypothalamus. The hypothalamus, in turn, transmits messages to the autonomic nerves controlling the body's involuntary functions, which include heart rate, blood pressure, breathing, digestion, temperature, sexual arousal, and immunity. As a result, a seemingly passive activity like guided imagery can bring about changes beneficial to physical health.

While guided imagery resembles other relaxation techniques that intervene in the autonomic nervous system, such as biofeedback training, it is distinctive in one regard. By releasing the imagination, it allows the person to get in touch with repressed emotions that may be at the root of his health problems. In finding a concrete image for a persistent problem, participants often bring troublesome needs and conflicts out into the open, where they can be resolved.

Practice

It is possible to learn guided imagery from a self-help manual or tape, but most people begin by working with a therapist at a doctor's office or health care center. The exact nature of the training depends on the individual's goals and the professional background of her therapist. Some therapists rely on a prepared script of healing images, whereas others encourage individuals to let their imaginations roam. Another major difference in approach concerns the use of imagery. In some techniques it is directed toward relaxation and healing. In a variant of guided imagery, known as Interactive Guided Imagery[SM], the emphasis is shifted away from creating ideal images to picturing symbolic scenes that may reveal hidden emotions. Given the many variants that are now available, it is advisable to ask a prospective therapist to explain the course of therapy before starting a training program.

Training generally involves learning a procedure to follow at home or work, two or even three times a day for five to twenty-five minutes. In many instances, the first steps of the procedure parallel those followed in meditation: the person withdraws to a quiet place, assumes a comfortable position, and turns her thoughts inward. But, unlike meditation, in guided imagery a person fashions an alternative version of her circumstances. Frequently, participants are instructed to imagine themselves mounting stairs that lead to a place where they feel secure and content, then to picture themselves gradually getting well. To exit from the imagery exercise they reverse the process, imagining themselves leaving the pleasant place, descending the stairs, and returning to normal activity.

When guided imagery was first introduced in American medicine, it employed aggressive images of combat between the forces of health and disease. Over the past decades researchers have discovered the importance of adjusting imagery to suit the individual's personality and have broadened the range of what is considered "imagery." Among participants without a strong visual sense, listening to music may take the place of imagining pictures. Another approach is "sensory recruitment." In this technique, rather than rely simply on one sense, individuals are urged to incorporate all the senses—sight, hearing, touch, smell, and taste—into their imagery exercises. This intensifies the impact of the healing messages that the autonomic nervous system sends to the immune system and other vital functions of the body.

Benefits

Daily practice with a routine of guided imagery has been used to relieve headaches and chronic pain. It has also helped people tolerate medical procedures, stimulate healing, and explore the emotions that may have caused an illness. Guided imagery can also give people a heightened sense of their own potential and encourage them to find creative solutions to personal and professional problems.

Resources

Academy for Guided Imagery
P.O. Box 2070
Mill Valley, CA 94942
Tel: 1-800-726-2070
Offers a training program in guided imagery for health professionals; also provides information about guided imagery, including a list of practitioners, books, and videotapes.

Exceptional Cancer Patients
1302 Chapel St.
New Haven, CT 06511
Tel: (203) 865-8392
Organization that maintains a referral list of imagery practitioners who work with cancer patients and offers books and tapes about guided imagery.

Health Associates, Inc.
P.O. Box 220
Big Sur, CA 93920
Fax: (408) 667-0248
Provides workshops on various uses of guided imagery.

Further Reading

Achterberg, Jeanne. *Imagery in Healing: Shamanism and Modern Medicine.* Boston: New Science Library/Shambala, 1985.

Borysenko, Joan. *Minding the Body, Mending the Mind.* Reading, Mass.: Bantam, 1988.

Rossman, Martin. *Healing Yourself: A Step-by-Step Program for Better Health Through Imagery.* New York: Pocket Books, 1989.

Siegel, Bernie. *Peace, Love, and Healing.* New York: Harper & Row, 1989.

Simonton, Carl, Stephanie Simonton, and Creighton Simonton. *Getting Well Again.* Los Angeles: Jeremy P. Tarcher, 1978.

Hypnotherapy

 Hypnotherapy is the use of hypnosis, trance states, and suggestion for therapeutic results. It is used to address a diversity of problems, including anxiety, phobias, and emotional problems, and to help break habits such as smoking. More and more doctors and dentists are incorporating hypnosis to help relieve pain and assist healing. It is also used to improve performance in sports activities, examinations, or public speaking and social activities. By inducing altered states of consciousness, hypnotherapists help clients use the resources of the unconscious mind to bring about psychological and physical benefits. Hypnotherapy asserts that the unconscious mind is a vast reservoir of learning and skills.

History

Franz Anton Mesmer (1734–1815), the father of hypnosis, is responsible for launching scientific investigation into trances. The German physician used auspicious passes of the hands, dramatic gestures, and magnetic apparatuses to induce sleeplike states in willing subjects. Mesmer termed the phenomenon *animal magnetism*, believing that a magnetic fluid had passed from his hands to the subject. In 1784 a commission for the Academy of Science in France (including Benjamin Franklin) was appointed to investigate Mesmer's practices and concluded, "Imagination is everything, magnetism nothing." However, future researchers would confirm the power of suggestion.

James Braid (1795–1860), a Scottish surgeon, used Mesmer's hand gestures to produce anesthesia in patients in his hospital in India, reducing his infection rate from 50 percent to 5 percent in the process. He coined the term *hypnosis*, shortened from

neuro-hypnosis, meaning "nervous sleep." Braid noted that a trance consisted of fixed and focused concentration that rendered a subject open to suggestion.

Auguste Ambroise Liebault (1823–1904) was the first to investigate hypnotic phenomena, founding the School of Nancy in France and developing the doctrine of suggestive therapeutics. Working under him as a professor of internal medicine, Hyppolyte Bernheim (1837–1919) established the foundation of our current understanding of hypnotic suggestion. Bernheim asserted that hypnosis is not a disorder of the nervous system, as many medical authorities of the day believed. It is instead a product of suggestion. He also believed that suggestion was a common occurrence in all interactions and not specific to a hypnotist's gestures.

One of the most famous suggestions in hypnotherapy comes from Émile Coué (1857–1926), another pupil of Liebault's. He thought that all suggestion is really self-suggestion. His exercise involved repeating the phrase, "Every day in every way I am getting better and better." He found that slowly repeated suggestions such as this could become absorbed into the unconscious and affect one's life. This is the basis for all the audiotapes in today's market promising reprogramming of the unconscious.

Sigmund Freud (1856–1939), although initially interested in the psychological use of hypnosis, abandoned it in treatment because he was not able to obtain successful trances in his neurology patients. He became more interested in the causes of neurosis and instead used free association for his "analytic inquiry." Freud's influence on the medical establishment's view of mental illness and its treatment set back the acceptance of hypnosis until Clark Hull, an American professor of psychology at the University of Wisconsin, published the book *Hypnosis and Suggestibility* in 1933. It describes some of the first experimental research on hypnosis.

A student of Hull's, Milton H. Erickson (1910–1980), who founded the American

Society for Clinical Hypnosis, is credited with bringing the techniques of hypnotherapy into mainstream medical and psychological practice and developing its most comprehensive form. Erickson stressed that hypnotherapy is most effective when it is part of a unique program of therapy, developed for each patient according to his situation or needs. He believed that hypnosis is a specialized form of communication in which both conscious and unconscious channels can learn. A patient's natural capacities and unique ways of learning and responding are utilized as part of the therapy. Rather than being controlled by suggestions, a patient is actively seeking solutions. In this model, indirect suggestions in the form of metaphors or stories are used in addition to direct and authoritative suggestions. This is intended to facilitate unconscious learning and bypass conscious imitation and resistance.

Theory

While the word *trance* may conjure up the idea of a zombielike state seen in so many Hollywood films, in reality we all experience different trance states every day. When we become absorbed in reading or watching television, we often shift into a trance state in which time is suspended, cares and worries are forgotten, or surrounding stimuli are tuned out. Intense trances can occur during meditation or prayer, or under states of extreme emotion, such as falling in love. More tranquil trances often are induced during procedures like relaxation training, guided imagery, or massage. Most therapeutic trances are relaxing but can also be arousing and invigorating.

A hypnotherapist induces trances to suspend the limitations of the conscious, analytical mind. This allows all the possibilities of a person's imagination and unconscious to solve, reinterpret, or reorganize an experience, issue, or problem.

Practice

Trances in and of themselves have little therapeutic value, but they greatly facilitate therapeutic goals. Unlike traditional psychotherapy, in which unconscious thoughts and impulses are brought to consciousness for analysis and understanding, in hypnotherapy the patient is trained in using trance to learn and practice new skills for alleviating symptoms or changing behavior. Suggestions may be incorporated unconsciously and can be brought to normal consciousness when that part of the mind is ready.

At the start of a typical session, the therapist first will ask questions about the client's problem and what he hopes to gain from the treatment. After discussing the problem, the procedure to be used, and the goals to be realized, the therapist then will explain what is to be done and answer any questions or concerns. A series of instructions will be provided that help guide the person into a relaxed trance state. Since hypnosis is a learned skill, the induction process is practiced slowly until the person feels comfortable and is able to relax and focus. Suggestions then are offered to help with the problem or issue at hand. As a person's conscious thinking is increasingly withdrawn from the outside environment and suggestions engage more and more of his inner awareness, the trance will become deeper. The goal is to allow one to experience an expanded awareness unhindered by ordinary limitations. In this state intuitive, instinctive, and imaginative thoughts and feelings are used to address the issue at hand. Most work is done in light or medium trances, but catalepsy, a condition in which the limbs stay where they are placed, often occurs. Unconscious hand levitation is a common technique for verifying and deepening the trance experience. The session is usually ended with suggestions to feel refreshed, alert, and completely ready for the rest of the day.

The induction procedure is often taught to the client so that it can be practiced at

> So far as I know hypnosis as a human activity has been used since the beginning of the human race.
>
> —*Milton H. Erickson*
>
> All suggestion is self-suggestion.
>
> —*Émile Coué*

home or used when needed, for example, in times of stress. Appropriate suggestions are prepared ahead of time. A person may rehearse by visualizing herself accomplishing a goal and feeling prepared. Another method of self-hypnosis is to repeat simple affirmations—for instance, "I will become naturally more confident as I practice these skills"—until they become absorbed into behavior.

Benefits

The uses of hypnosis in psychological therapy are well known. People may enter hypnotherapy to gain greater self-confidence for dealing with problems and difficulties. Hypnosis is also used to produce relaxation and relieve anxiety. Learning how to control emotions, impulses, and urges brings greater self-control and mastery. These results occur from most hypnotherapy interventions, even when the focus or problem is quite specific.

Common issues addressed by hypnosis include smoking, overeating, insomnia, and fears such as of flying, public speaking, or performing in sports or examinations. The range of problems is expanding as scientific knowledge about unconscious communication and motivational processes increases.

In medical settings, more and more hospitals are employing hypnotherapists to help create optimal conditions for patient re-

covery and health. For decades, hypnotherapy has been used successfully to manage pain and stress, often in preparation for childbirth and surgery. Migraines, respiratory conditions, ulcers, and arthritis are some of the medical conditions commonly treated.

Those interested in pursuing hypnotherapy should take certain precautions. While inducing trance is easy and can be learned by anyone, only trained practitioners with the appropriate licensing, experience, and knowledge in psychology and physiology should be consulted. Investigate the hypnotherapist's background, credentials, and education and experience. The American Society of Clinical Hypnosis and the Milton H. Erickson Institutes in the United States set the guidelines for proper training and certification for hypnotherapists. The International Medical and Dental Hypnotherapy Association, the Society for Clinical and Experimental Hypnosis, and the American Association of Professional Hypnotherapists are also long-standing associations with much experience in all aspects of hypnotherapy. Finally, be aware of the limitations of hypnosis. It is not a cure-all, and its effects depend completely on the abilities and limitations of the client. Skilled hypnotherapists utilize a client's internal resources but do not replace a person's own skills and capacities. It is highly individual. Avoid practitioners who make exaggerated claims and promise all-purpose cures. While hypnotherapy is a powerful tool, it cannot solve every problem.

—*Oscar A. Gillespie, Ph.D.*

Resources

American Association of Professional Hypnotherapists
4149-A El Camino Way
Palo Alto, CA 94306
Tel: (650) 323-3224
Web site: www.aaph.org

American Board of Hypnotherapy
202 East McFadden Ave., Suite 100
Santa Ana, CA 92705
Tel: 1-800-872-9996
Web site: www.hypnosis.com
Provides information on hypnosis practitioners and training programs, and holds regional workshops for professionals and laypeople throughout the year.

International Medical and Dental Hypnotherapy Association
4110 Edgeland, Suite 800
Royal Oak, MI 49073
Tel: (248) 549-5594; 1-800-257-5467

The Milton H. Erickson Foundation, Inc.
3606 N. 24th St.
Phoenix, AZ 85016
(602) 956-6196
Presents the National and International Erickson Congresses and publishes a newsletter that includes information on training programs. Separate Erickson Institutes and Societies can be found in major cities in the United States and several other countries.

The New York Milton H. Erickson Society for Psychotherapy and Hypnosis
440 West End Ave., No. 1C
New York, NY 10024
Tel: (212) 873-6459
Provides a 100-hour comprehensive training program (chartered by the Board of Regents of New York State) in Ericksonian approaches in psychotherapy and hypnotherapy and a referral service for the New York tristate area.

The Society for Clinical and Experimental Hypnosis, Inc.
111 N. 49th St.
Philadelphia, PA 19139
Publishes *The International Journal of Clinical and Experimental Hypnosis.*

Further Reading

Cheek, David B., and L. M. LeCaron. *Clinical Hypnotherapy.* New York: Grune and Stratton, 1968.

Hammond, D. Corydon, ed. *Hypnotic Suggestions and Metaphors.* New York: W. W. Norton, 1990.
Hunter, Marlene Elva. *Creative Scripts for Hypnotherapy.* New York: Brunner/Mazel, 1994.
Lynn, Steven Jay, and Judith W. Rhue, eds. *Theories of Hypnosis: Current Models and Perspectives.* New York: Guilford Press, 1991.
Phillips, Maggie, and Claire Frederick. *Healing the Divided Self: Clinical and Ericksonian Hypnotherapy for Post-traumatic and Dissociative Conditions.* New York: W.W. Norton, 1995.
Rowley, David T. *Hypnosis and Hypnotherapy.* Philadelphia: Charles Press, 1986.
Rosen, Sydney. *My Voice Will Go with You: The Teaching Tales of Milton H. Erickson.* New York: W. W. Norton, 1982.
Yapko, Michael D. *Trancework: An Introduction to the Practice of Clinical Hypnosis.* New York: Brunner/Mazel, 1989.

Interactive Guided Imagery^{SM}

Interactive Guided Imagery^{SM} is a method of using the mind to support healing and growth. An expert employs certain techniques to help a person enhance her awareness of unconscious images and learn to effectively interact with them. With the aid of a guide, clients use Interactive Guided Imagery sessions to learn to relax, relieve stress, enhance body-mind communication, sharpen intuition, and become more effective at reaching goals. It mobilizes the latent, innate healing abilities of the client to support rehabilitation, recovery, and health.

History

The practice was founded by Martin L. Rossman, a medical doctor, and David E. Bresler, a health psychologist. Both had been independently researching clinical applications of body-mind effects in health since the late 1960s. In 1982 Rossman cocreated the Power of Imagination Conference, where leading clinicians and researchers introduced the practical applications of imagery work to more than 1,400 health professionals nationwide. Frequent requests for clinical training led to the creation of "clinical guided imagery" courses taught by Rossman and Bresler throughout the United States from 1982 to 1989. In 1989 Rossman and Bresler founded the Academy for Guided Imagery. The academy's mission was expanded in 1995 to include teaching the public and organizations to work with the imagery methods that had been refined over the years.

Practice

A session begins with a simple relaxation technique used to help a client focus her attention inward. The guide will then teach skills to help with problem solving, conflict resolution, goal setting, stimulating healing responses in the body, or using personal strengths and resources most effectively. Participants are fully aware of their guide's suggestions and questions, and are engaged in an active dialogue at all times. In one typical technique, a client is asked to close his eyes to allow the mind to present a picture representing the experience of his problem. The client may then be guided in an imaginary dialogue with this image to explore and reveal its meaning and relevance. These images can provide information not only about the problem, but also about the client's beliefs, hopes, expectations, fears, resources, and solutions. The imagery process is used to reveal the client's intuitions about a problem and its solution.

The guide works to make a person become more aware of her own thoughts, feelings, and body responses, allowing her to have more control of how she feels. Many Interactive Guided Imagery self-care techniques can be learned from books, home

study programs, and tapes. A certified guide can assist a person with these approaches.

Benefits and Risks

Interactive Guided Imagery seeks to help a person learn to relax mentally and physically, relieve pain or other physical symptoms, stimulate healing responses in the body, solve difficult problems, resolve emotional issues, and envision and plan for the future. It may be used for self-care or by physicians, psychotherapists, nurses, and other professionals.

The technique can pose certain risks when used by poorly trained personnel. There is a possibility of uncovering traumatic insight or overwhelming effects. A certified Interactive Guided Imagery guide is trained and prepared to help prevent this whenever possible, and to help a person work through it, should it occur.

—*MARTIN ROSSMAN, M.D.*

Resources

Academy for Guided Imagery
    P.O. Box 2070
    Mill Valley, CA 94942
    Tel: 1-800-726-2070
    Fax: (415) 389-9342
    Sponsors professional training conferences, seminars, and retreats, and produces educational books and tapes to teach imagery skills to professionals, businesses, and the general public.

Further Reading

Bresler, David. *Free Yourself from Pain.* New York: Simon & Schuster, 1979.
Rossman, Martin. *Healing Yourself: A Step-by-Step Program for Better Health Through Imagery.* New York: Pocket Books, 1989.

Psychoneuro-immunology

Psychoneuroimmunology, commonly referred to as PNI, is the study of how thoughts and emotions may affect the body's immune system. The immune system is the body's elaborate and varied defense mechanism that fights against disease and illness. Advocates of this discipline have observed that the quality of a person's mental state, when improved through humor, positive thinking, and relaxation, can improve the body's ability to fight disease. Accordingly, stress, grief, and pain are seen to cause the body's defenses to weaken. Many supporters promote the use of relaxation techniques as a preventive measure for ensuring physical well-being. Some also see these techniques as a part of treatment for patients with chronic illnesses.

History

For most of the twentieth century, science has taught that the nervous system, including the brain, and the immune system function independently of each other. The body's ability to fight disease was thought to be beyond our conscious control. In the 1960s several researchers suggested that there is actually a complex network linking these two systems. Nerve cells, for instance, penetrate into the principal organs of the immune system, including the thyroid, spleen, and lymph glands, where lymphocytes, or disease-fighting cells, reside until they are called into action. Researchers also discovered that the chemicals nerve cells use to communicate with one another lock on to the membranes of lymphocytes. Thus, the information that the brain is sending and receiving is also shared with the immune system.

The idea of a connection between the nervous and immune systems gained attention after an experiment in 1975 appeared to confirm that the mind could affect physical health. Researchers fed rats saccharin-flavored water along with a drug that suppressed their immune functions. Later, when the rats were given the saccharin-flavored water without the drug, the researchers found that the rats' immune systems did not recover. As a result, the rats became ill and some died. Researchers believed that the rats had learned to associate the sweet water with the effect of the drug, thus proving that a thought or mental association could alter an animal's immune system. This experiment inspired similar studies that concluded that mental attributes, such as attitudes, sensations, memories, and emotions could change the immune system's ability to resist infections.

These early experiments developed into the field of study known today as PNI. Much of current PNI research investigates the physical effects of stress. Some researchers believe that stress, especially over long periods of time, can weaken the body's ability to recover from illnesses. To find out the physical effects of stress, researchers have tested the concentrations of lymphocytes in people's bodies while they were experiencing stressful situations. In one of these experiments, widowers were tested during the months following the deaths of their wives. The widowers' immune systems were found to be functioning less well than those of men who had not suffered the loss of their partners. In another experiment, medical students' immune systems appeared to weaken before they took an exam. As a result of these studies, some researchers claim that reducing stress can boost a person's immune system.

The case of noted journalist and commentator Norman Cousins changed the way many people viewed the relationship between body and mind. In 1976 Cousins was diagnosed with ankylosing spondylitis, a

Research has revealed some startling findings that may explain how emotions and stress can change a person's immune system:

- Early in the U.S. space program, NASA found that astronauts had reduced white blood cell counts after returning from space. Many scientists believed that it was a result of the stress of reentry into Earth's atmosphere.
- Subjects who viewed a film of Mother Teresa ministering to the poor were found to have increased levels of immune chemicals in their saliva.
- Women with breast cancer who attended support groups tended to survive longer than women who faced the illness alone.
- People who experienced the stress of being responsible for the care of another person were found to have fewer infection-fighting cells, suffer more upper-respiratory infections, and take longer to heal wounds.

severe, crippling disease of the spine. No known therapy offered any real promise for recovery. Cousins decided to confront his gloomy future with humor—consisting of an intense diet of movies featuring Laurel and Hardy, the Marx Brothers, and other famous comedians—and by prescribing for himself large doses of vitamin C. After months of laughter and good feelings, his debilitating spinal condition disappeared. Cousins went on to live fourteen more years and wrote a book, *Anatomy of an Illness as Perceived by the Patient: Reflections on Healing and Regeneration*, detailing his personal path to recovery. His story led many people to believe that positive thinking may help the body's ability to heal.

Applications

Some health care workers have begun to consider findings from PNI research when designing new therapies. Biofeedback is used to relieve stress in an attempt to reduce its burdens on the immune system. Guided imagery techniques are being used to direct the immune system responses to certain areas of the body. People with chronic illnesses are often encouraged to join support groups in which they can share their experiences, unburden themselves of fear, and draw strength and positive encouragement from others. All of these contribute to easing emotional strain, and possibly to improving the chances for recovery. The lessons learned from PNI research may also help explain other models of healing, such as Chinese acupuncture and Native American shamanism.

PNI is a recent and widely debated field of study. Not all researchers are convinced that the physical effects of stress or trauma are significant beyond extreme or chronic cases. It is far too simple to say that thinking positive thoughts will make us healthy and that negative thoughts will make us sick. Sudden and rapid recoveries like Cousins's are very uncommon. PNI is intended to enhance, not replace, the physical treatment of illnesses.

—LEONARD WISNESKI, M.D.

Resource

Integral Health Foundation
    4300 Crossway Court
    Rockville, MD 20835
    Tel: (301) 871-8384
    Promotes a greater understanding of the integral nature of the spirit, mind, and body in the healing process through interdisciplinary cooperation in research, education, and practice.

Further Reading

Benson, Herbert. *Timeless Healing: The Power and Biology of Belief.* New York: Simon & Schuster, 1994.

Cousins, Norman. *Anatomy of an Illness as Perceived by the Patient: Reflections on Healing and Regeneration.* New York: W. W. Norton, 1979.

Locke, S., and D. Colligan. *The Healer Within.* New York: Dutton, 1996.

Ornstein, R., and D. Sobel. *The Amazing Brain.* New York: Simon & Schuster, 1987.

PART 5

Sensory Therapies

AROMATHERAPY

BATES METHOD

BEHAVIORAL VISION
THERAPY

EYE MOVEMENT
DESENSITIZATION
AND REPROCESSING

FLOWER REMEDIES

HYDROTHERAPY

LIGHT THERAPY

SOUNDING

TOMATIS METHOD

Sensory therapies use one of the five senses to adjust chemical or other imbalances within the body that may be the cause of physical or psychological problems. While the name *sensory therapies* generally refers to those methods that work with the senses of sight, sound, or smell, this section also includes some disciplines that work with the senses of taste or touch. There are also many body-mind disciplines that work with the kinesthetic sense, or sense of body movement. These disciplines can be found throughout this book under Subtle Energy Practices, Mind/Body Medicine, Yoga, Martial Arts, Massage, Acupuncture and Asian Bodywork, Movement Therapy Methods, Somatic Practices, Expressive and Creative Arts Therapies, and Body-Oriented Psychotherapies.

Whereas the idea of treating physical and psychological problems by manipulating the senses is ancient, most of the methods described in this section were developed in the twentieth century by Western physicians who often worked outside or on the fringes of accepted allopathic medical practice. Through their pioneering work many sense-organ exercises and treatments, often involving special equipment or combined with more traditional psychotherapeutic practices, were developed. Many of these methods are prescribed as part of naturopathic cures. They have been effective in treating a wide variety of specific physical or emotional ailments such as post-traumatic stress disorder, nearsightedness, hearing loss, chemical addictions, depression, anorexia, and bulimia, while offering interesting and effective practices to strengthen the immune system and reduce the many harmful effects of stress on the body and mind.

Sensory Therapy:
Practices Ancient and Modern

Many diverse cultures, including Native American, Indian, Chinese, and Egyptian, used sensory therapies such as aromatherapy and hydrotherapy for healing the body and mind. Living in concert with the world around them, these cultures recognized the healing potential of plant essences, which they used to create pungent or sweet-smelling cosmetics, medicines, and incense. Water, one of the most basic ingredients necessary for life, was used for therapeutic baths, as an elixir, and in purifying rituals.

The ancient Greeks and Romans also made use of these natural methods of life enhancement, health maintenance, and healing. Hippocrates (c. 460–377 B.C.E.), often called the father of modern medicine, was known to have prescribed both hydrotherapy and sunlight (the most basic form of all light therapy) for many conditions. The Romans constructed bathhouses for relaxation, hygiene, and recreation, much like the health clubs of today.

Hydrotherapy has been used fairly constantly throughout Western history. Spas were built throughout Europe in the eighteenth century in places such as Spa, Belgium; Baden-Baden, Germany; and Vichy, France, where people went to "take the waters."

Sensory Therapies in Western Medical Practice

At the beginning of the nineteenth century, sensory therapies grew more popular and more abundant in use. Vincent Priessnitz (1799–1852), an Austrian peasant, intuitively used hydrotherapy to heal his broken ribs. Father Sebastian Kneipp (1821–1897), a German priest, used hydrotherapy for a variety of ailments. In France in the mid-1800s, ophthalmologist Emile Javal (1839–1907) was designing eye exercises as an alternative to the destructive eye surgery practices of the day. These exercises became the basis of present-day behavioral vision therapy.

By the early twentieth century, sensory therapies had become an accepted part of Western medical practice. Father Kneipp's methods, which came to be known as naturopathy, spread throughout Europe and America through the work of Benedict Lust, a German American cured of tuberculosis by Kneipp in 1892. The sun cure, the therapeutic use of sunbathing, was used in many hospitals and sanatoriums, including the prestigious Charing Cross Hospital in London.

Many doctors began to experiment with these drug-free, nonsurgical methods, developing deeper insights into the connections between the senses and the mind. In the 1930s Edward Bach, a British physician, began experimenting with methods of imbibing plant essences to alleviate the psychological problems he observed as the precursors and hindrances to healing of the physical ailments presented by his patients. The thirty-eight remedies and methods he discovered are the basis of present-day flower remedies.

Pharmaceuticals Overshadow Sensory Therapies

After 1928, with the discovery of penicillin and other powerful antibiotics, the Western medical establishment began to lose interest in sensory therapies. The newly discovered drugs worked quickly and were thought to be more effective than the slower-working sensory therapies. As pharmaceutical research exploded, scientists manufactured a multitude of synthetic drugs that were applied to numerous physical and psychological illnesses.

Through the mid–twentieth century, interest in sensory therapies was kept alive by curious and dedicated individuals such as the American physician Harry Spitler. Spitler expanded the range of light therapy by exploring the effects of various colored lights on the emotions. In the 1950s Alfred Tomatis (1920–), a French physician, discovered that the ability to speak is directly related to the ability to hear and that both abilities affect creativity, motivation, and the ability to learn. His series of exercises, known as the Tomatis method, helps people regain the abilities to listen and concentrate.

A Revival for Sensory Therapies

In the 1960s a confluence of forces in science and culture sparked a resurgence of interest in sensory therapies, as well as in other holistic health and living practices. Many people were becoming disillusioned with conventional medicine and its increasing reliance on pharmaceutical solutions, which often create dangerous side effects and debilitating conditions. The social revolution of the sixties brought a greater awareness of the value of the senses in living life to the fullest. Many people, young and old, began turning to more natural sources of healing.

With the arrival of the twenty-first century, scientists and healers in many areas are continuing to explore the ways in which we can use the senses to affect our physical and emotional functioning and enhance our experience of life. Today a wide variety of sensory therapies are used individually or combined with other natural healing modalities such as bodywork and massage, psychotherapy, diet, and movement practices to heal specific injuries and conditions, to alleviate the detrimental effects of stress, and to improve the quality of life.

The methods in this section share many philosophical beliefs with the other body-mind disciplines presented in this book. They all see human beings as complex organisms of interconnected aspects, complete with their own self-healing/self-regulating mechanisms. Illness, whether viewed as a chemical imbalance or as a breakdown in an interconnected process involving body and mind, is believed to be continually perpetuated by a malfunction or block in the self-regulating mechanism. The goal of each of the methods described in this section is to remove blocks in the self-regulating mechanism and bring the body and mind back into balance.

Because advocates of sensory therapies view human beings as an integral part of nature, they believe the means to remove these blocks, or stimulate the self-healing mechanism, can be found in natural elements and processes. What distinguishes these methods from any other holistic healing modalities is their use of the sense organs—eyes, ears, nose, taste buds, and skin—as the primary entry point to the interconnected systems of body, mind, and spirit.

Western Science's Theories

Although human beings have reaped the benefits of sensory therapies for centuries, advances in scientific research in the latter part of the twentieth century have given the Western medical community new information about the connections among the senses and other systems of the body.

Today scientists have identified that the limbic system, which controls heart rate, blood pressure, breath rate, and hormone levels, is highly sensitive to odors and also stores emotional memories. It is believed to be the system activated through aromatherapy and the use of flower remedies. The nervous system, with its thousands of receptors on the surface of the skin and access to every organ of the body, is thought to be the primary system activated through the many external forms of hydrotherapy. Light therapy seems to achieve its effects through the endocrine system. This system is stimulated when light- and color-sensitive photoreceptors in the eyes convert sunlight into electrical impulses, which are sent along the optic nerve to the brain.

Although this information may be reassuring to some, it is admittedly sketchy to others, and few advocates of sensory therapies would aim to convince a prospective practitioner of a method's efficacy based solely on current Western scientific knowledge. But with ever-greater interest in drug-free, nonsurgical methods of health maintenance and healing, and ever-greater development of scientific research methods, it may not be long until the many healing effects of these methods are fully understood.

—*Nancy Allison*, CMA

Further Reading

Bates, William H. *The Bates Method for Better Eyesight Without Glasses.* New York: Henry Holt, 1940.

Buchman, Dian Dincin. *The Complete Book of Water Therapy.* New Canaan, Conn.: Keats Publishing, Inc., 1994.

Devi, Lila. *The Essential Flower Essence Handbook.* Carlsbad, Calif.: Hay House, Inc., 1996.

Dewhurst-Maddock, Olivea. *The Book of Sound Therapy: Heal Yourself with Music and Voice.* New York: Simon & Schuster, Inc., 1993.

Kelville, Kathi, and Mindy Green. *Aromatherapy: A Complete Guide to the Healing Art.* Freedom, Calif.: The Crossing Press, 1997.

Kennedy, Teresa. *Sensual Healing: An Elemental Guide to Feeling Good.* New York: M. Evans and Company, Inc., 1996.

Scheffer, Mechthild. *Bach Flower Therapy: Theory and Practice.* Rochester, Vt.: Healing Arts Press, 1988.

Aromatherapy

 Aromatherapy is a branch of herbal medicine in which aromatic plant extracts are inhaled or applied to the skin as a means of treating illness and promoting beneficial changes in mood and outlook. Though aromatherapy and herbal medicine use many of the same plants, in aromatherapy the plants are distilled into oils of exceptional potency. As much as 3,000 pounds of a plant may be consumed in the production of 1 pound of "essential oil."

The therapeutic power of such oils is generally attributed to their ability to influence the workings of the limbic system, the "switchboard" in the brain that coordinates mind and body activity. When a small amount of oil is rubbed into the skin or inhaled, it sets off a chain reaction that leads to rapid, profound alteration in memory, heart rate, and other bodily processes. Most recipients choose oils that promote relaxation, but certain oils can boost energy, and others are thought to have pharmaceutical properties.

The 1990s saw an explosion of scientific interest in all aspects of aromatherapy. It is, however, an ancient mode of medicine that can be traced back to the dawn of civilization.

History

In ancient Egypt, extracts of plants were mixed with animal oil to form aromatic balms thought to be of inestimable worth in proper care of a person's whole being, mind, body, and soul. The balms were rubbed into the skin and hair for medicinal as well as cosmetic purposes and burned in religious rituals at temples and tombs. The practice of mummification was itself a type of aromatherapy, since the body was preserved and purified through the systematic application of balms.

Although the ancient Greeks and Romans did not practice mummification, they employed aromatic balms much as the Egyptians had. Balms were regarded as medicine, as luxurious items of personal care, and as offerings in religious rituals. Renaissance paintings that depict the Three Wise Men presenting gifts of frankincense and myrrh to the infant Christ are an example of the ancient ritual use of aromatic balms.

Modern aromatherapy is based on the research of a French chemist, René-Maurice Gattefosse, who recognized the healing powers of the substances routinely made into perfumes. In 1928 he published a paper that gave the medicinal use of plant oils a name, "aromatherapy," as well as introducing a set of principles. These principles were developed by a handful of French and English scientists, most notably Marguerite Maury and Jean Valnet, who compiled data and published a number of books, including Valnet's classic, *The Practice of Aromatherapy*. But awareness of the benefits of aromatherapy was confined to European circles until the advent of holistic medicine swept it into prominence in the United States.

By 1990 aromatherapy had sparked a nationwide boom in the sale of incense, scented candles, and bath oils and became a popular adjunct of massage and stress-management programs. Today Egyptian, ayurvedic, Chinese, and Native American practices are being studied with a view toward scientific adaptation. Drug-free treatments for shingles and herpes have already been developed, and there are indications that essential oils can also be helpful in treating colds and similar airborne infectious diseases, arthritis, and muscle disorders.

Theory

Aromatherapy is based on the belief that plants, particularly flowers and herbs, have healing properties that can be obtained by distilling the plants into fragrant oils. The aroma of the oils is by no means simply an attractive extra, like the candy coating on a bitter pill. The limbic system of the brain is highly sensitive to odors and routinely encodes them into patterns of associations and memories that are ever present within the unconscious. Because the limbic system is also a "switchboard" controlling heart rate, blood pressure, breathing, and hormone levels, aroma provides a subtle yet effective way to induce beneficial changes in the vital functions of the organism.

When essential oils are rubbed into the skin, the power of their fragrance is thought to be increased by their ability to penetrate bodily tissue and swiftly enter the bloodstream. In the case of eucalyptus, the action is said to be anti-inflammatory in nature. Other oils are believed to have antiviral, antibacterial, or detoxifying powers.

Approximately three dozen essential oils are now in common use among aromatherapists. Though the oils can be administered separately, a typical treatment entails a blend of oils made to suit the physiological and psychological needs of the individual. It is for this reason that aromatherapy is often described as both an art and a science. The rules governing the mixing and application of the plant extracts must be interpreted in a way that is sensitive to the person's inner and outer conditions.

Practice

Aromatherapy can be performed either by a practitioner who is likely to specialize in both aromatherapy and traditional herbal medicine, or by a massage therapist who includes aromatherapy in his regimen. It is also possible to approach aromatherapy as home care, using products purchased at a holistic health center or ordered from an aromatherapy institute. Generally speaking, beginners are advised to consult an expert before embarking on aromatherapy.

Once the appropriate essential oils have been acquired, they are either inhaled or applied to the skin through one of several methods. The oil can be put on a piece of cotton that is held close to the nose and sniffed. Diffusers that disperse the oil into the air are equally effective.

The manner in which the oils are applied to the skin depends in part on the nature of the problem being treated. Herpes lesions respond to direct application of oil, whereas relief from stress customarily requires soaking in bathwater containing some essential oil. When the oils are incorporated into massage, they are always mixed with a carrier lotion such as jojoba.

Benefits and Risks

Aromatherapy can bring relief from stress and promote a sense of well-being that activates the organism's capacity for self-healing. It has also been used effectively in the treatment of burns, insect bites, bruises, disorders of the skin ranging from acne to herpes, indigestion, colds, flu, and immune deficiencies.

As a precaution, no aromatherapy treatment should ever involve more than a few drops of essential oil. Overdoses may cause severe toxic reactions. A physician's guidance is required if the oil is to be placed on the tongue or swallowed.

Resources

Aromatherapy Seminars
   3379 S. Robertson Blvd.
   Los Angeles, CA 90034
   Tel: 1-800-677-2368
   Offers a variety of educational services in aromatherapy, including introductory and advanced training programs, correspondence courses, and videotapes.

National Association for Holistic Aromatherapy
   P.O. Box 17622
   Boulder, CO 80398-0622
   Tel: (303) 258-3791

Provides courses in aromatherapy and a nationwide referral service for aromatherapists.

The Pacific Institute of Aromatherapy
P.O. Box 6842
San Rafael, CA 94903
Tel: (415) 479-9121
A research and teaching institute that offers individual and group courses in aromatherapy.

Further Reading

Lavabre, Marcel. *Aromatherapy Workbook.* Rochester, Vt.: Healing Arts Press, 1990.

Rose, Jeanne. *The Aromatherapy Book: Applications and Inhalations.* Berkeley, Calif.: North Atlantic Books, 1992.

Tisserand, Robert. *Aromatherapy to Heal and Tend the Body.* Santa Fe, N.M.: Lotus Light Press, 1988.

Valnet, Jean. *The Practice of Aromatherapy.* Rochester, Vt.: Inner Traditions, 1990 (first published 1977).

Bates Method

 The Bates method is a system of holistic eye care that uses mental and physical exercises, rather than corrective lenses, to improve chronic problems of vision. It is named after its founder, the American ophthalmologist William Bates (1860–1931), who challenged the medical establishment by ascribing poor sight to habitual misuse of eye muscles caused ultimately by emotional stress. Bates believed that damaging habits could be unlearned through application of a daily routine of exercises designed to relieve tension in the eye muscles and teach the eyes to function in a relaxed, natural way. Contemporary vision training makes extensive use of these exercises.

History

Bates was a prominent ophthalmologist in New York City when he began to doubt the fundamental principles of his profession. Problems of vision were generally considered hereditary or part of the aging process and treated with prescription glasses, which did little to halt, let alone reverse, the weakening of vision. Though contemporary vision training incorporates many new techniques, it is based on Bates's approach and makes extensive use of the exercises he devised. These have also been an important resource for airline pilots and athletes seeking to strengthen their eye-brain coordination.

After several years of research, Bates published a controversial book, *The Bates Method for Better Eyesight Without Glasses* (1920), in which he argued that the standard treatment not only was based on false premises but actually damaged patients' ability to recover. Glasses, Bates reasoned, reinforced bad use of eye muscles, caused initially by psychological tension, and destined their wearers to a lifetime of impaired vision. The remedial exercises recommended by Bates proved to be as controversial as his attack on prescription glasses and found little support in professional circles.

Nonetheless, the Bates method did attract followers and had some notable successes. One of these was the British writer Aldous Huxley. In an essay on his experiences with the treatment, Huxley contended that questions concerning the "orthodoxy" of the Bates method were misinformed. It is, he explained, "a method of education, fundamentally similar to the method of education devised and successfully used by all the teachers of psychophysical skills for the last several thousand years."

Practitioners believe that the Bates method is a pioneering form of biofeedback and stress-reduction training. In addition, Bates is notable as one of the first doctors to recognize the relationship between vision and emotional disturbance, an insight of vast significance to fields ranging from special education to sports to the study of art.

Theory

According to Bates, "we see very largely with the mind and only partly with the eyes." This hypothesis led Bates to regard vision as inherently individual and variable: mood, memory, health, and circumstances play a role in what and how a person sees.

His primary concern was the functioning of the six muscles controlling the shape of the eye. In his opinion, they determine the eye's ability to focus and therefore constitute the all-important link between mind and vision. Accumulated tension in any of these small muscles could gradually weaken vision, producing nearsightedness, farsightedness, astigmatism, or a condition such as lazy eye. Conversely, Bates argued that releasing tension and encouraging the muscles to regain their innate flexibility and strength could improve poor vision.

Bates's understanding of vision is based on the behavioral model of health, also crucial to the Alexander technique, which credits the organism with the ability to heal itself once "blocks" in its natural operation are removed. To this end he formulated a set of eye exercises, commonly referred to as the Bates method, which he believed could "re-educate" the muscles of the eye.

No doubt, the most surprising of Bates's training exercises is one that turns the vision test chart into a memory device. By memorizing the letters and numbers on the chart, trainees simultaneously sharpen their acuity of vision and assume mastery of a source of anxiety. Most of the exercises were designed to stop the habitual staring Bates identified as a prime symptom of "blocked" vision. In "shifting," the trainee learns to look "through" objects, while in "swinging," they move their eyes in accordance with a rhythmic, side-to-side swaying of the body.

Practice

Treatment is available from optometrists who are specialized in vision training. Programs of therapy are adjusted to meet individual need and are likely to include recently developed techniques or updated versions of the Bates exercises. In most cases therapy entails several months of weekly training sessions and faithful performance of a routine of daily exercises at home, school, or work.

Benefits and Risks

The Bates method is credited with dramatic improvement in the vision of many people required to wear corrective lenses because of a common vision problem. By relieving a key pocket of stress, it is also thought to enhance the individual's sense of well-being and sometimes can speed recovery from other disorders.

The method, with or without a comprehensive vision training program, should not be considered an appropriate treatment for cataracts, glaucoma, or other diseases of the eye. Anyone with these or related problems is advised to consult a licensed ophthalmologist.

Resource

College of Optometrists in Vision Development
  P.O. Box 285
  Chula Vista, CA 91912
  Tel: (619) 425-6191
  Fax: (619) 425-0733
  A professional organization for optometrists specializing in the Bates method and other techniques of vision training.

Further Reading

Bates, W. *The Bates Method for Better Eyesight Without Glasses.* New York: Henry Holt & Co., 1987 (first published 1920).

Cheney, E. *The Eyes Have It: A Self-Help Manual for Better Vision.* York Beach, Maine: Samuel Weiser, Inc., 1987.

Behavioral Vision Therapy

 Behavioral vision therapy is an optometric specialty that uses a visual training regimen to improve vision by strengthening the vital link between the mind and the eye. In contrast, surgery for eye muscle problems targets the physical structure of the eye while neglecting the mental aspects of seeing, and therefore may produce less-than-desirable results. Behavioral optometrists consider environmental factors that affect vision as well as psychological and physiological factors that may contribute to—and result from—vision difficulties. With vision training, significant improvements in social, academic, and athletic skills can be achieved.

History

In the mid-1800s, after witnessing the horrible outcomes of eye surgery for both his father and sister, the French ophthalmologist Emile Javal (1839–1907) developed a scientific and nonsurgical method of visual rehabilitation known as orthoptics. Orthoptics was designed to treat improper eye alignment, specifically crossed eyes (inward turn), wall eyes (outward turn), and lazy eyes (visual impairment not correctable by glasses). Modern vision therapy, an advanced form of the orthoptic eye exercises developed by Javal, deals with a much wider variety of visual and perceptual problems while also considering their effects on behavior and performance. By the twentieth century the practice of orthoptics had progressed significantly in England and France.

The dawn of orthoptics in the United States occurred in 1912. This was the result of the publication of a comprehensive text on stereoscopic, or three-dimensional, eye exercises by David Wells, an ophthalmologist at Boston University Medical School. A large part of this classic text is devoted to the treatment of eye muscle problems that are hard to diagnose because they are not as easily recognized as crossed eyes or wall eyes, which have a definite observable cosmetic component. Wells believed that subtle eye problems were more common than the visibly obvious eye turns. Wells proposed the idea that having a single unified vision of the world through two eyes is an important and complex psychic ability, and that "its inefficiency could result in an inability to fix one's mind on study and reading." Wells also strongly felt that the clinical significance of common eye problems was largely ignored by practicing ophthalmologists. Many modern practitioners of vision therapy feel that this is still a problem among ophthalmologists.

The Optometric Extension Program (OEP), postgraduate study dedicated to education and research in vision, was established in 1928. OEP represented the earliest organized approach to orthoptics within the optometric profession, and it is still a vital force in the field of behavioral vision care today. A leading figure in OEP, A. M. Skeffington, broadened the orthoptic approach, giving it a much more holistic base. He introduced the idea that eye muscle and focusing deficiencies, rather than developing spontaneously, may evolve as a person grows and adapts to their environment. Skeffington and other behavioral optometrists also introduced the revolutionary concepts of reducing and controlling nearsightedness and improving focusing ability through vision training.

Theory

Modern vision therapy is based on the concept that vision is a dynamic process made up of numerous skills that can be learned through training. In addition, vision is a process influenced by emotions, intellect, posture, breathing, physiology, visual working habits, lighting conditions, diet, and our own styles of visual perception. An expanded, humanistic approach to vision further maintains that total visual performance cannot be adequately reduced to a single measurement such as 20/20. More traditional methods measure visual performance by reading charts at a distance of 20 feet, assessing the ability to focus on stationary images directly ahead. The rating 20/20 is equated as "perfect vision." It has never been scientifically or clinically validated that 20/20 endows us with the ability to see with comfort, efficiency, meaning, or while in motion. As the educational consultant Sally Brockett has written, "When we speak of vision, we are referring to the ability of the brain to organize and interpret information seen so it becomes understandable or meaningful. Even individuals with good eyesight (20/20 acuity) can have undiagnosed vision problems that make it difficult to correctly comprehend the visual message." Although testing for 20/20 is clinically valid, this measurement is only a partial assessment of an extremely complex process. According to behavioral optometrists, traditional eye care methods—those represented by the simple chart test—need to be supplemented by more dynamic approaches to testing and enhancing visual performance.

Practice

Participants in a behavioral vision therapy program have all aspects of their visual performance tested and trained in an "eye gym," which has an almost carnival-like appearance. It consists of walking rails, balance boards, trampolines, eye exercise equipment, metronomes, focusing charts, special training lenses and prisms, strobe lights, and other light-therapy devices. This equipment is used to improve visual comfort, efficiency, and performance. Exercises vary in difficulty and frequently involve several different kinds of sensory information presented simultaneously to the patient. For example, an individual may stand on a balance board and attempt eye-hand coordination tasks while trying to perform in time with a metronome. The exercises are repeated and, over time, increase in difficulty until the individual gradually enhances his neurological response related to vision and establishes good habits.

Visual biofeedback is commonly incorporated into treatment, giving the individual a physiological readout of current performance levels. Often people are unaware of the extent, nature, or even presence of eye problems. Feedback indicators show blurring, doubling, or vanishing of an image. Training techniques are designed to isolate and highlight symptoms of eye dysfunction, enabling the individual to better recognize, understand, and respond to the specific features of her vision problems. The individual is taught to send a conscious message to the eyes to restore the clarity, singleness of vision, or presence of the image. This practice strengthens the eye and brain connection and can improve performance in most cases. An example of an optical device used for a biofeedback session might be a pair of glasses with one red lens and one green lens. An individual wearing these glasses and looking at a beam of light should perceive only a single light that is a red-green mixture resulting from the brain's combination of sensory input received through the red lens and the green lens. In contrast, an individual who perceives two separate lights, one red and one green, has double vision. Alternatively, the person who perceives only one colored light, either red or green, is relying primarily on one eye to see. Now the individual has concrete, understandable feedback that something is wrong and can start working on consciously changing the incorrect response. Through practice, the proper response may become naturally and unconsciously incorporated into the individual's daily performance. Depending on the individual's level of performance during a treatment session, home exercises are usually prescribed.

Conditions Helped by Behavioral Vision Therapy

Conditions that might bring you to a behavioral optometrist include persistent eye strain, blurring or double vision, headaches, short attention span, learning problems or reading discomfort, lazy eye at any age, eye muscle problems, depth perception difficulties, or worsening eyesight. Behavioral optometrists can offer alternative therapies if you are having eye or vision problems and the only solution offered by other doctors is another pair of glasses, or you are told that you have 20/20 vision and thus there is nothing wrong with your eyes. Behavioral optometrists cite examples in which proper assessment and treatment of vision problems have helped children with behavior problems participate productively in the classroom, improved the performance of top athletes, and given children the confidence to take part in social activities that previously might have drawn attention to their vision difficulties.

—DR. JOSEPH SHAPIRO, OPTOMETRIST

Resources

American Optometric Association
243 N. Lindbergh Blvd.
St. Louis, MO 63141
Tel: (314) 991-4100
Fax: (314) 991-4101
Professional society of optometrists. The association will provide referrals to behavioral optometrists on request.

The study of developmental vision, that is, the study of the development of the faculty of sight, emerged in the 1950s. The Gesell Institute of Child Development in New Haven, Connecticut, sponsored controlled studies of children and served as a training ground for optometrists in applied research. Working on the premise that newborn children do not have the visual abilities of adults, researchers at the Gesell Institute tested the eyesight of infants over a period of time in order to identify the components involved in the development of vision.

College of Optometrists in Vision Development
P.O. Box 285
Chula Vista, CA 91912
Tel: (619) 425-6191
Fax: (619) 425-0733
Organization for optometrists involved in orthoptics and optometric vision therapy. It publishes the quarterly *Journal of Optometric Vision Development*.

Optometric Extension Program Foundation
1921 E. Carnegie, Suite 3L
Santa Ana, CA 92705
Tel: (714) 250-8070
Fax: (714) 250-8157
Arranges conferences and seminars and publishes the bimonthly *Journal of Behavioral Optometry*.

Further Reading

Beverstock, Caroline. *Your Child's Vision Is Important*. Newark, Del.: The International Reading Association, 1990.

Brockett, Sally. "Vision Therapy: A Beneficial Intervention for Developmental Disabilities." Web site: www.autism.org/visual/htm.

Cohen, Neville S., and Joseph L. Shapiro. *Out of Sight and into Vision*. New York: Simon & Schuster, 1977.

Dawkins, Hazel Richmond, et al. *The Suddenly Successful Student: A Guide to Overcoming Learning and Behavioral Problems.* 2nd rev. ed. Santa Ana, Calif.: Optometric Extension Program, 1990.

Flax, Nathan, ed. *Vision Therapy and Insurance: A Position Statement.* New York: State University of New York/State College of Optometry, 1986.

Keogh, Barbara, and Michelle Pelland. "Vision Training Revisited." *Journal of Learning Disabilities,* vol. 18, no. 4, April 1985.

Marcus, Steven E., and Arthur S. Seiderman. *20/20 Is Not Enough: The New World of Vision.* New York: Knopf, 1989.

Toufexis, Anastasia. "Workouts for the Eyes." *Time,* February 13, 1989.

Wells, David Washburn. *Stereoscopic Treatment of Heterophoria and Heterotropia.* New York: E. B. Meyrowitz, 1912.

Eye Movement Desensitization and Reprocessing

 Eye movement desensitization and reprocessing (EMDR) speeds recovery from a traumatic event by separating upsetting memories into basic parts. The therapy typically involves simple exercises such as using the eyes to track a rapidly moving object. While discussing the upsetting events, these eye movements create a reaction in the mind, desensitizing the brain to the disturbing sensory and emotional aspects of a memory and allowing the sufferer to begin reprocessing that trauma in the present. Traditional psychotherapy is then used to help the client digest the trauma and store it. While the mechanics of EMDR are not fully understood, it has gained respect for its application in cases of posttraumatic stress disorder (PTSD), a common condition among Vietnam veterans and rape victims. It can also be used to help process less acute traumas such as negative childhood experiences, which can lead to poor self-esteem and unhappiness.

History

EMDR emerged from the experiences of Francine Shapiro, Ph.D. While taking a walk in 1987, Shapiro noticed that disturbing thoughts she was having sometimes disappeared suddenly. When she consciously brought these thoughts back, they held none of the previous "hot" or negative weight. She later realized that at the time of her original thoughts, her eyes had spontaneously begun a rapid back-and-forth motion. Shapiro theorized that the removal of the upset from the memory might be linked to that movement, and tested her theory as treatment for PTSD. Initial success in small, controlled studies encouraged her to pursue further research and to found the EMDR Institute. Since 1990, more than 22,000 therapists worldwide have been trained in this method.

Theory

EMDR helps to reprocess memories that were not properly handled by the brain when they initially occurred. EMDR theory asserts that the brain handles memory as a package of five distinct information components: the picture or image, the thought or auditory bundle, an emotional feeling, a physical sensation, and the belief about oneself that results from the event. This information is perceived via the senses as what we see, hear, smell, touch, and taste. Under normal circumstances, the brain metabolizes, or processes, these five types of information by talking, thinking, and dreaming about them. Through these activities, the brain sorts the information, storing the valuable aspects for easy retrieval and discarding smaller, insignificant bits of data.

In traumatic situations, however, this natural process does not always function properly. A malfunction may leave the information in a distressing, "undigested" state. The mind then locks all five types of information together, surrounding the resulting lump with negative emotional energy. Thus, the event becomes a blockage in the mental storage system. Any attempt to access information from the event stirs the negative energy surrounding it. In severe cases, this negative energy overwhelms and debilitates the sufferer. The normal processes of thinking, talking, and dreaming are inadequate ways of handling these blockages. Just as a cut will not properly heal until the splinter is removed, the body's normal processes can, at best, work only around a damaged memory bundle.

EMDR may act as a more intense version of rapid eye movement (REM) sleep, harnessing the body to effect a change in the mind. The mechanics of EMDR and REM sleep are similar. During REM sleep, a dreamer's eyes move rapidly from side to side. Shapiro believes that this eye movement stimulates links between the two sides of the brain. Because each side serves a different role—the left side is the positive, analytical side, while the right side is the less linear, more sensory-oriented side—the link through REM seems to help information pass between the two sides and be processed. Hence, REM is one catalyst for natural memory "digestion."

Normal REM sleep, however, cannot penetrate particularly severe hurts. As the patient's unconscious seeks to access the memory through REM sleep, the sleeper's mind re-creates the painful negative sensations that occurred at the time of the hurt. Once awake, the right and left sides of the brain are no longer able to continue their information processing. The hurt remains locked in the body and mind.

Just as a car engine must be properly warmed up to tackle steep hills, an activity of the body—eye movement—"warms" the brain to the task of unraveling even the densest ball of hurt. It is believed that the conscious rapid eye movement powerfully ignites one side of the brain, then the other in rapid succession, until finally both sides churn together. Once warmed like this, the subconscious is empowered to process the hurt without undue discomfort to the patient. The splinter being thus removed, normal healing begins.

Practice

A typical EMDR session lasts ninety minutes. The patient is asked to think about the disturbing event. The practitioner then asks the patient to follow the therapist's fingers or a light bar with his eyes. The patient continues thinking of the memory as the practitioner moves her fingers or pointer rapidly from side to side. Upon stopping, the practitioner and patient discuss any information or revelations that occurred while the patient's eyes were moving. For most people, the traumatic event feels inexplicably less traumatic and more clear or more distant. The sufferer can finally talk with some detachment about the event, which allows the healing process to begin.

Benefits and Risks

In many case studies, EMDR has helped victims of PTSD and other anxiety-related disorders cope with their conditions. The therapy is still largely unproved, however, and does not work with all patients. Ideally it should be performed in comfortable, stress-free situations; and it does not affect all people in the same way. Additionally, EMDR should be performed only by a trained and licensed and/or certified psychotherapist. While the therapy may reduce the emotional attachment surrounding an event, the patient is still left with factual memories of the unpleasant event, which are best processed through the therapeutic skills of a trained professional.

—BARBARA PARRETT, RN, M.S.

Resources

EMDR Institute, Inc.
   P.O. Box 51010
   Pacific Grove, CA 93950-6010
   Tel: (408) 372-3900
   Web site: www.emdr.com
   Provides information on EMDR.

Further Reading

Parnell, Laurel. *EMDR: The Revolutionary New Therapy for Freeing the Mind, Clearing the Body, and Opening the Heart.* New York: W. W. Norton & Co., 1997.

Shapiro, Francine. *EMDR: Breakthrough Therapy for Overcoming Anxiety, Stress, and Trauma.* New York: Basic Books, 1997.

———. *Eye Movement Desensitization and Reprocessing: Basic Principles, Protocols, and Procedures.* Guilford, N.C.: Guilford Press, 1995.

Flower Remedies

 Flower remedies are liquid preparations made from the flowering heads of plants and trees. They are used to deal with emotional and psychological difficulties such as fear, lack of self-confidence, jealousy, anger, and resentment, which are believed to be one of the root causes of physical disorders.

These remedies are not chosen according to physical ailments, but instead are selected based on emotional and psychological difficulties and on personality and behavioral traits. Once administered, it is believed that flower remedies trigger a mechanism within the brain that stimulates the body's internal healing processes, eventually resulting in a healthier emotional, psychological, and physical state. Flower remedies have been used successfully not only on humans but also to deal with negative emotional and behavioral traits in animals.

History

In the early 1930s Edward Bach (1880–1936), a young British physician, discovered that many of his patients displayed various emotional and psychological difficulties prior to the onset of physical disease. He also found these same problems would complicate the disease once it manifested, thereby making treatment more difficult. The doctor's prior experience with pharmaceutical drugs and their side effects convinced him that the answer could be found in nature, not in the laboratory. Bach left his medical practice and began researching his theories by experimenting with various species of plants.

Believing the greatest healing value resides in the flowering heads of plants and trees, the doctor began developing ways to prepare and administer them. Flowers were picked at various times in their blooming cycle and floated in a bowl of freshly obtained spring water in direct sunlight. Other flowers were gathered and prepared by boiling in water. These preparations were then administered in minute doses according to the emotional and psychological profile of the patient. After years of research, thirty-eight flowering plants, trees, and special waters were found to have a profound positive effect on a wide range of emotional and psychological difficulties. In the last few decades several companies and researchers have produced these same thirty-eight flower remedy preparations under different brand names, and have produced other flower remedy preparations from newly discovered flowering plants found in other parts of the world.

Why people use flower remedies: You are very depressed when someone close to you dies, and you personalize the situation by asking, "Why did life take this person from me?"

Though there is no scientific explanation for what we call the soul, for our purpose we may say that the soul is a part of a person that is transcendental and connected to a higher order of reality. Being visionary, the soul understands that there is no death, that the basis of all living things is energy, which you cannot destroy. From this internal conflict, a schism develops, and this is where Edward Bach had his most profound insights. He found that the first sign of this schism is the onset of a specific emotional or psychological difficulty. In the example of the loss of a loved one, you might feel resentment developing—resentment toward life for having been unfair, for having taken away someone you dearly loved.

Bach proposed that the manifestation of this resentment directly reflects the conflict between the personality and the soul, and is the first sign that you have fallen out of harmony within yourself. If left untreated, this disassociation results in physical symptoms and ailments. You might not realize that your illness is a direct result of this disassociation.

A flower remedy would relate to the emotional state of mind that you are in and bring about a sense of well-being. It is also believed to trigger a mechanism that stimulates your internal healing system, thereby alleviating the physical symptoms that resulted from the conflict between the personality and the soul.

Deeply visionary, Bach wrote: "All emotional, psychological, and physical disorder grows out of a conflict between our personality and our Soul." He believed we should regard illness as a signal that we are out of harmony within ourselves.

Over the years scientists have examined how negative thoughts and emotions affect our health. Their studies show that if an emotional difficulty is not resolved within a reasonable period of time, generally from six months to a year, serious internal problems and eventually physical disease can develop. Early stages may see the development of functional difficulties, which include predisposition to colds and other infections, sexual dysfunction, headaches, fatigue, allergies, and digestive problems. These problems, among others, are the first physical warning signs that we are out of harmony within, and if underlying psychoemotional and spiritual conflicts are not resolved, physical disease might result. At this point the physician is generally consulted. To this

Bach wrote: "The main reason for the failure of modern medicine is that it is dealing with results, not causes . . . . Disease will never be cured or eradicated by present materialistic methods for the simple reason that disease in its origin is not material, [but the] ultimate result produced in the body, the end product of deep and long-acting forces."

Practice

Flower remedies are easy to choose and use. Ellon, Inc., a major international supplier, provides a free self-help questionnaire on choosing and applying the remedies.

Remedies may be taken any number of ways—directly from the concentrate bottles under the tongue, by mixing several drops in a drink and sipping at intervals, or by mixing several drops in a 1-ounce dropper bottle with water and consuming it over a period of time. For people with alcohol sensitivities (most flower remedy preparations contain some alcohol as a preservative), these remedies can also be applied directly from the bottle to the temples or wrists, behind the ears, or under the arms. This can also be an effective way of administering flower remedies to infants and small children.

Flower remedies are known to have a unique and personal effect on each person taking them. Remedies are taken until difficulties are resolved, until there is a lifting of the negative emotional state, or until overreactive personality traits are stabilized. In general, most people can resolve difficulties within one to twelve weeks, although some may take longer. Once these difficulties are resolved, the remedies may be discontinued. Often, however, one can experience a "peeling" effect, where one or more emotional difficulties are resolved and other underlying emotions emerge. In these and other instances, new remedies may be chosen as needed by consulting the self-help questionnaire.

Benefits

Since the mid-1930s, the thirty-eight flower preparations have been used successfully by countless physicians and others to deal with a wide range of difficulties that include but are not limited to fear, anxiety, uncertainty, indecisiveness, envy, jealousy, and lack of self-confidence. They have also been used to deal with the stress associated with everyday problems, such as financial difficulties, relationship problems, day-to-day worries, periods of transition, and job-related tensions. Additionally, preparations of these flowers have proven effective in dealing with stress-related hyperactivity in children, dieting and eating problems, learning difficulties, sleeping problems, and the trauma of divorce and other loss.

—*LESLIE J. KASLOF*

Resources

Ellon, Inc.
 193 Middle St., Ste. 201
 Portland, ME 04101
 Tel: 1-800-423-2256
 Produces and distributes worldwide the thirty-eight flower preparations. Carries a full line of flower remedy product information. Also provides an extremely useful self-help questionnaire for choosing the thirty-eight flower remedies.

Flower Essence Society
 P.O. Box 459
 Nevada City, CA 95959
 Tel: (916) 263-9162
 Disseminates various information about flower remedies. Sells its own line of flower essences and imports and distributes other lines of flower remedies.

Further Reading

Bach, Edward, and F. J. Wheeler. *Bach Flower Remedies.* New Canaan, Conn.: Keats Publishing, 1979.
Kaslof, Leslie J. *The Traditional Flower Remedies of Dr. Edward Bach: A Self-Help Guide.* New Canaan, Conn.: Keats Publishing, 1993.
Vlamis, Gregory. *Flowers to the Rescue.* New York: Thorsons, 1986.

Hydrotherapy

 Hydrotherapy is the treatment of injury or disease with the application of water in one of its three forms: steam, liquid, or ice. It may be used as either hot or cold applications alone, or by alternating hot and cold in contrasting applications. Hydrotherapy exerts its effects both locally and at sites away from its application. Its distant effects are mediated through a reflex arc that is a normal function of the nervous system. An example of this reflex action would be the effect of hydrotherapy on the liver. An application of heat over the liver will not heat the liver itself, but through the reflex arc, there will be a vasodilation of the liver as if it were heated directly.

Hydrotherapy may be used to aid in the treatment of addiction through detoxification treatments or to aid in the general mental and physical health of a person by encouraging relaxation, increasing energy level or vitality, and strengthening the immune and other total body systems.

History

Hydrotherapy has been employed throughout the world, from earliest recorded history to the present. The Egyptians, Babylonians, Greeks, Chinese, Native Americans, and numerous other cultures have used water for therapeutic purposes. Baths, saunas, mineral soaks, flushes, irrigations, steams, and compresses are just some of the ways water has been used for healing purposes. The Greek physician Hippocrates (c. 460–377 B.C.E.) employed hydrotherapy in the treatment of fevers, ulcers, hemorrhages, and other medical and surgical conditions. The Roman baths are a prime example of the social, hygienic, and medical uses of hydrotherapy.

Modern hydrotherapy owes much to several practitioners of the art. Some were trained physicians, while others were lay practitioners who learned more by experience than training. A nineteenth-century Austrian peasant, Vincent Priessnitz (1799–1852), is said to have treated his own broken ribs with cold water applications, and soon began treating others with great success. German priest Father Sebastian Kneipp (1821–1897) was cured of tuberculosis after he had begun immersing himself in cold water a few times a week. His book *My Water Cure* (1890) is a classic in the field of

hydrotherapy. William Winternitz (1834–1912) was a prominent physician who was the first to demonstrate that hydrotherapy exerts its greatest influence on the nervous system. John Harvey Kellogg (1852–1943) established the Battle Creek Sanitorium in Michigan, where hundreds of patients were treated with hydrotherapy, diet, and exercise. Kellogg wrote *Rational Hydrotherapy* (1900), which remains the most comprehensive text ever written on the subject of hydrotherapy and includes more than 1,100 pages of text and illustrations.

Today hydrotherapy is used as either a primary or supplemental therapy by a number of physicians, physical therapists, and psychologists to treat a wide range of conditions, including stress, AIDS, addictions, and allergies.

Theory

Hydrotherapy recognizes the interrelatedness of the mind and body. Although most hydrotherapy treatments aim to relieve a physical condition, the theory supporting the treatment is based on the knowledge that the state of the body affects the state of the mind. The chemicals, nutrients, or toxins that affect both the mind and body are messengers that communicate vital information connecting the major organs and systems of the whole person. Hydrotherapy directly stimulates these messengers.

External hydrotherapy—the application of water to the outside of the body—is divided into three types: hot water, cold water, and contrast. Hot water stimulates the immune system to release white blood cells that remove toxins from the blood. It also relaxes muscles and soothes nerves. Nerves are responsible for sending all messages from the brain to other areas of the body and, therefore, play an important role in our emotional and mental as well as physical conditions. Cold water counteracts swelling and inflammation by constricting the blood vessels. Contrasting applications of hot and cold water stimulate the endocrine and adrenal glands, reduce congestion, and improve organ functioning.

Water with a high content of certain minerals can provide additional benefits. Water high in sulfur, for example, can help ease the effects of arthritis, rheumatism, and skin diseases. Bicarbonated spring water has been used in the treatment of allergies.

Internal applications of hydrotherapy may also be made. These may be as simple as drinking water to relieve dehydration or as complex as the application of internal irrigations. Internal irrigations of hydrotherapy are frequently used to dislodge unwanted material from the area being irrigated. Ear lavage is used to clean earwax from the external ear canal, whereas enema or colonic irrigation is used to eliminate dry, hard fecal material from the colon. It is, therefore, possible, using internal application, to take advantage of the thermal, chemical, and/or mechanical properties of water.

Practice

There are countless forms of hydrotherapy, including baths and soaks, steams and saunas, irrigations and flushes, and wraps and compresses. The chemical properties of water allow it to be used to dissolve and remove unwanted materials from the body. This might be done by immersion in a tank of hot water, allowing water-soluble substances to dissolve from the skin. It may also be used in irrigations applied to the body. The chemical properties of water are also helpful in dissolving and applying desirable compounds, such as Epsom salts, to the body. Both internal and external applications may be made using herbal teas and other infusions, such as echinacea or goldenseal.

Water's thermal properties make it ideal for adding heat to or removing heat from the body. It can raise a low body temperature or reduce a fever. Hydrotherapy can also aid in relieving the heat from inflammations, such as those that might occur from a sprained ankle, or to add heat to relieve muscle spasms. In addition, water has been found to alleviate the stresses and strains of everyday life, as well as treat emotional and mental disturbances by soothing the nervous system.

The mechanical properties of water, in the form of sprays and showers, can be stimulating to various parts of the body. Immersion in water can exert pressure to help relieve swelling, provide buoyancy to counteract the effects of gravity—easing pain and improving movement—and provide resistance for exercise. For people whose general body condition is so poor that "on-land" exercise programs prove impossible, hydrotherapy can create a physical environment in which progress can be made, thus stimulating the patient's motivation—an important emotional component of the healing process.

Benefits and Risks

Hydrotherapy treatments strengthen the body's own functions and defense mechanisms. The treatments work with the body and the mind, enabling the return of balance and allowing healing to occur.

When applying hydrotherapy treatments, care must be taken with the elderly and the very young, both of whom often have a diminished ability to maintain their body temperature and therefore can be heated or chilled too much. Persons with diminished sensation or poor circulation should also be treated with great care since it is possible to burn or freeze tissue without their being aware.

—DOUGLAS C. LEWIS, ND

Resources

American Association of Naturopathic Physicians
    2366 Eastlake Ave., Suite 322
    Seattle, WA 98102
    Tel: (206) 323-7610
    Provides referrals nationwide to health care professionals who practice hydrotherapy.

Bastyr University Natural Health Clinic
    1307 N. 45th St., Suite 200
    Seattle, WA 98103
    Tel: (206) 632-0354
    A teaching and treatment clinic for the use of hydrotherapy.

National College of Naturopathic Medicine
    11231 S.E. Market St.
    Portland, OR 97216
    Tel: (503) 255-4860
    Offers referrals to naturopathic doctors as well as training in naturopathic medicine.

Further Reading

Boyle, Wade, and Andre Saine. *Lectures in Naturopathic Hydrotherapy.* East Palestine, Ohio: Buckeye Naturopathic Press, 1988.

Croutier, Alev Lytle. *Taking the Waters.* New York: Abbeville Press, 1992.

Moor, Fred B., et al. *Manual of Hydrotherapy and Massage.* Boise, Idaho: Pacific Press Publishing Association, 1964.

Ruoti, Richard, David Morris, and Andrew Cole. *Aquatic Rehabilitation.* Philadelphia: Lippincott, 1997.

Thrash, Agatha, and Calvin Thrash. *Home Remedies.* Seale, Ala.: Thrash Publications, 1981.

Light Therapy

 Light therapy is a general term for therapies that use the entire electromagnetic spectrum or specific wavelengths of light to treat physical and emotional problems. Although light therapy draws on ancient ideas about the healing powers of sunlight, it is in many ways a new field, one in which clinical research is continuing and therapeutic applications are still being determined. There are many variations of light therapy. A therapist may direct solid or strobelike flashes of light into a client's eyes or onto parts of the body. Different types of light, including full-spectrum, ultraviolet, infrared, colored, and laser, are being tested for their ability to treat a wide range of conditions, including depression, insomnia, fatigue, premenstrual syndrome, psoriasis, jaundice, learning difficulties, and addictions.

History

From ancient to modern times, sunlight has played a central role in the cure of disease. The use of light in modern medicine began in the early eighteenth and nineteenth centuries as scientists discovered the component frequencies of sunlight and observed its effects on animals and humans. In 1703 English physicist Sir Isaac Newton chronicled his pioneering experiments with sunlight in his book *Optiks.* He was the first to show that sunshine's white light, when passed through a prism, divides into seven wavelengths of the visible color spectrum—red, orange, yellow, green, blue, indigo, and violet. In the early 1800s two German physicists, John Herschel and Johann Ritter, discovered that the sun also emitted light outside the visible spectrum. Sunlight contains infrared light rays with longer wavelengths and lower frequencies than visible light, and ultraviolet rays with shorter wavelengths and higher frequencies. In 1870 scientists proved that sunlight kills bacteria and other microorganisms. The first surgical theaters used ultraviolet lights to effectively and inexpensively reduce airborne microorganisms by 50 percent. Danish physician Niels R. Finsen received the 1905 Nobel Prize in medicine for establishing that visible wavelengths of blue-violet and invisible ultraviolet, when isolated and focused on the body, could cure tuberculosis of the skin and other infectious conditions, such as measles and scarlet fever. Finsen also effectively treated smallpox by using red light (filtered sunlight or artificial light that excludes the heating rays of infrared and the burning rays of blue-violet and ultraviolet). Psychiatric applications of light therapy began in the 1880s, when mental hospitals in Europe and South America routinely calmed agitated patients with artificial blue light and energized depressed and unresponsive patients with red light applied through the eyes and on the body.

Throughout the opening decades of the twentieth century, therapeutic sunbathing, a method known as the "sun cure," was a widely prescribed medical treatment for tuberculosis, cholera, viral pneumonia, bronchial asthma, gout, jaundice, and severe wounds. At the same time, advances in the design of electric lighting made it possible for hospitals in America and Europe to have heliotherapy wards that used artificial light for the treatment of cardiovascular and degenerative disorders.

After the development of the first antibiotics in 1938, interest in light therapy and other natural healing methods waned. However, in the 1940s Harry Spitler, a medical doctor and an optometrist, contributed to the development of light therapy with his investigation of syntonic optometry. The term *syntonic* comes from a Greek word meaning "to bring into balance." Spitler's treatment used rhythmic flashing of colored light into the eyes to improve visual acuity and coordination as well as energize and relax the autonomic nervous system. The patient's re-

sponse varied with different flash rates and colors. He found that warm colors—red, orange, and yellow—were invigorating, while cool colors—green, blue, and violet—were relaxing. Spitler's pioneering work demonstrated that light entering the eyes profoundly impacts the autonomic nervous system and the endocrine system, balancing important hormones and brain chemistry.

Current investigations into therapeutic potentials of light were touched off in 1983 by psychiatrist Norman Rosenthal's study of winter depression, or seasonal affective disorder (SAD). He and his coworkers at the National Institute of Mental Health and more than two hundred medical colleges around the world showed that regular exposure to full-spectrum (artificial lighting that has all the colors of sunlight) fluorescent light alleviates the symptoms of SAD in 80 percent of people. People with SAD begin to experience symptoms at the onset of autumn, usually in September, as the days become shorter and darker. Rosenthal's technique is called bright-light therapy, as it uses therapeutic doses of light more than twenty times brighter than typical indoor lighting. Bright-light therapy has been used by NASA to adjust the daily rhythms of space shuttle astronauts and by mental health professionals to help people cope with shift work, jet lag, addictions, and various psychiatric conditions.

Basic Principles

Major physiological processes in the brain and body are switched on and off by the presence or absence of natural or artificial light. Biochemical processes triggered by light include the production of vitamin D, the inhibition of melatonin (a hormone that affects mood), and the stimulation of serotonin and norepinephrine (brain chemicals that influence mental alertness and well-being). Light-sensitive cells in the eyes called photoreceptors convert sunlight into electrochemical impulses, which are transmitted through the optic nerve to brain centers that affect vision and activate the endocrine system. Many functions necessary for growth and well-being—breathing, sleeping, blood pressure, body temperature, appetite, moods, mental acuity, and the immune system—are governed by the endocrine system and hence are affected by natural light.

Evidence also suggests that proper quantities of visually perceived light are needed to maintain healthy functioning of various parts of the brain: the cerebral cortex, which controls motivation, learning, and creativity; the limbic system, which stores emotional impressions of the world; and the motor cortex and the brain stem, which coordinate body movement and the maintenance of life.

Practice

There are many different ways that light may be used in therapy. Goals and techniques will differ with each procedure. A therapist may direct the light into a person's eyes or on other body parts, and the light shown may be in strobing flashes or as solid light. The benefits may be both physical and psychological. Several common forms of light therapy utilize full-spectrum or specific frequencies of colored light.

Neurosensory Development.
For the last twenty-five years, optometrist John Downing has researched, applied, and extended Spitler's theories and formulated a form of light therapy called neurosensory development. Like Spitler, Downing promoted the therapeutic use of strobing colored light. A typical session begins with a discussion of the participant's medical and optometric history to determine the program and therapy. Light is administered with a device invented by Downing called the photron ocular light stimulator. It uses a combination of twelve colored-glass filters, from red to violet, placed in front of a special full-spectrum xenon light with an adjustable

strobe capable of flashing from 1 to 60 cycles per second.

To determine a program of therapy, the patient is classified as either a slow or fast neurological type, and then the colors and flash rates on the photron are adjusted to counteract and balance the person's neurological tendencies. For example, blue, indigo, and violet, which tend to slow down and relax, are flashed slowly (six to twelve times a minute) into the eyes of a fast neurological individual. Conversely, a slow neurological individual is treated with rapid flashes (thirteen to sixty times per minute) of red, orange, and yellow. The typical course of treatment entails twenty or more half-hour sessions of light therapy.

These techniques lead to an increase in the patient's visual field and to a reduction of his blind spot, indicating that more light energy is reaching the visual cortex and other key brain structures. Besides visual enhancement, the types of individuals who appear to be helped by neurosensory development are those with chronic fatigue, menstrual difficulties, thyroid problems, insomnia, depression, and mental inefficiency.

Brief Strobic Phototherapy.
Like neurosensory development, this method also uses the photron. However, the treatment goal is different. It is used to help the client access her thoughts and feelings and work on the emotional components of physical illness. Brief strobic phototherapy (BSP) was pioneered by Jacob Liberman, an optometrist, and Steven Vazquez, a medical psychotherapist. In this system the psychotherapist uses strobing colored light to facilitate awareness and resolution of the client's thoughts, feelings, and memories.

Generally the therapist chooses a color and flash rate that is emotionally evocative and uncomfortable to the client. Various colors tend to access different psychological content and are selected according to the client's objectives. This stimulation facilitates a participant's awareness of unresolved, unconscious thoughts, feelings, and sensations. At the start of a typical session, the therapist uses flashes of colored light to put a person into a trancelike state. Then the client engages in a variety of psychological techniques to help facilitate emotional processing, such as talking, deep breathing, eye movement, awareness of physical sensations, and recollection of dreams. The rhythmic colored lights stimulate brain wave patterns that evoke different states of consciousness. Clients look into the light and can easily and rapidly see their unconscious material projected before them. By selecting specific colors and specific strobe rates, desired results can be targeted. BSP seeks to release repressed traumas or other memories and emotions that may be the root cause of illness. It may be part of treatment for various psychological problems, including depression, anxiety, panic attacks, obsessive-compulsive disorder, addiction, eating disorders, closed brain injuries, and dissociative identity disorder.

Bright-Light Therapy.

This common form of light therapy was developed in the 1980s to treat SAD. More recently this therapy has been successfully applied to a wide variety of psychiatric conditions, including sleep difficulties, food and substance addictions, jet lag, Alzheimer's disease, and attention deficit disorder in children.

The treatment itself is used either under professional guidance or for self-care applications for less serious stress symptoms. The light is usually viewed at home with a portable light box designed to fit on a desk or table. Sitting with her head and upper body facing about 3 feet from the light box, the participant focuses her eyes on a surface illuminated by the light, not on the light itself.

The full-spectrum fluorescent light may be as much as twenty times stronger than normal room light and is usually most effective when it replicates the quality of natural light just before dawn or sunset. The intensity of the light and the scheduling and length of exposure are determined on a case-by-case basis. Daily exposure in the early morning for thirty minutes to several hours is often recommended, and an additional late-afternoon session may be prescribed. Bright-light therapy is usually confined to the fall and winter months, when SAD patients experience severe depression, lethargy, fatigue, decreased energy and activity level, anxiety, irritability, lowered sex drive, avoidance of social activities, sadness, concentration and sleep difficulties, interpersonal difficulties, carbohydrate and sweet cravings, and weight gain. Bright-light therapy is usually discontinued in the spring as the days get longer and brighter. Once a satisfactory regimen is established, it must be maintained to receive maximum benefits. Bright-light therapy relieves the symptoms of SAD; it does not cure the disorder.

Colorpuncture.

This discipline uses a light pen to apply different frequencies of visible light on the acupoints and meridians, where needles are placed in a traditional acupuncture treatment. This procedure was developed by German naturopath Peter Mandel in the early 1970s. A colorpuncture therapist balances one's vital energy by either stimulating or sedating it with light. Different colors have different effects. Warm colors such as red and yellow are used to add energy, while cool colors such as green and blue are used to subtract energy. A therapist may monitor the status of a client's energy flow before and after treatments by taking his pulse or by examining a Kirlian photograph, a black-and-white image in which the body's radiating energy appears. Colorpuncture is often used in place of acupuncture, especially on children or adults who are frightened by needles. It has the same applications as acupuncture, including the treatment of respiratory and gastrointestinal infections, neurological and muscular difficulties, visual and learning problems, and pain. It may be used for stimulation of the immune system and as adjunctive therapy for those with mental disorders and addictions.

There are many other medical applications of light, including ultraviolet (UV) sterilization of human blood (photoluminesence) and the UV treatment of psoriasis and infant jaundice. The photodynamic treatment of cancer employs light to activate cancer medications and guide them to diseased tissue. Some types of light therapy, such as bright-light therapy, are becoming more popular in the medical community and may be used either alone or in combination with psychiatric medication. Others, such as syntonic optometry, neurosensory development, and brief strobic photostimulation, are gaining acceptance.

Benefits and Risks

In more than two decades of experimental trials, bright-light therapy, neurosensory development, BSP, and colorpuncture have been consistently found to be safe and effective when used under the supervision of a competent and licensed health professional. However, overexposure to bright full-spectrum light can produce negative side effects, including eye irritation, headaches, insomnia, and agitation. These can be decreased by reducing exposure time and by sitting farther from the light source. Strobic colored light stimulation can temporarily stimulate a "healing crisis," a temporary exacerbation of old emotional conflicts or physical difficulties in the process of releasing old traumas.

Each individual's reaction to light through the eyes and on the body is unique. One in three thousand people can experience photosensitive seizures brought on by flashing lights such as those found in video games, televisions, and nightclubs. Individuals with a history of severe emotional difficulties or visual pathology should not begin phototherapy without consulting a licensed health care professional.

—Dr. Brian J. Breiling

Resources

College of Syntonic Optometry
Betsy Hancock, DO
21 E. 5th St.
Bloomsburg, PA 17815
Tel: (717) 784-2131
Organization of optometrists who incorporate syntonic light therapy into their work; offers a referral service.

Health Institute of North Texas
P.O. Box 820963
North Richland Hills, TX 76182
Tel: (817) 268-7050
Fax: (817) 285-7729
e-mail: Vazquez@txcc.net
Holistic treatment center, founded by psychologist Steven Vazquez, offering treatment and education on BSP.

Society for Light Treatment and Biological Rhythms
10200 W. 44th Avenue, No. 302
Wheatridge, CO 80033-2840
Tel: (303) 424-3697
Fax: (303) 422-8894
e-mail: sltbr@resourcenter.com
Web site: www.websciences.org/sltbr
Publishes newsletter on medical research on the use of full-spectrum and colored light.

Universal Light Technologies
P.O. Box 520
Carbondale, CO 81623
Tel: 1-800-81-LIGHT
Fax: (303) 927-0101
Web site: www.ulight.com
Organization founded by optometrist Jacob Liberman that offers treatment and education with strobic colored light and other modes of light therapy.

Winter Depression Program
Columbia Presbyterian Medical Center
722 W. 168th St.
New York, NY 10032
Tel: (212) 960-5714
Web site: www.cet.org/cet1996

Clinical program for treatment of SAD headed by Michael Terman, a pioneering bright-light researcher; also provides information and referrals for light therapy.

Further Reading

Breiling, Brian, ed. *Light Years Ahead: The Illustrated Guide to Full Spectrum and Colored Light in Mindbody Healing.* Berkeley, Calif.: Celestial Arts Press, 1996.

Liberman, Jacob. *Light: Medicine of the Future.* Santa Fe, N.M.: Bear & Co, 1991.

Mandel, Peter. *Practical Compendium of Colorpuncture.* Bruchal, Germany: Energetik Verlag, 1986.

Rosenthal, Norman. *Winter Blues: Seasonal Affective Disorder: What It Is and How to Overcome It.* New York: Guilford, 1993.

Sounding

 Sounding, originally known as toning, is a discipline that developed from the belief that being heard is one of the greatest needs of all people. Often we cannot find the right words that allow others to understand exactly what we mean. Sounding strives to improve how people use their own voice and listening abilities to help them express what is not spoken and understand what prevents them from feeling in communication with the world.

History

Sounding was developed by Don Campbell as a result of nearly fifteen years of studying voice. Focusing on how sound and music affect learning and health, he created a series of exercises meant to improve how people communicate with themselves and the world around them. In 1988 he founded the Institute for Music, Health, and Education in Boulder, Colorado, and served as its executive director until 1995. Campbell has written several books and produced cassette tapes that describe his theories and outline a program of sounding exercises. He has traveled to forty countries teaching musicians, teachers, physicians, therapists, and business trainers the basic principles and exercises of sounding. Sounding is now being used in hospitals, schools, and educational centers throughout the world to release stress.

Theory

According to Campbell, the voice is the first real tool we have to bring attention to ourselves, tell the world we need something, or show how happy we are. The first sounds we make as infants are coos and woos. There are hums and giggles, slides and wild curves that our voices project to let our parents know that we are experiencing pain, pleasure, or self-discovery. A lot of sounds that little children make are actually pleasurable sounds, although that *squeak* and *wreak* may drive others in the room crazy. Once we get to school, we are told to sit down, be quiet, and earn our education. To be unable to express our thoughts freely with the safety of being understood and heard is inhibiting to our minds, bodies, and emotions.

Campbell believes one of the great purposes of education is that we learn to express our thoughts. Sometimes our thoughts come out in creative art forms such as music, dance, and painting. Other times our expression comes in writing and not speech. But it is our speech that allows the world community and our social peers to know immediately what we are thinking. Yet we are taught that we do not want the world to know everything we are thinking. So we put on a mask, a persona, or a personality that keeps our inner thoughts from going to the outside world. When we do not learn to express ourselves and sound our minds and bodies, by the time we are finished with col-

ASound Therapy Exercise
Put your hand to your cheek and begin to hum: *hmmmmmmmmmmmmm.* That does not seem to be a great earth-shaking event. But if you close your eyes and put both hands on your cheeks and repeat the same hum for a long breath, you will realize that both your cheeks are vibrating. If you bring one hand to the center of your chest and another hand to the top of your head, you are going to feel different vibrations.

Each vowel has altogether different places where it massages the body. Toning, or sounding, is literally the only way you can massage your body from the inside out.

Begin to experiment with different vowel sounds. The *ah* is very relaxing and may make you groggy or sleepy. The *eh* is charging and brings your attention to center. The *ee* is very sharp and works almost like sonic caffeine on the body. The *hmm* allows you to feel your body very effectively. The *ouu* is a soothing, cool sound. Prolonging these sounds for five to ten minutes while sitting down with your eyes closed brings your body into alignment. This is not so metaphysical. It is actually quite physiological. Your brain waves balance left and right, your skin temperature increases, your muscles relax, your breathing increases, and your heartbeat stabilizes. It is a very healthy oasis in the middle of a busy day.

lege, we have spent a life in tension and repression, and actually have harmed our bodies by not releasing our sounds and our inner thoughts.

Learning to speak our minds, to become aware of our bodies, and to let our emotions tell the truth is a lifelong education. Learning to speak involves learning to listen. Listening is not just hearing. It is the ability to focus on outside information and attend and reach out to the world. By improving our own listening to the point that we genuinely realize that other people may not have the right words or the right timing to best communicate with us, we develop a little more patience.

Practice

Sounding is a way in which you can bring about changes in your vocal production, self-expression, and listening abilities by spending just five to eight minutes releasing sounds from your body. It is important to remember that just a gentle hum while driving the car or even while reading and studying is used to provide an enormous release of energy. Toning, which actually means elongating vowel sounds with a relaxed chin and jaw, relaxes the whole body and mind. In six weeks of humming or toning, Campbell believes a person can awaken to a new world of inner massage and vibration.

As a clinician, Campbell has worked with thousands of people to release their voices by toning. As Campbell states: "The left brain may think this is overly simple and perhaps trivial. But the rest of the brain and the body enjoys the vibration and expression."

Sounding is used as a complementary therapy to a variety of different physical and emotional therapies. Because the exercises can be fitted to the participant's schedule of treatment, sounding is often used as a warm-up exercise in schools, clinics, and hospitals for other activities or therapies.

Benefits

Practitioners believe that one of the strengths of sounding is that everyone can use it by just relaxing his or jaw. Whether you are a nurse, doctor, therapist, or teacher, going back to our primal, natural sounds can tap into elegant, natural pathways to enlighten our minds and bodies.

—FROM AN INTERVIEW WITH DON CAMPBELL

Resource

Mozart Effect Center
    P.O. Box 4179
    Boulder, CO 80306
    Tel: (303) 440-8046
    Web site: www.mozarteffect.com
    Provides information on sounding, including the cassette *Heal Yourself with Your Own Voice* (Sounds True, 1991) and *The Power of Music* (5 tapes, Nightingale Conant, 1995).

Further Reading

Campbell, Don G. *Introduction to the Musical Brain*. St. Louis, Mo.: MMB Music, Inc., 1983.
———. *The Roar of Silence*. Wheaton, Ill.: Quest Books, 1989.
———. *100 Ways to Improve Teaching Using Your Voice and Music*. Tucson, Ariz.: Zephyr Press, 1992.
———. *The Mozart Effect™*. New York: Avon Books, 1997.
Campbell, Don G., and Chris Brewer. *Rhythms of Learning*. Tucson, Ariz.: Zephyr Press, 1991.

Tomatis Method

 The Tomatis method is a form of sound therapy discovered by Dr. Alfred Tomatis in the early 1950s. It is not a therapy for individuals who are severely hearing-impaired; instead, it is meant for individuals who have lost the ability to listen clearly to the world around them. The therapy works to overcome various health problems that can affect the ability to listen and communicate with others, such as childhood ear infections, stress, accidents or traumas, or major lifestyle disruptions. Considered a type of listening training, Tomatis therapy is accomplished with the aid of an electronic ear, a specialized device that trains the ear to block out disorder and static. The Tomatis method is also used to improve vocal ability, heighten creativity and concentration, improve reading levels, and lessen stress in both children and adults.

History

Alfred Tomatis was born in 1920 in Nice, France. He studied to be a doctor of medicine specializing in troubles of the ear and language. During his early twenties, he worked for the French Ministries of Labor and War and the French Air Force. As one of his duties, he investigated hearing loss among factory workers who constructed aircraft. At the same time, he treated a European opera singer who had lost the ability to sing in tune. When Tomatis compared the test results for both the laborers and the singer, he found the same kind of hearing loss. From those results, he realized that the ear and voice are connected. "The voice can produce only what the ear can hear," Tomatis said.

From his experiments, Tomatis developed a device called the electronic ear, which improves listening, learning, and language by re-educating the ear. The electronic ear exercises the muscles of the middle ear. Special headphones make it possible to sense vibrations through bones and increase the ear's frequency ranges to sound.

Tomatis then developed a new discipline he called audio-psycho-phonology, or APP. It is a science that acknowledges the connection between ear, voice, and psychology. It deals with the functional, social, and psychological factors that impact listening, communication, language, motor control, learning, and health.

Tomatis has published fourteen books and more than fifty articles that document his research and the neurophysiology and psychology of listening. Three of his books have been translated into English: *The Conscious Ear, The Ear and Language,* and *Education and Dyslexia.*

Philosophy

The Tomatis method makes a crucial distinction between listening and hearing. Listening is defined as the active ability, intention, and desire to focus on sounds we want to analyze and to reject the ones we do not want. Hearing is simply the passive reception of sound. Listening is a skill that can be both lost and recovered. Our ability and desire to listen can be poorly developed, diminished, or even halted at any stage of our lives. If a person has difficulty listening to the world around her, this dysfunction could result from a health problem like childhood ear infections, accident, trauma, a major lifestyle disruption, or stress. With the help of the electronic ear, the ability (or disability) to listen is something that can be identified, improved, and/or corrected.

By training the ear and the mind to listen, the Tomatis method is expected to improve one's motivation to communicate and learn.

Practice

The program begins with an initial assessment, followed by a consultation to review the results and the recommendation of a specific program. Once the listening training begins, the individual listens for two hours each day. A typical program includes intensive sessions (one session per day for fifteen days, eight days, and eight days with breaks of three to six weeks separating the intensives). Longer programs are recommended when severe or long-standing problems exist.

One of Tomatis's experiments involved children with learning disabilities. During these tests, he re-created for these children the sound of a mother's voice to her unborn child. When one autistic child who hadn't spoken since he was four began to babble like a ten-month-old infant, Tomatis realized how significant his method was.

The Tomatis method is provided over an intense but relatively short time span. Sounds are presented through special headsets with bone and air conduction. First, the listener does passive sessions of hearing sounds modified by the electronic ear. The types of sounds used in this phase may include Mozart, Gregorian chant, and the filtered voice of the patient's mother. As soon as the foundation and desire for language and learning appear, active sessions of repeating sounds (humming, words, phrases, and sentences) and reading aloud begin. A microphone connected to the electronic ear allows the patient to listen to his own voice. While listening, children and adults are encouraged to draw or paint, do puzzles, play games, or relax.

Each listener receives a reassessment and consultation at the start and end of each intensive to monitor changes and allow for the program to be adjusted based on the listener's progress. Parents report on the changes they observe in their children. Adults provide reports on changes they observe in their own voices, listening, stress levels, creativity, attention, organization, spatial awareness, posture, ability to tune out distractions, desire to express themselves, musical ability, and reading ability. Other structured and unstructured behavioral observations during the program provide feedback, as do the reports of any other professionals working with the individual, such as speech pathologists, psychologists, teachers, physicians, and occupational therapists.

Benefits

The Tomatis method can be helpful for people of all ages with many types of problems, including those involving learning, language, social interaction, attention deficit, voice, speech, motor control, dyslexia, balance, posture, rhythm, and low motivation. Tomatis found that these types of disorders are almost always affected by sound stimulation.

—Dr. Billie Thompson

Resources

Sound Listening and Learning Center (Tomatis Center)
    2701 E. Camelback Road, Suite 205
    Phoenix, AZ 85016
    Tel: (602) 381-0086
    Fax: (602) 957-6741
    e-mail: drbthmpsn@aol.com
    Provides information on Tomatis training and qualified practitioners.

Sound Listening and Learning Center
    200 E. Del Mar, Suite 208
    Pasadena, CA 91105
    Tel: (626) 405-2386
    Fax: (626) 405-2387
    Refers practitioners and disseminates information regarding the Tomatis method.

Further Reading

Tomatis, A. A. *The Conscious Ear.* Rhinebeck, N.Y.: Station Hill Press, 1991.
———. *The Ear and Language.* Norval, Ontario: Moulin Publishing, 1996.

PART 6:

Subtle Energy Practices

Subtle energy therapies are bodywork methods that share the belief that our physical bodies are surrounded by and imbued with an energetic essence invisible to the naked eye. Nevertheless, the state of this essence is thought to be the primary cause of health and disease. Practitioners of subtle energy therapies use a variety of techniques to perceive blocks in the flow of this energy and work to alleviate them.

These therapies are part of a larger group of practices that have come to be known collectively as *bodywork*, a term that describes a wide variety of methods that use touch to improve awareness of feelings and sensations in the body, improve physical functioning, relieve pain, and encourage relaxation. Many disciplines in this book may be included in the category of bodywork: see under Massage, Skeletal Manipulation Methods, Acupuncture and Asian Bodywork, Movement Therapy Methods, and Body-Oriented Psychotherapies.

In addition to the energetic bodywork practices traditionally associated with the title "subtle energy therapy," this section also includes nonbodywork practices such as feng shui and magnet therapy. Feng shui is based on observation of subtle energy in one's environment. Magnet therapy focuses on electromagnetic energy surrounding and infusing the body, and works with this energy in much the same way subtle energy practices work with subtle energy.

DO-IN

FENG SHUI

MAGNET THERAPY

POLARITY THERAPY

QIGONG

REIKI

SHEN®

THERAPEUTIC TOUCH

The Life Force: A Worldview

The concept of an energetic life force has a long and honored tradition throughout the world. It is the basis of ayurvedic, Asian, Western esoteric, and many modern therapeutic health care practices.

Throughout time the energetic life force has been known by many different names around the world. The Sanskrit word *prana* means "breath," and refers to both the material air taken into the lungs and the metaphorical breath, or energy, of life. In this way *prana* is similar to the Judeo-Christian concept of "breath" as the essence of life described in the Hebrew Bible. God breathes life into Adam, thereby changing him from inert clay into the first living man.

Chi or *qi* is the Chinese word used to describe the subtle energy permeating the body. In the Chinese model *chi* moves through the body in a series of invisible channels known as meridians. The meridians touch every organ of the body, regulating the flow of *chi*. *Ki* is the Japanese name for *chi*.

The energetic life force has gone by many names in Western scientific health models. The Greek physician Hippocrates (c. 460–377 B.C.E.), the father of orthodox, or allopathic, medicine, recognized an invisible life force, which he described as the body's own internal healing and balancing mechanism. He believed that the proper role of the physician is to do only what is necessary to aid this invisible healing energy.

From the first through the fourth century C.E., Gnostic Christian sects in Greece and the Roman Empire practiced religious healing rituals based on the belief that the divine spirit of Christ literally existed in each person. Variations of these practices, relying on touch methods of healing, survive to this day and have been incorporated into contemporary subtle energy therapies such as reiki and therapeutic touch.

Samuel Hahnemann (1755–1843), a German physician working in the latter part of the eighteenth century, developed the health care modality called homeopathy based on his belief in a dynamis, or vital force. Like Hippocrates, Hahnemann believed that this invisible energy was the primary healing and life-giving agent of the body.

Another German physician, Wilhelm Reich (1897–1957), working in the early nineteenth century in Europe and the United States, combined elements of Sigmund Freud's groundbreaking psychological theory with his own research into the nature of neuroses and other diseases to create medical orgonomy. Reich believed the entire universe was pulsating with an invisible life energy, which he called orgone, that was to some extent the cause of all health or disease. Contemporary subtle energy therapies such as SHEN® and polarity combine various cultural and historical beliefs about the energetic life force with Western psychological and physical modalities to improve and maintain the physical, psychological, and spiritual dimensions of life.

Locating and Alleviating Blockages

The techniques developed to encourage the balance and flow of subtle energy throughout the body are as numerous and creative as the human imagination. They include physical exercises and breathing practices such as those found in yoga and t'ai chi, meditation methods, herbal remedies such as those emphasized in ayurvedic and traditional Chinese medicine and homeopathy, and massage techniques such as those used in acupressure and shiatsu. Most of the specific subtle energy therapies included in this section use techniques similar to forms of massage or bodywork except that they generally rely less on physical manipulation and more on very light touch, which is used to perceive and reorganize the body's internal and external energy fields. Some methods such as qigong or do-in rely on methods of manipulating subtle energy, including self-massage, massage by others, dietary and herbal practices, and movement exercises. Magnet therapy, a Western approach to manipulating electromagnetic energy, considered by some to be the physical explanation of subtle energy, doesn't use touch at all, but relies on the force of the positive and negative pulls of strategically placed magnets. Feng shui, the ancient Chinese method of environmental and spatial design, harmonizes the flow of subtle energy within a person with the flow of that energy in the environment by carefully attending to the various shapes and materials in a landscape, house, or room.

Subtle Energy and Western Science

Advanced scientific research on the effects of subtle energy is taking place at the Menninger Foundation. Researchers there have observed and witnessed seemingly miraculous feats attributed to subtle energy but have yet to prove the existence of subtle energy within the known physical field as Western science understands it. The Institute of Noetic Sciences also studies subtle energy and is working toward explaining it in Western scientific terms. Advanced research by many physicists suggests similarities between Western scientific wave/particle and energy theories of the nature of matter and the ancient subtle energy theories. Therefore, subtle energy therapies may require a leap of faith for some, but for others they may represent the cutting edge of body-mind-spirit healing today.

—*NANCY ALLISON, CMA*

Resources

Institute of Noetic Sciences
    P.O. Box 909
    Sausalito, CA 94966
    Tel: (415) 331-5650
    Organization that studies the mind, consciousness, and human potential. Also organizes lectures and conferences, publishes books and journals, and offers research grants.

Menninger Foundation
    P.O. Box 829
    Topeka, KS 66601-0829
    Tel: (913) 273-7500
    Training and research center for mental health professionals. The foundation studies conventional and unconventional methods of treating mental illnesses.

Further Reading

Manning, Clark A., and Louis J. Vanrenen, eds. *Bioenergetic Medicines East and West: Acupuncture and Homeopathy.* Berkeley, Calif.: North Atlantic Books, 1988.
Claire, Thomas. *Bodywork: What Type of Massage to Get and How to Make the Most of It.* New York: William Morrow and Company, Inc., 1995.

Do-In

 Do-in is the Japanese name for an ancient exercise system that brings the mind and body into concert with the inherent, natural rhythms of human life. This self-help program, which includes self-acupressure, massage, breathing techniques, and physical exercise, enhances the flow of vital life energy in the body. Do-in, however, is more than just relearning ancient lessons. It is the art of unlearning the artificial habits that we are taught in modern life and returning to an earlier, more instinctual life.

History

The first mention of do-in appears in the most famous medical treatise of ancient China, *The Yellow Emperor's Classic of Internal Medicine,* or *Nei Ching.* This third-century B.C.E. book alludes to the legend in which men and women lived as gods, enjoying a healthy, long life with incredible physical, mental, and spiritual powers. According to the medical sage Chi Po, the people of this time lived in a balance typified by the two complementary energies of life, yin and yang. Through mental discipline and careful attention to diet and other bodily needs, these people were able to live in harmony with nature and thus attain health and longevity.

As men and women moved into civilized communities, these natural ways of eating and living were forgotten. The special powers that do-in exercises (which resemble yoga postures, breathing, and meditative practices) were believed to have brought—extra-long life and the ability to raise the dead, walk on water, foresee the future, communicate telepathically, and control the weather, among others—were lost as well.

According to do-in lore, Taoist sages in the mountains of India, China, Korea, and Japan preserved the ancient forgotten movements and practices. These sages, or *sen-nin,* developed systematic teachings and exercise routines to help regain, develop, and maintain physical health and sharp, quick minds. These regimens, known as do-in in Japan and *tao-yin* in China, were then written or told to others. New forms developed in response to the changing needs of the people. Chi kung (or Qigong) and t'ai chi ch'üan, which share many similarities to the original do-in routines, can be viewed as later forms of do-in. Many other Asian disciplines, including yoga, karate, judo, aikido, and kung fu, also make use of basic theories of do-in.

Michio Kushi, a pioneer of the American natural foods movement, first introduced do-in to the United States. As part of macrobiotics, Dr. Kushi's system for practicing a more natural and balanced lifestyle, do-in exercises are used to complement a natural diet of grains, beans, vegetables, and other natural foods.

Theory

Several years ago researchers filmed the movements of sleeping patients at night. Afterward, when the tapes were sped up, the tossing and turning of the participants in fact resembled a carefully choreographed dance. Practitioners of do-in describe this "dance" as an instinctual version of do-in, carried out by the subconscious mind during sleep.

The movement of humankind toward civilization was a movement away from a more natural life. As people were forced to live according to a "civilized" schedule and ignore the body's urges to eat, sleep, and exercise at will, the visceral, instinctual nature of people was suppressed and weakened. Natural movements were suppressed and forgotten, but practitioners believe they remain in all of us. Thus, do-in movements do not need to be taught so much as released.

Practice

Do-in comprises a regimen of many different exercises. Do-in practices include self-massage and self-acupressure techniques, stretching and twisting movements, breathing exercises, meditation and visualization techniques, dancelike movements and routines to ease specific ailments, the use of special sounds, and healing with the palms.

These practices can be done at any time of the day. Certain exercises are suggested for morning or evening practice. Loose cotton clothing is recommended. It is best to practice in a well-ventilated and well-lit room. When possible, practice outdoors is recommended.

Benefits

In do-in and other Eastern healing arts, the body is viewed as having antennae that pick up energy and vibration from one's surroundings. Do-in helps "tune" these antennae. By practicing the various techniques of do-in, the body is able to pick up, circulate, and accumulate more energy from the environment. Once collected, this subtle energy flows throughout the body, rejuvenating and enlivening the organs, tissues, cells, and systems. Thus, do-in is doubly beneficial. Even as the body becomes healthier through this newly collected energy, a healthier body is better equipped to perform do-in.

Do-in movements mimic the body's own rhythms such that all people will recognize them. Still, instruction is encouraged to achieve proper technique and emphasis.

—*JOHN KOZINSKI*

Resources

John Kozinski Seminars
   P.O. Box 526
   Becket, MA 01223
   Tel: (413) 623-5925
   e-mail: kozinski@berkshire.net

For the *sen-nin*, do-in involved eight to ten hours daily of rigorous exercise under the guidance of an experienced teacher. In order to follow this extreme lifestyle, the *sen-nin* lived in the mountain regions and followed a special diet consisting of wild plants, and including grains, seeds, fruits, and bark. Later, aspects of the practice were incorporated into Chinese t'ai chi ch'üan, as well as acupuncture and acupressure.

Provides information about "Energy Healing," a seminar that features do-in.

Kushi Institute
   P.O. Box 7
   Becket, Massachusetts 01223
   Tel: (413) 623-5925
   Do-in forms are an integral part of seminars at this macrobiotics center. The Kushi Institute can also help locate do-in courses at other macrobiotics centers throughout the United States and Canada.

Further Reading

Hua Ching, Ni. *Attune Your Body with Dao-In.* Santa Monica, Calif.: SevenStar Communications, 1994.

Kushi, Michio. *The Book of Do-In.* Tokyo: Japan Publications, 1986.

———. *Forgotten Worlds.* Becket, Mass.: One Peaceful World Press, 1992.

Feng Shui

 Feng shui is the ancient Chinese philosophy and spiritual practice of arranging environments, based on the idea that all living things in the universe are affected by the forces of nature in their environments. Practitioners believe that by properly designing certain environments, they can direct the energy in all living things, known as *chi*, in a way that promotes harmony, prosperity, and good health.

History

The practice of feng shui began in China more than three thousand years ago. It was first used to locate grave sites that would bring good luck for the spirit of the deceased and descendants who believed their ancestors' spirits continued to affect them. Farmers later used it to find the best locations to plant crops and build homes. They studied the land to observe how the forces of nature, particularly those of wind and water, interacted. By observing the natural properties of the land and how it was shaped by the forces of nature, they tried to discern how the *chi* was flowing in that area and how they could interact with it to achieve favorable results for their crops. Later, villages, towns, and cities were built using these principles. Europeans first learned about feng shui practices in the nineteenth century through British missionaries' accounts of Chinese society and beliefs.

In early Chinese societies, feng shui was practiced by experts in astrology, numerology, and supernatural forces. These respected individuals came to be known as geomancers. When a person wanted to build a home, farm, road, or temple, or find a grave site, a geomancer was consulted for his understanding of feng shui. He would make important decisions about the proper location and design to ensure the most beneficial flow of *chi.*

The social importance of feng shui persisted in China until the late 1960s, when the Cultural Revolution was launched. The movement abolished many elements of traditional culture, including feng shui. Although it has remained popular in Hong Kong, its practice in China is only recently being restored, as many in China have been hesitant to accept its principles and practices. The suppression of feng shui in China prevented it from being integrated with contemporary beliefs and needs, making it appear archaic and superstitious. However, as a growing number of designers and architects in Asia and in the United States discover these traditional practices, the popularity of feng shui is being renewed and spread worldwide.

Principles

According to traditional Chinese philosophy, the Earth emanates an energy called *chi,* which if weakened or interfered with could be devastating to a person or community. According to this philosophy, *chi* moves through every object, creature, and space like the flow of blood through the body or a river through a landscape. Feng shui is used to ensure that buildings are placed and interior environments are designed in a way that does not aggravate or disrupt this flow of energy.

This view of the relationship among human beings, vital life energy, and their environments is based primarily on two Chinese concepts: the Tao, and yin and yang. The Tao, which may be translated as "the path" or "the way," refers to the constant patterns of change in the basic elements of nature, of which human beings are an intrinsic part. This concept is the core of Taoism, a religion characterized by its reverence for nature. According to Taoism, human beings should seek to observe patterns of nature, such as the changing seasons or transitions between night and day, and put their lives in a harmonious relationship with these patterns. Resisting the natural course of the Tao will only cause difficulties and misfortune.

The movement of the Tao is imaged as a constant dance between yin and yang, the two basic complementary energies in nature. Yin energy is characterized by its dark, cool, caring, and receptive properties. Taoists observe yin energy in water; soft, flowing fabrics such as silk; and cool colors such as blues and purples. Yang energy is characterized by its light, warm, straight, and active qualities. Wind, wood, straight objects such as knives or swords, and vibrant saturated colors such as reds and yellows exhibit higher degrees of yang energy.

According to the principles of feng shui, a healthy environment will acknowledge the Tao by a harmonious balance of yin and yang energy and unobstructed pathways for the *chi* to flow between them. The building will be situated in the landscape with respect to the flow of wind and water. Interiors will be created by the careful selection and placement of walls, doorways, and windows in order to respect the flow of *chi* and the balance of yin and yang in the building materials. Finally, the colors and materials of the objects in a room will also be selected with respect for the balance, harmony, and flow of the forces of nature.

To design a home or office properly according to the principles of feng shui, the design, materials, and function of every area should be adjusted to match the occupants' needs with the ba-gua. The ba-gua is an eight-sided "compass" that matches a specific color and human need or desire with each of the eight directions according to principles derived from ancient Chinese astrology, geometry, and mathematics. The ba-gua is used to identify areas where the flow of *chi* or the balance of yin and yang creates favorable or unfavorable conditions. Yang is most concentrated in the south, and yin is most concentrated in the north. The eight directions of the ba-gua and the associated colors and human needs are as follows:

South *(Li):* fame, red
Southeast *(Hsun):* wealth, purple
East *(Jen):* family, green
Northeast *(Gen):* knowledge, blue
North *(Kan):* career, black
Northwest *(Chyan):* helpful people/travel, gray
West *(Dwei):* children/future/creativity, white
Southwest *(Kuen):* marriage/relationship, pink

For spaces that do not align easily with the ba-gua, feng shui details a set of "cures" to remedy disturbances to the flow of *chi*. There are eight basic cures:

- *Light.* In addition to electric lights, this category consists of objects capable of light reflection and refraction, including mirrors, leaded glass, and crystals. Mirrors are frequently used in rooms designed according to feng shui. They may be aimed to deflect the flow of *chi* away from an area or used to enhance *chi* by reflecting a pleasing image.
- *Sound.* Sound is thought to set static *chi* in motion. A room is filled with sound to radiate the *chi* throughout the space. Sound may be produced by wind chimes, bells, or recorded music. Wind chimes are often used by feng shui to draw good *chi* from outside into a home.
- *Living items.* These include plants, trees or flowers (real or realistic), aquariums, and fishbowls. Plants are used to generate *chi*. Fish symbolize money, and fishbowls are often used in homes and business settings to bring wealth.
- *Moving objects.* Moving objects are used to stimulate *chi*. Motion may be produced by mobiles, fountains, windmills, whirligigs, or windsocks. Objects that are naturally powered, such as these, are preferred.
- *Heavy objects.* Heavy objects have the opposite effect of moving objects. They are used to introduce stillness in areas where *chi* moves too quickly. These may be large stones, heavy furniture, or statues.

- *Electrically powered objects.* The electricity that powers televisions, computers, stereos, or air conditioners affects the flow of *chi.* Since the energies may conflict, a space designed according to feng shui will proportion the use of electricity to balance the two energies. When properly distributed, electricity may also stimulate *chi.*
- *Straight lines.* These are usually bamboo flutes but may also include swords, scrolls, and fans. The straight lines in these objects are used to direct *chi* to a desired location. Flutes are popular cures because they may be arranged to resemble the octagonal shape of the ba-gua.
- *Colors.* Colors are used for their symbolic value within the ba-gua. When designing a room, a person may emphasize the colors that correspond to a desired direction.

Practice

Feng shui may be used to determine the proper placement of a building in a landscape or to design the interior and exterior walls, doors, and windows of a building. It is also often used to design individual rooms in a way that will benefit the people who use them. The ba-gua is used to identify the direction that represents a principle, such as knowledge or fame, that a person wants to change. Then, feng shui cures are used to stimulate the flow of *chi* in that area. For example, a person who wants to design a room to benefit her family will see that "family" is located in the east on the ba-gua. She will see if any barriers are cutting off the flow of *chi* to the east in the room. The ba-gua associates the color green with the family, so the room will be designed with green objects. A plant may be placed next to the east wall to further stimulate the *chi.*

A person may be able to use feng shui without hiring a consultant. There are a number of how-to books on feng shui that offer some basic lessons. However, those who want to employ more complex aspects of feng shui should consult an expert. When people consult feng shui experts to design their homes, they may be asked about their

According to feng shui, it is important that furniture and objects are properly placed in each room. There are specific guidelines for essential parts of a home, including the entrance, the bed, and the kitchen.

- *Entrance.* Designing a house with feng shui requires careful consideration of the entrance, since it is where *chi* enters the building. Traditionally, homes designed with feng shui will have southern entrances, since that is the direction in which the most favorable energy is thought to flow. One should be careful that the *chi* is not hindered by an obstacle blocking the front door, such as a tree or another building.
- *Bed.* One of the most significant placements in a home designed with feng shui is the location of a bed. The location of one's bed is thought to affect one's health and marriage. A properly positioned bed will give a person "command" of the bedroom door. A person is never to have his back to the entrance. When a person is in bed, he should face the doorway, but should not be in direct line of it. The ba-gua is often used to help determine the proper location of a bed.
- *Kitchen.* Homes designed with feng shui often have kitchens in the southern or eastern side of the house, since these directions represent fire and wood on the ba-gua. Small spaces and sharp corners should be avoided since they inhibit the flow of *chi.* A proper kitchen will be designed to allow the chef to see the kitchen's entrance and be prepared when a person arrives.

lives and what they would like to enhance or change. The practitioner and client will go through each of the client's rooms and discuss positioning of important objects such as the bed, desk, couch, artworks, plants, and colors to create the best possible environment to enhance or change the desired aspect.

Benefits

Although feng shui can be used simply to bring beauty and serenity to an environment, it is also used to bring benefits to many aspects of a person's life. A person who wants to improve his fortune in business, relationships, or family may use feng shui to be sure that *chi* is flowing properly in the corresponding directions of his home or business environment.

Today feng shui is used in both personal and professional settings. Several companies in the United States and Asia use feng shui to design office spaces, hoping to increase their fortune in business. Service industries like restaurants and hotels have used feng shui to make clients feel more comfortable and willing to spend more money. As its popularity grows, feng shui is changing the way that many people view the relationship between a person and his surroundings.

—MARILYN SALTZMAN

Resources

Yun Lin Temple
    2959 Russell St.
    Berkeley, CA 94705
    Tel: (510) 841-2347
    This organization offers courses in feng shui throughout the United States.

Further Reading

Rossbach, Sarah. *Feng Shui, the Chinese Art of Placement.* London: Century Hutchenson, 1987.

———. *Living Color: Master Lin Yun's Guide to Feng Shui.* New York: Kodansha International, 1994.
Skinner, Stephen. *The Living Earth Manual of Feng Shui.* London: Arkana, 1989.
Spear, William. *Feng Shui Made Easy.* San Francisco: Harper San Francisco, 1995.

Magnet Therapy

Magnet therapy, also called magnetotherapy, refers to the practice of applying a magnetic field to the body for the treatment of physical and emotional disorders. It can relieve discomfort, pain, or swelling, and has been used to treat both acute injuries, such as cuts and burns, and many chronic conditions, most notably arthritis. Some experts say magnet therapy is useful in treating depression and such mental disorders as hallucinations and delusions. Experts are not clear on why magnet therapy works, but most agree that it has been used effectively to treat diseases and ailments such as arthritis, sprains, torn ligaments, headaches, certain types of insomnia, and environmental stress. Placing the magnets directly over the area of pain can help diminish the pain from these afflictions.

History

Several books have been published over the last few decades in which the authors make reference to magnet therapy being used in times prior even to the development of acupuncture. If true, this would make the use of magnets for healing purposes one of the oldest of all therapies. Some advocates believe magnets have been used to treat pain by such ancient cultures as the Egyptians, Hebrews, Arabs, Indians, and Chinese. There are even reports of a natural magnetic material called lodestone being ground up and used as a potion as far back as 100,000 years ago. Whether these modern-day historical accounts of ancient magnet therapy are true or not, it does not diminish the fact that, at the present time, the use of magnets for therapeutic purposes is enjoying a renewed interest and an increase in popularity.

Philosophy

There are many theories about the mechanism of magnet therapy, but no one knows for certain how it works. Some theorists speculate that the local application of magnetic fields increases blood flow through the capillaries, which brings more oxygen and nutrients to the tissues. Others have suggested that the magnetic fields alter nerve function, muting the transmission of pain impulses from an area of the body that hurts. Some practitioners insist that the biomagnetic north pole, or negative pole of the magnet, somehow changes the acid-base balance of certain fluids in the tissues, making the area under the north pole magnets more alkaline. One expert theorizes that the "vector potential" and "curl" of the magnetic field may have important effects on enzyme function.

Magnets have both a negative, or north, and a positive, or south, pole. There are two different ways of naming the poles of the magnet. For purposes of what some people call biomagnetic therapy, the poles should be named as follows: the north pole of a magnet is the one that will attract the arrowhead or pointer of a compass; the south pole repels the arrowhead. Many magnetotherapists believe the negative pole has a calming effect on the body, whereas the positive pole causes stress. Being exposed to the positive pole for too long can have a deleterious effect. Proponents of so-called unipolar magnetic therapy believe it is primarily the biomagnetic north pole, or negative pole, that should be oriented to face the body, and that the south pole should always face away from the body. Other magnet therapists hold that bipolar therapy, which exposes the body to both north and south magnetic poles arranged in some sort of spatial pattern, helps to heal the body better than unipolar magnet therapy.

Practice

The magnetic field can be produced by permanent magnets, or electromagnets utilizing pulsed or alternating electrical currents traveling through a coil of wire. The permanent magnet-type devices come in a large variety of shapes and sizes. They can be as simple as a single, large, flat magnet, or as complex as a custom-fitted, contoured, cloth-covered pouch containing many small, flat, circular, or rectangular magnets. A common method is simply placing magnets over, near, under, or on an area of the body that hurts. In most types of magnetic products, many small, flat, circular, or rectangular magnets are placed so that all the magnets are oriented with the north pole facing toward the body and the south pole facing away from the body.

These devices produce a magnetic field of several dozen to several hundred gauss at the surface of the body where they are applied. A gauss is a unit of magnetic flux density or magnetic field strength. For comparison purposes, the magnetic field of the Earth that causes a compass arrow to point north is about half a gauss. In contrast, the magnets used in most permanent magnet devices are usually about 700 gauss or more.

Depending on the condition of the individual, the magnets may be applied several times a day or for days or weeks at a time. Some people may prefer to sleep on a magnetic bed or mattress pad. For others, magnet therapy may involve hours of treatment at a magnetic therapist's office, usually using pulsed-magnetic fields.

Benefits

Most people who have tried magnet therapy have experienced positive results, though they agree that more research is needed to understand how the therapy works. There have been tens of thousands of anecdotal reports that either bipolar or unipolar magnet therapy has relieved the pain or discomfort of such conditions as arthritis, fibromyalgia, rheumatism, gout, back pain, shoulder pain, carpal tunnel syndrome, bedsores, ulcers, diabetic neuropathy, trigeminal neuralgia, and toothache. In addition, magnetic field therapy has been applied in cases of acute injuries such as sprains, strains, torn ligaments, and soft-tissue injuries, including smashed thumbs, pinched fingers, insect bites, burns, scrapes, cuts, and bruises.

One benefit of magnet therapy is that foreign substances are not introduced into the body. In the long run, this might prove safer than over-the-counter medications and other treatments.

—Dr. John Zimmerman

Resources

Bio-Electro-Magnetics Institute
    Dr. John Zimmerman, President
    2490 W. Moana Lane
    Reno, NV 89509-7801
    Tel: (702) 827-9099 (best time to call is 8–10 A.M. Pacific time)
    Offers resources and information on magnet therapy.

North American Academy of Magnetic Therapy
    Cindy Kornspan, National Secretary
    28240 Agoura Road, Suite 202
    Agoura, CA 91301
    Tel: (818) 991-5277 or 1-800-457-1853
    Professional organization for practitioners of magnet therapy.

Further Reading

Becker, Robert O., and Andrew A. Marino. *Electromagnetism and Life.* Albany, N.Y.: State University of New York Press, 1982.

Becker, Robert O., and Gary Seldon. *The Body Electric: Electromagnetism and the Foundation of Life.* New York: William Morrow & Company, 1985.

Burke, Abott George. *Magnetic Therapy.* Oklahoma City: Saint George Press, 1980.

Hanneman, Holger. *Magnet Therapy.* New York: Sterling Publishing Company, 1983.

Philpott, William H. *Biomagnetic Handbook.* Choctaw, Okla.: Enviro-Tech Publisher, 1990.

Washnis, George J., and Richard Z. Hirack. *Discovery of Magnetic Health.* Rockville, Md.: Nova Publishing Co., 1993.

Polarity Therapy

Polarity therapy is a holistic method of healing that acts on the field of bipolar energy surrounding and animating the body. It assumes that illness is caused by an imbalance or block in the field, and through touch, diet, exercise, and counseling attempts to realign balance and recharge the overall level of energy. Although the principles of polarity therapy were formulated in the twentieth century, they incorporate the teachings of several ancient traditions of medicine, particularly the ayurvedic tradition of India. Proponents view it as a means of alleviating chronic physical problems, forming healthy habits in everyday life, and enhancing other modes of medical treatment.

History

Polarity therapy was developed by Randolph Stone (1890–1981), an American who was initially trained as a chiropractor and later as an osteopathic physician and naturopath. During the 1920s Stone realized that modern Western medicine could not explain the health benefits resulting from chiropractic techniques of applying direct manual pressure to parts of the body. With chiropractic techniques as a basis, he embarked on a global study of medicine that entailed voluminous reading and campaigns of travel to observe healers at work preparing medications and treating patients. Attempts to gather knowledge into universal systems were common in the twenties.

The Swiss psychoanalyst Carl Jung was integrating the world's symbols into a system of psychology, and Stone endeavored to make a comparable grand synthesis of healing traditions. He studied ayurvedic medicine in India; acupuncture, acupressure, and herbal medicine in China; and the modes of healing used in the West prior to the scientific revolution. By the 1940s he was convinced that medicine did have a central universal principle—the concept of a bipolar life force—and could be unified into one coherent system of precepts and techniques.

The final work of defining the system was carried out in Stone's private practice in Chicago and in a writing project that he started in 1948 and completed in 1970. Even staunch advocates of polarity therapy acknowledge that *Health Building* and *Polarity Therapy,* Stone's major treatises, are difficult reading and have numerous inconsistencies and ambiguities. This has left his teachings open to wide interpretation and has resulted in various approaches to treatment.

Nonetheless, Stone is recognized as an important pioneer in holistic medicine. His principles and techniques have served as a catalyst for research into non-Western medicine as well as an effective therapy in their own right. Polarity therapy is now available throughout the United States and is offered by practitioners required to meet standards for practice established by the American Polarity Therapy Association in 1987.

Theory

Stone believed the body is animated by a three-dimensional field of pulsating energy called *chi* in Chinese tradition and *prana* in ayurvedic medicine. When the energy flows outward, it is considered positive, and when it contracts backward, it is considered negative. There is no moral connotation to the distinction, but Stone followed ayurvedic teaching, which maintains that complex, dynamic interplay of the positive and negative currents determine the particular character of every portion of the human organism. Further, he held that the polarized energy pervades the cosmos, pulsating in patterns that can be correlated with the patterns it assumes in the human body. Like the ayurvedic masters, Stone approached the human being as a microcosm of the larger macrocosm, the universe. "As within, so without" was one of his favorite sayings.

Polarity therapy focuses on the connection between the energy structures of the five elements distinguished in ayurvedic tradition (ether, air, fire, water, and earth) and five of the energy centers in the body known as chakras in Eastern thought. Each element-chakra unit is associated with a quality of energy, an organ of the body, and a bodily function. The entire element-chakra series is found acting together in every human being, usually in a way that features some imbalance. The imbalance is regarded as the key to unlocking the mysteries of individual personality and health. If, for example, the air-chakra correspondence is dominant, mental activity is presumed to be the person's great strength and potential weakness. She will have unusual intellectual powers that pose no problem so long as efforts to redress the imbalance are made. Otherwise, the excess air energy will disrupt the flow of energy and cause an illness to occur in the upper chest and lungs, where the air-chakra is located.

Microcosmic energy movement is the main diagnostic and therapeutic tool of polarity therapy. Through observation and touch, the practitioner assesses the functioning of the element-chakra system, then proceeds to correct any dangerous disequilibrium. Manual pressure is applied on or around the chakras in order to balance the energy flow, and often a regimen of corrective exercises and diet is prescribed. Because the person's entire being, mind and body, is at stake, Stone believed polarity therapy should also address troublesome personality traits.

Practice

A polarity therapy session lasts an hour to an hour and a half. It generally begins with a discussion of the patient's health history, lifestyle, and therapy goals. During the course of the interview, the practitioner pays close attention to vocal changes, gestures, and aspects of posture indicative of the patient's element-chakra system. The assessment continues after the patient, still fully dressed, lies on a treatment table and bodywork starts. The practitioner is trained to use his hands as a type of magnetic transmitter of energy. In the opening phase, the hands cradle the patient's head, then move to other sites on the body, all the while picking up

various qualities of pulsation. After contact, a diagnosis is made and the practitioner uses more touching to harmonize the positive and negative charges of energy throughout the body.

The practitioner always employs both hands for treatment and draws on a repertory of more than twenty movements that include gentle to vigorous holding, vibrating, and rocking motions. A session may include stretch releases of the neck and spine; cranial balancing; work on reflex points in the ears, hands, and feet; connective tissue strokes; and strokes that connect the chakras. During these movements the type of touch may vary from light and balancing to stimulating to deep and dispersing. No two sessions are ever alike because ongoing energy assessment of the patient determines the sequence of movements and type of touch.

As the bodywork proceeds, the patient may become deeply relaxed, see dreamlike images, or feel a release of emotion and the need to talk about past traumas and current problems. The conclusion of the session depends on the practitioner. Some focus primarily on the bodywork, while others emphasize the importance of supporting the bodywork with diet, exercise, and

The standards of practice established by the American Polarity Therapy Association (APTA) require that a practitioner complete more than 615 hours of study in bodywork, exercise, nutrition, anatomy, communication skills, professional ethics, and energy evaluation. Practitioners are registered at two levels: associate polarity practitioner (APP) and registered polarity practitioner (RPP). APTA publishes a directory of registered polarity practitioners and trainers.

In choosing a practitioner, be sure to take into account both your personal needs and the qualifications of the practitioner. The practitioner you choose should be nationally registered with APTA. Registered practitioners are required to meet basic standards after which their training may vary based on school emphasis, postgraduate training, and additional degrees/specialties in other fields. Many practitioners are qualified in other disciplines such as medicine; chiropractic, osteopathic, and naturopathic practice; nursing; massage; psychology; and social work. Many polarity practitioners work for one hour and charge between $50 and $100 per session. Practitioners with additional training and degrees may work differently and charge more based on their expertise.

psychological counseling. The diet pre-scribed is usually vegetarian and may include a preliminary regimen to detoxify and cleanse the body. The exercises, based on yoga routines, involve squats, stretches, rhythmic movements, deep breathing, and utterance of the sound *Ha!* Like the other components in polarity therapy, the counseling is designed to promote freedom and balance in the patient's energy field.

Benefits

Polarity therapy acts as a tonic that brings relief from specific problems such as digestive disorders and produces an overall sense of well-being, increased energy, and serenity in the patient. Though it should not be regarded as a substitute for medical diagnosis and therapy, it can accelerate the effects of conventional treatments for major illnesses and promote recovery from surgery. As a holistic system of health care, polarity therapy can also provide guidelines for regulating everyday habits so as to strengthen the body's resistance and achieve inner harmony with one's sense of self and one's feelings.

—*JOHN BEAULIEU, ND, PH.D.*

Resources

American Polarity Therapy Association
   2888 Bluff St., Suite 149
   Boulder, CO 80301
   Tel: (303) 545-2080
   Fax: (303) 545-2161
   Sets standards for certification in polarity therapy, maintains a list of certified polarity therapy practitioners, and provides information about the theory and practice of polarity therapy.

Further Reading

Beaulieu, John. *Polarity Therapy Workbook.* New York: BioSonic Enterprises, 1994.

Stills, Franklyn. *The Polarity Process: Energy as a Healing Art.* Dorset, England: Element Books, 1990.
Stone, Randolph. *Health Building: The Conscious Art of Living Well.* Sebastopol, Calif.: CRCS Publications, 1987.
———. *Polarity Therapy.* 2 vols. Sebastopol, Calif.: CRCS Publications, 1987.

Qigong

Qigong is the most popular method of disease prevention in China. It means, literally, "energy cultivation," and is an ancient system of exercise, breathing techniques, self-massage, and meditation designed to purify, gather, and circulate life energy, called *qi.* Many studies in China and the United States have shown that practicing qigong improves health, increases vitality, and can reduce pain, anxiety, and depression. Qigong emphasizes strengthening the immune system and treating problems when they are subclinical—that is, before they produce obvious symptoms. However, qigong is also a method of disease treatment. It has been found effective for disorders such as hypertension, headaches, bronchitis, asthma, ulcers, arthritis, chronic pain, and some forms of cancer. The patient learns self-healing skills and how to take greater charge of his own health. Instead of shifting all responsibility into the hands of a physician, the qigong patient cooperates in the healing process.

The Chinese word *qi,* pronounced "chee," means "vital breath" or "life energy." According to Chinese medicine, health is the result of an abundance of clear flowing *qi.* Disease is caused when the body's reserves of *qi* are depleted through physical, emotional, or environmental stress, or when the *qi* is stuck and unable to flow. Stagnant *qi,* like stagnant water, is a breeding ground for disease. When *qi* flow is blocked, some areas of the body have too much energy or a yang condition, creating tension, congestion, and inflammation. Other areas have too little energy or a yin condition, creating weakness and conditions such as poor digestion and anemia. When the *qi* is completely gone, the body is dead.

History

Qigong began many thousands of years ago in the healing dances of ancient Chinese shamans. For instance, in the third millennium B.C.E., a bear-masked shaman would lead a dance to cleanse a village before the new year. This evolved into the philosophy that movement and exercise could also cleanse and refresh the body. According the Chinese doctor Hua Tuo (110–207 C.E.), "A door hinge won't rust as long as it is used." Similarly, physical movement stimulates internal movement of *qi*.

The practice of controlling *qi* through movement and exercise was originally called *dao-yin*, which means "leading and guiding the *qi*." In 1973 archaeologists discovered the first written record of these exercises in a text called *Dao-yin Tu*, "Dao-yin Illustrated," in a tomb near the city of Changsha. The *Dao-yin Tu*, dated approximately 168 B.C.E., showed forty-four seated and standing figures in various qigong postures. Short captions under several of the figures indicated the disease that the particular posture or exercise was designed to treat. The figures were from all walks of life—rich and poor, farmer and bureaucrat, man and woman, young and old.

By the second century C.E., qigong was a popular healing therapy practiced by a broad segment of Chinese society. Later centuries produced a wealth of practical and philosophical literature on qigong. Most early texts are found in the *Taoist Canon*, the 1,120-volume collection of Taoist religious works. Taoists had a great interest in qigong

because it includes meditation techniques that cultivate tranquil self-awareness and a feeling of harmony with nature and the cosmos. Most modern qigong texts are written by doctors rather than Taoists. In this century the practice of qigong was not encouraged by the Communist regime in China until the late 1980s, when it was adopted as a sanctioned method of disease prevention. Throughout the 1990s qigong has experienced a huge resurgence in popularity, with more than 90 million practitioners in China and several thousand in the United States.

Basic Principles

Qigong has three principal applications. Medical qigong is qigong for improving health. This is further divided into self-healing qigong, made up of exercises and meditations, and a method of healing patients called external *qi* healing. An external *qi* healer attempts to transmit healing energy by holding her hands either a few inches above or lightly on a diseased area. This method is similar to therapeutic touch practiced by many nurses in the West. Spiritual qigong, the second major application, uses meditative practices, such as abdominal respiration and mental quiet, to develop a serene and hardy spirit immune to stress and worry. Martial arts qigong, the third application, emphasizes dynamic qigong exercises that improve balance, coordination, strength, and stamina to make the body more resistant to injury. Martial arts qigong can improve performance in any sport, increasing power in a tennis serve, a swimmer's stroke, or a boxer's punch.

There are thousands of qigong styles. Some are named after legendary or actual founders; others are named after animals that the exercises imitate (for instance, crane style, five animal frolics, turtle breathing); and some describe health benefits (inner nourishing, tendon strengthening, relaxation, improving vision). Many are identified by philosophical principles: wisdom (zhi-neng) qigong, primordial (hun yuan) qigong, inner elixir qigong. Most qigong exercises are gentle, fluid, and graceful. Some styles, such as taiji quan (t'ai chi ch'üan), look like dance, consisting of many postures linked one to the next, like a flowing stream. In the past many styles were taught to only a small, select number of students or to family members. Today several qigong schools have millions of followers, with branches in major Chinese cities. Students generally select one or two qigong styles according to their interests, health needs, and teacher availability.

The foundation of all qigong practices is correct posture. Practicing the qigong posture is, of itself, good qigong. Stand with feet parallel, shoulder-width apart. Your knees should be slightly bent. Feel the weight of your body dropping down through the feet and into the ground. You are like a tree with deep roots. The abdomen is relaxed rather than unnaturally held in. The chest is also open and relaxed, neither depressed nor distended. The back is straight. Imagine that your tailbone is being pulled slightly down and your head lifted up, as though held like a puppet on a string. The entire spine feels stretched open. Your shoulders are relaxed rather than lifted in an "uptight" posture. The shoulders drop straight down, neither pulled back nor slouched forward. The fingers are gently extended, as if water were streaming out the fingertips. The mouth is lightly closed. Your eyes are open, gazing softly into the distance. The whole body is as relaxed as possible. If you need only 5 ounces of strength to stand, do not use 6! The extra ounce creates unnecessary effort and stress.

While holding this stance for a comfortable length of time—generally about five to ten minutes—observe your breath. The most natural and healthiest way of breathing is to allow the abdomen to gently expand as you inhale and retract as you exhale. Think to yourself, *My breath is slow, long, deep, smooth, and even.* Let the breath move at its own pace. Do not pull the breath in; do not push

it out. Let nature's wisdom work without interference. As you continue standing, notice how the fingers begin to tingle from improved circulation. You may also feel a pleasant sensation of warmth, stability, and inner strength. These are signs that the *qi* is both gathering and circulating.

Benefits

It is recommended that qigong be practiced daily before breakfast. The morning is called the "springtime of the day," the best time to plant seeds of new growth. The guiding principles in qigong are practice, patience, and moderation. Qigong is a lifetime discipline. It is possible to reap benefits after only a few lessons or to continue gathering *qi* for a lifetime. Practice, but not to excess. If there is pain, there is no gain, because pain inhibits learning and personal growth. Qigong students should not seek quick results but rather slow, steady progress. The body is an energy garden that must be tended and nurtured daily. According to the ancient Chinese philosopher Mencius, you cannot make wheat grow more quickly by pulling on the stalks!

—*KENNETH S. COHEN, M.A.*

Resources

American Foundation of Traditional Chinese Medicine
　505 Beach St.
　San Francisco, CA 94133
　Tel: (415) 776-0502
　Publishes a quarterly newsletter, *Gateways;* offers a referral service and international listing of classes; and sponsors continuing education programs.

The Qigong Institute
　561 Berkley Ave.
　Menlo Park, CA 94025
　Promotes education, research, and clinical work. Offers lectures and demonstrations and sponsors a qigong science program.

The Qigong Research and Practice Center
P.O. Box 1727
Nederland, CO 80466
Tel: (303) 258-0971
Offers training classes and conducts research into the efficacy of qigong.

Further Reading

Cohen, Kenneth S. *The Way of Qigong.* New York: Ballantine Books, 1997.

Eisenberg, David. *Encounters with Qi.* New York: W.W. Norton & Co., 1985.

Jiao Guorui. *Qigong Essentials for Health Promotion.* Beijing: China Reconstructs Press, 1988.

Wang, Simon, and Julius L. Liu. *Qi Gong for Health and Longevity.* Tustin, Calif.: The East Health Development Group, 1994.

Qi: The Journal of Traditional Eastern Health & Fitness. Anaheim Hills, Calif.: Insight Publishing. 1-800-787-2600 (lists many qigong schools).

Distributors of Books, Videos, and Audiocassettes

Dragon Door Publications. 1-800-247-6553, (612) 645-0517.

Redwing Book Company. 1-800-873-3946, (617) 738-4664.

Sounds True. 1-800-333-9185, (303) 449-6229.

Wayfarer Publications. (213) 665-7773.

Reiki

 Based on ancient Buddhist teachings, reiki is a mode of healing that uses hands-on touch to strengthen energy on the physical, intellectual, emotional, and spiritual planes. Reiki (pronounced "RAY-key") combines two Japanese words: *rei*, referring to the vital force that pervades the entire cosmos, and *ki*, referring to the life force that animates every individual being. In reiki treatment, universal and individual energy are aligned and balanced through the application of gentle hands-on touch to en-

ergy pathways of the body. Since no medication is ever prescribed, reiki is widely regarded as one of the most natural of all holistic systems of healing. Benefits range from reduction of stress to quantum healing, including recovery from acute and chronic conditions. It is often used as an adjunct to medical treatment in order to gain relief from the trauma of illness and to accelerate healing.

History

Until recently reiki has been taught through oral tradition, making it difficult to be precise about either the early development of reiki or many of its tenets. It may be the world's oldest system of healing, with origins that reach back to the dawn of civilization. There is agreement that after antiquity, knowledge of the original system was lost until a Japanese man, Mikao Usui (1865–1926), rediscovered it in the second half of the nineteenth century.

Usui transcends the categories Buddhist, Christian, scholar of theology, teacher, holy man, and charismatic healer. Oral tradition holds that the path that led him to reiki started at a Christian seminary in Kyoto, sometime around 1850, when a student asked Usui why he was willing to explain Christ's spiritual teachings while saying nothing about his miraculous powers of healing. Though simple, the question raised fundamental problems about the relationship of body, mind, and spirit in Western and Eastern religion. To resolve the question, Usui resigned his post in Kyoto and embarked on a quest that took him to the graduate school of the University of Chicago and eventually back to Kyoto to a Zen Buddhist monastery. By this time his research was concentrated on the earliest records of Hindu and Buddhist belief, and at the monastery he came upon ancient sutras (Buddhist teachings written in Sanskrit) that gave him an insight into the principles he had been pursuing.

A deeply spiritual man, Usui knew his understanding of the sutras would be incomplete so long as it remained on the intellectual level. After studying the texts, he ascended the sacred mountain Kuriyama and fasted and meditated for twenty-one days. Early on the morning of the twenty-first day, he had a vision in which a brilliant light struck him between the eyes, exploded into tiny colored bubbles, then gave way to a number of gleaming Sanskrit characters. Usui believed this vision initiated him into the ancient system of reiki and empowered him to revive its methods of healing. Upon returning to Kyoto, he brought about cures that were considered miraculous. He traveled throughout Japan and attracted a devoted following.

Shortly before his death, Usui passed the reiki teachings to Chijuro Hayashi, who founded the first reiki clinic. One of the patients cured in Hayashi's clinic during the 1930s was Hawayo Takata, a Japanese American woman. She studied reiki with Hayashi, became his successor in 1941, and in the 1970s traveled throughout North America, offering reiki treatment and the combination of training and initiation needed to become a reiki practitioner. Takata is responsible for transforming reiki into an internationally known mode of healing with a network of professional organizations. Many advanced practitioners are now qualified to provide treatment. In addition, a number of massage therapists, nurses, and other health care professionals incorporate aspects of reiki into their repertory of techniques. Today many reiki master-instructors are qualified to provide instruction in the Usui system of natural healing as well as offer treatment.

Philosophy and Methods

Reiki is based on a belief that the individual is animated by a vital energy emanating from the life force of the universe and falls ill if the flow of energy is weakened. Further, it is believed that everyone is born with the ability to access this universal energy. Opening pathways of healing using universal energy is reiki's central objective. To learn the procedures for self-treatment and treating others using the Usui system, a would-be practitioner must himself receive an "attunement." This attunement can be given only by an experienced reiki master instructor in a ceremony of initiation. Though no religious dogma is involved in reiki, Usui's teachings require that the ceremony be administered in a sacred manner. Sanskrit symbols from Usui's vision on Mount Kuriyama serve as the formulaic key to knowledge. Hands-on touch is the key component in the opening of an individual's energy transfer ability.

Reiki's attunements/initiations and symbols may confound rational explanation, but practitioners and masters are content simply to trust in their beneficial workings. Most practitioners and masters emphasize that hands-on touch of energy pathways in the body has been a means of therapy used around the world for millennia. They deliver reiki through hand patterns and positions that relate to the major organs and systems of the body, assisting the flow of energy through these systems. It follows that if reiki normalizes the flow of energy to the entire system, it would generate profound physical and emotional benefits, improving the entire organism's resistance to stress and disease.

Practice

Although reiki treatment may vary based on the practitioner's level of experience and the recipient's needs, it generally takes the form of a bodywork session that lasts from an hour to an hour and a half. During the bodywork the recipient remains fully clothed and lies on a massage table, first in a supine, then in a prone position. Sometimes ambient sounds of a relaxing type accompany the treatment: music or recordings of pleasant sounds in a natural environment such as a stream of water. The recipient may express preferences for such things.

Reiki bodywork should not be confused with massage. The hands-on touch is gentle and aims not to manipulate tissue, but rather to transmit universal life force to the recipient. The practitioner uses both hands, palms down, fingers held together, and proceeds in a pattern over the recipient's body. After the front surface has been treated, the client turns and treatment continues on the back. Each positioning of the hands is maintained for three to five minutes without any movement of the fingers or change in the initial gentle touch. Practitioners may use twenty or more hand positions in any single session.

Experience of reiki bodywork differs from person to person; each client's perception of how the energy transfer feels will vary. A slight warmth or tingling coming from the hands of the practitioner may be felt, or his hands may feel cool. In some instances recipients doze or go into a threshold condition between sleep and full consciousness. Most find reiki relaxing and refreshing. The full effects of treatment may be experienced immediately or not until several days after a session. It is recommended that first-time recipients receive three or four treatments as close together as the recipient can manage in order to deepen the process of healing. The number and timing of subsequent treatments depends on the nature of the recipient's condition.

Hands-on bodywork has become standard in reiki practice, but touch is not necessary to the healing process. According to Usui, the channeling of the universal life force can be achieved through mental and manual focus that is effective even over long distances, which is learned as an advanced technique. After attunement/initiation, it is suggested that reiki be used as a mode of self-care as well as care for others.

Benefits

Practitioners believe reiki gives recipients a sense of trust and overall well-being. It is particularly beneficial in the treatment of

Reiki Training
Reiki instruction has three degrees, or levels. In first-degree, or level I, training, the participant receives attunement from a reiki master. She also learns techniques for administering self-care. In second-degree, or level II, training, the participant receives further attunements of energy from a reiki master. She also embarks on the study of the ancient symbols and sounds Dr. Usui recovered from the sutras, learning to apply them to the healing process. Third-degree, or level III, training provides the participant with yet another attunement and final study of the ancient symbols and sounds used in reiki. Practitoners with third-degree training are called reiki masters, and are the only ones able to offer level I and II instruction.

stress and stress-related illnesses. Reiki is also considered helpful in treating patients with debilitating diseases because the technique supplies energy and strengthens the immune system. While reiki is not a religious system, it often becomes a potent stimulus to self-healing and spiritual growth.

—ELAINE J. ABRAMS, REIKI MASTER-INSTRUCTOR

Resources

The Reiki Alliance
P.O. Box 41
Cataldo, ID 83810
Tel: (208) 682-3535
Fax: (208) 682-4848
A professional organization comprised of credentialed Usui system reiki masters.

The Reiki Alliance Europe
  Honthorststraat 40 II 1071 DG
  Amsterdam, Netherlands
  Tel: (20) 6719276
  Fax: (20) 6711736
  The European headquarters of the Reiki
  Alliance.

Further Reading

Brown, Fran. *Living Reiki: Takata's Teachings.* Mendocino, Calif.: LifeRhythm, 1992.

Haberly, Helen J. *Reiki: Hawayo Takata's Story.* Salem, Ore.: Blue Mountain Publications, 1990.

Sharamon, Shalila, and Bodo Baginski. *Reiki: Universal Life Energy.* Trans. Christopher Baker and Judith Harrison. Mendocino, Calif.: LifeRhythm, 1988.

SHEN®

 SHEN®, which stands for specific human energy nexus, is a relatively recent approach to body-mind health and wellness that is concerned with how the body deals with repressed emotion. SHEN techniques release trapped emotional trauma from specific areas by focusing energy on the biofield that surrounds and permeates the human body. The release and resolution of these emotions is meant to reestablish normal functioning of the affected organs and balance emotional and physical forces in the body.

History

SHEN's basic concepts were developed by scientist Richard R. Pavek after he retired from a career in business in order to become an alternative medical and health practitioner. In 1977 he began formulating his original concepts about emotions and their effects on the body and the mind from observations made during his own experimentation with hands-on healing techniques.

To Pavek, emotions were far more significant in determining our health than was then presented in the medical and psychological textbooks. While the textbooks were teaching that emotions occurred in the brain and were unimportant by-products of mental activity, he, along with many other scientists, physicians, and psychologists, believed emotions were far more complex and often played a dominant role in our lives. When we have an emotion, we feel it in our bodies, our bodies react to it, and our minds cannot easily make it go away. Because emotions were not readily controlled by the brain, they were not directly produced by the brain. It followed that emotional empowerment is as important to how we live our lives as intellectual development is.

As he began to determine the effects emotions had on the body, Pavek noticed a relationship between the locations of painful emotions and the physical disorders with which they were associated. For example, he realized that anger and fear, emotions associated with eating disorders, are experienced in the same region of the body that contains the digestive organs. This relationship was the same for long-term grief and heart disorders, and for shame, guilt, and the dysfunctions they produce. Pavek conceived that the organs in that region of our bodies must be adversely affected by those emotions because they are experienced there. Somehow, emotions were controlling the body.

The last part of the puzzle fell into place when Pavek noticed that if one felt painful emotions, such as fear, grief, and shame, the body would clench around the locations where they were felt. Subsequently, the emotion would be trapped inside that location. He reasoned that the physical tension that trapped the emotion interfered with normal flow of blood and other nutrients and prevented the physical organs in the region from functioning normally. With these principles established, Pavek began developing the SHEN techniques now being used to release trapped emotional trauma within the recipient's body. He demonstrated that release and resolution of these emotions does reestablish normal functioning of the organs.

Practice

A unique hands-on process, SHEN does not use physical pressure or manipulation. Instead, it uses the biofield that surrounds and permeates the human body. This field was first identified in ancient times and has been used in healing ever since. In some forms of biofield treatment, the *qi* (pronounced "chee"; it is the Chinese name for the energy that makes up the biofield) from the practitioner's hands is applied to the body, either in direct contact with the skin or through clothing. In other forms the hands are placed close to but not touching the body. SHEN practitioners use both forms, but most of the time their hands are in contact with the body through clothing.

During the SHEN session the recipient reclines, fully clothed, on a hammocklike frame or a table similar to a massage table, but with twice as much padding. The recipient is encouraged to relax while the practitioner places her hands in a rationally planned sequence of several positions around the regions in the body where, according to Pavek's theories, we mainly experience or feel the individual emotions. These are the heart, the upper abdomen, the lower abdomen, and the groin. The recipient often feels tingles or warmth as the *qi* between the practitioner's hands flows through his body. Often the client drifts into a light sleep state, similar to what one experiences just before falling fully asleep or just before becoming fully awake.

In this state, emotionally charged, dreamlike images often emerge. Sometimes memories of forgotten, painful emotional events from earlier portions of one's life come to the surface and are relived. Whenever emotions come to the surface in a SHEN session, they are experienced in a different way than we usually experience them. Instead of being driven to physically respond to, or act out the effects of the emotion, the person strongly feels the emotion in one of the emotion regions. This occurs in a way the person can handle and absorb. Very often these feelings are understood and resolved when they are recalled in a SHEN session. Recall of previous emotional states and the resolution of troubling emotions are the hallmarks of the SHEN session; emotional empowerment is its intent.

Certified SHEN practitioners and interns can be found throughout the United States, Canada, and many European countries. More are being trained in a comprehensive professional training program that is currently available in several countries.

Benefits

SHEN is greatly beneficial with all physical conditions where unpleasant or painful emotions are major factors. These include conditions that have often been slow to respond to conventional medical or psychological treatment methods. Among these are anorexia, bulimia, compulsive behaviors, disturbed childhood sleep patterns, emotional depression, emotionally upset digestion, migraines, panic attacks, severe premenstrual and menstrual distress, all types of posttraumatic stress disorders, and recurrent nightmares.

Besides being instrumental in causing physioemotional disorders, our emotions often interfere with our thoughts. As a result, we find ourselves unable to think clearly and often end up at cross purposes with our best and most desired interests. SHEN has been proven to be a safe and reliable process that is extremely beneficial in resolving unpleasant and detrimental emotional states that undermine rational thinking and normal psychological development.

SHEN's singular techniques are unusually effective because they are based on conventional physics rather than on the metaphysical principles used in the past. Through a series of careful experiments, Dr. Pavek has been able to show that the biofield is regulated by the same patterns of arrangement that oversee all other moving fields in nature: electricity, magnetism, oceanic currents, and weather currents. SHEN practitioners learn to apply the *qi* between their hands to the recipient according to these patterns in ways that produce the greatest effect.

By clearing out the old, crippling, and injurious emotional energy, SHEN paves the way for emotional empowerment.

SHEN is helpful in dealing with grief and feelings of humiliation, and in resolving troublesome dreams. In addition, it has been extremely beneficial in promoting and accelerating recovery from alcohol and drug addictions and from childhood and adult physical, sexual, and/or emotional abuse. It is often successful where more conventional methods and approaches have failed to foster psychological and behavioral change, or real emotional empowerment and true personal growth.

—RICHARD PAVEK

Resources

The International SHEN Therapy Association
3213 W. Wheeler, No. 202
Seattle, WA 98199
Tel: (206) 298-9468
Fax: (206) 283-1256
A not-for-profit corporation founded in 1990 with the goal of expanding and promoting SHEN throughout the world. It is charged with the responsibility of maintaining and administering uniform worldwide standards for certified SHEN practitioners, for maintaining an internship training program, and for examining and granting certification to interns.

SHEN Therapy Centre
26 Inverleith Row
Edinburgh EH3 5QH
Scotland
Tel/fax: 0131-551-5091
Information about practitioners and training in the United Kingdom.

SHEN Therapy Centre
73 Claremont Park, Circular Road
Galway, Ireland
Tel: 91-525-941
Fax: 91-529-807
Provides information about practitioners and training in Ireland.

The SHEN Therapy Institute
20 YFH Gate 6 Road
Sausalito, CA 94965
Tel: (415) 332-2593
Fax: (415) 331-2455
Provides information about SHEN research and development, as well as training in the United States and Canada.

Therapeutic Touch

Therapeutic touch is an approach to healing that assesses and balances the energy field that surrounds and penetrates the body with the goal of supporting an individual's own potential for self-healing. Therapeutic touch, or TT as it is affectionately known to practitioners and devotees, is a contemporary interpretation of a number of ancient healing practices, one of which is the laying on of hands.

History

TT was developed in the 1970s by Dolores Krieger, Ph.D., RN, a nurse healer and research scientist at New York University, in collaboration with Dora Kunz, a clairvoyant. Both were interested in studying various healers to uncover any underlying principles that might form a common basis for healing. They also wanted to know if these principles might be taught to other people for use in healing. The pair did indeed find certain fundamental principles, and from their research therapeutic touch was developed. Krieger maintains that healing is a natural human potential that can be learned by virtually anyone.

Theory

The practice of TT is based on the assumption that the human being represents an open energy system, and that this system is bilaterally symmetrical. The practitioner feels for areas of imbalance in the receiver's field, such as areas of temperature difference (hot or cold), pressure, tingling, or other sensations. These sensations are cues that an area is out of balance. Once the practitioner has gained a snapshot "feel" for the client's energy field, he then works to rebalance the field.

The practitioner clears areas of imbalance by gently brushing away any places of congestion, in a movement known as "unruffling." The movement looks almost as though the practitioner is using his hands to iron out wrinkles in the space around the receiver's body. Energy is then transferred to any areas in the receiver's field that may feel as though they lack energy. The practitioner does this by holding his hands a few inches from the receiver's body, and sending energy through the palms to the receiver until the receiver's energy field feels as though it has "filled up."

Some people may think therapeutic touch sounds like hocus-pocus, and the practice has, in fact, been the subject of intense scientific scrutiny. One of Krieger's most important contributions to the field of healing has been her commitment to subjecting TT to academic research. Therapeutic touch has been the subject of no less than twenty-seven doctoral studies, fifteen postdoctoral studies, and innumerable master's theses—plus two National Institutes of Health (NIH) grants and eighty-three articles in five countries. TT is taught at more than eighty colleges in the United States and in seventy foreign countries.

The method is practiced by a large and devoted following, many of whom are nurse healers. As the practice grows, however, many other health professionals and laypersons are discovering its many benefits. It is one bodywork practice that is easy for laypersons to learn to use with family members and friends. In fact, the foundational techniques can be learned in a one-day workshop. Even children can be taught to do TT.

Practice

A typical TT treatment lasts about twenty to thirty minutes. The receiver remains dressed in street clothes, and is generally seated on a stool or straight-backed chair, facing sideways, with the back exposed for treatment. If this position is uncomfortable or unsuitable because an individual has difficulty sitting, treatment can be performed with the receiver lying on a comfortable padded surface.

The practitioner begins by quietly centering, or focusing his thoughts, and requesting that the receiver do the same. Centering calms the mind and enables both practitioner and receiver to access deep inner resources that are powerful forces in healing. While centered and attuned to the receiver, the practitioner assesses the receiver's field. The practitioner does this by gently, rhythmically, and rapidly passing his hands, palms facing the receiver, about 4 to 6 inches over the receiver's body. The practitioner then proceeds to clear areas of imbalance and transfer energy as needed to the receiver's field.

Benefits

Studies have shown that TT is effective at inducing relaxation, diminishing pain, alleviating anxiety, and accelerating healing. Receivers report various sensations during treatment, such as tingling, heat, and other effects. They often say they feel both relaxed and energized. Therapeutic touch is especially recommended for acute conditions, such as infections, wounds, and sprains.

Because therapeutic touch is gentle and the practitioner often does not even touch the body, there are very few situations in which it cannot be used. Treatments should be shorter and gentler for infants, the elderly, women who are pregnant, seriously ill people, and individuals with head injuries.

—THOMAS CLAIRE, M.S., L.M.T.

Resources

Nurse Healers–Professional Associates, Inc.
  P.O. Box 444
  Allison Park, PA 15101-0444
  This organization, to which Dr. Krieger gave all her original TT materials, can help you find more information on therapeutic touch.

Pumpkin Hollow Foundation
  RR 1, Box 135
  Craryville, NY 12521
  Tel: (518) 325-3583 or (518) 325-7105
  Offers the only year-round setting in which a full program of TT classes from beginning to advanced is available.

The Therapeutic Touch Network (Ontario)
  P.O. Box 85551
  875 Eglinton Ave. West
  Toronto, ON M6C 4A8
  Canada
  Tel: (416) 65-TOUCH
  Provides information about Canadian programs and practitioners.

Further Reading

Claire, Thomas. *Bodywork: What Type of Massage to Get—and How to Make the Most of It.* New York: William Morrow, 1995.

Krieger, Dolores. *Accepting Your Power to Heal: The Personal Practice of Therapeutic Touch.* Santa Fe, N.M.: Bear & Co., 1993.

———. *The Therapeutic Touch: How to Use Your Hands to Help or to Heal.* New York: Prentice Hall, 1979.

Macrae, Janet. *Therapeutic Touch: A Practical Guide.* New York: Knopf, 1987.

PART 7:

Massage

Massage is one of the oldest methods of healing the body, mind, and spirit. The instinct to console one another through touch is perhaps as old as humanity itself. According to the seminal study *Healing Massage Techniques: Holistic, Classic, and Emerging Methods* (1988) by Francis M. Tappan, the first cave dwellers probably rubbed their bruises and aches by instinct, the same way many other animals touch and groom one another. Humans recognized the therapeutic power of touch early on by observing its physical and psychological benefits. Many different massage techniques have evolved out of that instinct, known today under the broad umbrella called massage therapy.

How Massage Therapy Developed

The use of massage as a therapeutic tool has been documented throughout history. In the Americas, massage and joint manipulation were used by the Maya, Inca, and other native peoples. Traditional African and Eastern cultures used sharp stones to scratch the skin's surface in a healing practice similar to Chinese acupuncture. Indigenous peoples of the South Pacific have their own forms of massage as well.

Although touch has been used as a method of folk healing in many cultures, the development of formal therapeutic massage is firmly rooted in China. Evidence of this can be found in *The Yellow Emperor's Classic of Internal Medicine*, which, according to legend, was written by the Yellow Emperor Huang-ti, who died in 2598 B.C.E. Two descriptive names were used in China for massage: *anmo*, meaning "press-rub," and *tui-na*, meaning "push-pull." According to the book *Fundamentals of Therapeutic Massage* by Sandy Fritz (1995), these methods involved kneading and rubbing down the entire body with the hands and using a gentle pressure and traction on all the joints. Acupressure, the ancient practice of applying hand and finger pressure to specific points on the body, came from Chinese

BOWEN TECHNIQUE

CONNECTIVE TISSUE THERAPYSM

CORE STRUCTURAL INTEGRATIVE THERAPY

INFANT MASSAGE

MUSCULAR THERAPY

MYOFASCIAL RELEASE

MYOFASCIAL TRIGGER-POINT THERAPY

REFLEXOLOGY

ROLFING®

ROSEN METHOD

ST. JOHN METHOD OF NEUROMUSCULAR THERAPY

SWEDISH MASSAGE

acupuncture—the practice of stimulating certain points along the body by inserting tiny needles.

Chinese massage techniques spread along trade routes to Japan and other Asian countries, including India, where to this day they have enjoyed respect for their therapeutic value. There is evidence in medical literature that massage was used as a respected element in ancient Egyptian and Persian medical practices. The "laying on of hands" and "anointing with oils" has been recorded in the writings of the early Hebrews and Christians; in fact, there is reference to these practices in the Book of Isaiah.

Massage was considered an integral part of ayurvedic medicine in ancient India. Alexander the Great (356–323 B.C.E.) was one of those responsible for bringing massage to the West. When conquering India, his troops were ravaged by fatal snake bites. The Indian physicians had developed advanced surgical techniques to treat snakebite, so Alexander replaced all of his Greek physicians with Indian physicians, and massage was incorporated into Greek medicine. Tschanpua—eventually known as shampooing—was a technique initially employed by Alexander's officers; it survived until the 1800s. Last used by the British Colonial Army, it was incorporated as a part of a greater health regimen that also involved bathing and the use of scented oils.

The ancient Greeks built great bathhouses, called thurmae, where exercise, massage, baths, and scholastic studies were available, much like modern-day health spas. Citizens visited the thurmae daily as a part of the "duty of health." Socrates, Plato, and Aristotle were all teachers at thurmae and also received massage there. The Greeks employed massage especially in conjunction with athletics; for example, an athlete would be massaged before taking part in the Olympic Games.

Hippocrates, often referred to as the father of modern medicine, lived in ancient Greece from about 460 to 377 B.C.E. He learned massage and gymnastics, developed his own method of medicine, and wrote prescriptions for massage and exercise. Many of his techniques have survived to this day.

The Romans learned massage from the Greeks. Massage and baths were used extensively throughout the Roman Empire (27 B.C.E.–476 C.E.), which covered most of Europe. Cicero wrote about receiving massage and attributed his health to it. Even Julius Caesar had himself "pinched all over" daily for relief of nerve pain and to treat his epilepsy.

After the fall of Rome and the barbarian invasions, the rise of monasticism helped to preserve written accounts of the use of massage in the West. The monks were both scribes and physicians. Although they were not medically trained as Roman physicians were, they carried on the practice of massage, exercise, and anointing with oils as a part of folk medicine. Eventually the monks abandoned the practice of medicine as well as massage, and as a result massage faded in Europe. During the Middle Ages, invasions and wars caused great political and social chaos throughout Europe. Communication among countries was lost. This contributed to the decline of medicine, massage, and medical advancements. At this time supernatural occurrences were often associated with massage, and according to some sources many healers were persecuted by the Church for having evil powers.

Change occurred once again after the Black Plague, which destroyed large populations in Europe. The period known as the Renaissance (fourteenth to sixteenth centuries C.E.) followed. Travel increased and communications were restored. People started learning about Arabic and Persian culture, where the Greco-Roman traditions of massage had thrived.

In the late fourteenth century, massage was first used in postsurgical recovery and was even considered a noninvasive type of surgery. Formal two-year medical training programs were established at universities across Europe, similar to the old Roman schools. A well-known French physician, Ambroise Paré (1517–1590), began using massage for postsurgical healing of wounds and joint stiffness. His ideas helped massage find acceptance in the medical community of the West and were passed on to other European physicians.

Massage was finally popularized in the West through the work of a Swede named Per Henrik Ling (1776–1839). A fencing master and gymnastics instructor, Ling is credited with the development of Swedish massage. After curing himself of rheumatism in his arm by the use of massage techniques, he developed a system that included massage and exercise, based on the new science of physiology. Because of his continual study and dedication, Ling's method eventually became known as "the Ling system" or the "Swedish movement treatment." In 1813 he established the Royal Gymnastic Central Institute, the first college to include massage in its curriculum. The school was popular around the world, and even the czar of Russia sent someone there to study. Through the writings and practice of Ling's students, his system became well known throughout Europe. Many new forms of massage are based on this standard form.

From 1813 to 1918 massage became quite popular as a medical treatment. Many spas were built all over Europe for the rheumatoid "cure." In the mid-1800s two Vermont physicians, Charles Fayette Taylor and George Henry Taylor, brought massage to the United States from Europe. However, after World War I its popularity declined once again with the rise in pharmaceutical drugs and new medical technologies.

This decline lasted through World War II, and massage did not appear again in medical literature until the late 1970s. Massage began to reappear in American popular culture in the 1960s after President John F. Kennedy emphasized the importance of physical fitness in preventive medicine. After the reopening of China to the West during the Nixon administration, American physicians traveled there to learn acupuncture and returned with the basics of acupressure and other Chinese massage.

Massage was a part of the new age movement that began with the hippie culture in the United States, but it was not taken seriously by the medical community until the 1980s, when studies were published describing the benefits of Eastern techniques for certain conditions. It gained popularity as a method of managing pain. On-site massage at the workplace became popular for work-related pain and stress management.

Sports massage has also flourished with the popularity of athletics. Practitioners in the twentieth century began to improve the practice of massage by combining techniques and adding their own insights. This synthesis of old and new methods contributed to the resurgence of therapeutic massage in the United States and throughout the world.

Basic Systems

Today there have grown several systems, or modalities, of massage. They can be divided into three different approaches:

- *Mechanical approaches* attempt to change the quality of muscles, tendons, and ligaments or blood and lymph flow by the direct application of force. Connective Tissue Therapy℠, myofascial release, Rolfing, and manual lymph drainage are some of the popular forms that fall in this category.
- *Movement approaches* focus on passively repatterning habits of moving the body for greater ease and relief. Neuromuscular facilitation and trigger-point myotherapy are good examples.
- *Energetic approaches* deal with influencing reflexes in the nervous system and balancing energy in the body. Shiatsu and many Eastern forms of massage, as well as polarity therapy, therapeutic touch, reiki, and Zero Balancing® deal with this approach. Because these methods use substantially different techniques than the first two approaches, they are dealt with in separate sections of this encyclopedia.

Many modalities, including medical and sports massage, may integrate all three approaches.

Massage aims to bring the participant's body, mind, and spirit into balance by encouraging the body's own healing potential. The body has the amazing ability to bring itself back to equilibrium through many built-in balancing mechanisms. When a harmful microorganism enters the body, one's temperature rises to kill the germ and then eventually returns to normal (98.6° F). Using a mechanical or movement approach, massage therapists determine where imbalances may lie in the structure of the body (perhaps very tight muscles) and support the body's return to a more balanced state (that is, encouraging the nervous system and musculature to let go of excess tension in over-contracted muscles). This is done by manipulating the soft tissues of the body—mainly muscles, tendons, and ligaments.

Because the body and its systems are quite complex, a certain level of understanding of energy-flow patterns, knowledge of anatomy and physiology, and competence is required in order to give an effective massage. Thus, many states in the United States require massage therapists to be licensed professionals who have completed a certain number of hours of specialized training in a certified school and abide by certain rules and ethical guidelines. This ensures the public a safe, quality service and is similar to other professions in the field of health science such as physical therapists, doctors, and chiropractors, who must also be licensed.

The requirements for licensure vary from state to state. Some states do not require a license at all; most states require between 500 and 1,000 hours of training in anatomy and physiology as well as massage technique. Ontario, Canada, requires extensive training of 2,200 hours, while British Columbia has a 3,000-hour curriculum. Recently in the United States, standards for national certification have been established to require at least 500 hours of training and the successful completion of a national exam.

Licensure has also helped to distinguish massage therapy from the business of prostitution, which sometimes shrouds itself under the veil of "massage." Therapeutic massage is a nonsexual health practice.

The Power of Touch

Massage is usually done with the hands, but elbows, forearms, knees, or feet may be used. The client may be clothed, as is the custom with Japanese shiatsu, which is done on the floor or a mat with the practitioner kneeling alongside the client and crawling along different parts of the body to administer pressure. Touch may also be administered directly to the skin and underlying muscles of unclothed clients, as in Swedish massage. Usually in these cases the client lies on a massage table and is draped with sheets and/or towels so that only the part of the body being worked on is exposed, and most often a cream, oil, or some form of lubricant is used on the skin.

A typical treatment session lasts about one hour. If one is going for medical massage for a specific injury, it may last only thirty to forty minutes. Thai massage sessions, which involve many elaborate stretches that the practitioner does for the participant, may last for two hours.

Benefits and Risks

There are many benefits to massage therapy. Above all, it is used to relieve pain. Psychologically, touch gives a message of caring, compassion, and support to a participant and can thereby help reduce stress and aid healing. Mechanically, it can alleviate muscle spasm and help increase flexibility. Physiologically, circulation of blood and lymph is increased, which helps deliver nutrients to all the cells of the body and also helps to remove the waste products of cells. Studies with AIDS patients have shown that massage therapy can help activate the immune system. Touch can have a soothing or stimulating effect on the nervous system. Furthermore, it heightens awareness of the body and its sensations, which supports the connection of body, mind, and spirit. Scientific research is currently being done at the Touch Research Institute in Florida to further investigate the effects of touch and therapeutic massage.

Despite all of these healing effects, there are times when massage therapy is not appropriate. Massage should not be administered if either the client or the practitioner is under the influence of certain types of drugs, such as cortisone treatments or mind-altering drugs. It should also be avoided if the client or the practitioner has a fever or a communicable disease such as the measles or influenza.

Cancer is another major contraindication. Many forms of massage therapy, especially Swedish, involve moving lymph fluid, which may cause the cancer to spread. If the participant has been diagnosed with any form of inflammation of the blood vessels (especially phlebitis) or with a blood clot, massage should not be done for fear of moving the clot where it may damage the heart or cause a stroke. Massage should be avoided locally if the participant has varicose veins, bruises, or open wounds. Liver problems and other inflammations of internal organs should be investigated with the client's doctor before massage is administered.

—KATIE SCOVILLE, WITH INFORMATION FROM AN INTERVIEW WITH RICHARD VAN WHY, PUBLISHER OF THE BODYWORK KNOWLEDGEBASE

Resources

American Massage Therapy Association
    820 Davis St., Suite 100
    Evanston, IL 60201
    Tel: (847) 864-0123
    Fax: (847) 864-1178
    Web site: www.amtamassage.org
    An organization that provides information and resources on massage therapy. Publishes the *Massage Therapy Journal.*

The American Oriental Bodywork Therapy Association
    Glendale Executive Campus, Suite 510
    1000 White Horse Road
    Vorhees, NJ 08043
    Tel: (609) 782-1616
    Fax: (609) 782-1653
    Web site: www.healthy.net/pan/pa/bodywork
    A national organization of bodyworkers in eleven different styles. It certifies practitioners, teachers, and schools throughout the United States. The organization enforces minimum entry-level standards (500 hours) for all types of Oriental bodyworkers. Currently represents about 1,200 members.

College of Massage Therapists of Ontario
    1867 Yonge St., Suite 810
    Toronto, Ontario M451Y5
    Canada
    Web site: www.cmto.com
    Organization that promotes the therapeutic use of massage in Canada.

National Certification Board for Therapeutic Massage and Bodywork
    8201 Greensboro Dr., Suite 300
    MacLean, VA 22102
    Tel: 1-800-296-0664
    Fax: (703) 610-9015
    Web site: www.ncbtmb.com
    Establishes and implements certification standards for massage therapists.

Further Reading

Fritz, Sandy. *Mosby's Fundamentals of Therapeutic Massage.* St. Louis, Mo.: Mosby-Year Book, Inc., 1995.
Lidell, Lucinda. *The Book of Massage.* New York: Fireside, 1984.
Tappan, F. M. *Healing Massage Techniques: Holistic, Classic, and Emerging Methods.* Norwalk, Conn.: Appleton & Lange, 1988.

Bowen Technique

 Bowen technique, or Bowtech©, is a system of muscle and connective tissue movements used to stimulate energy flow and restore the body's self-healing resources. A Bowtech specialist uses a series of gently rolling movements to manipulate a client's connective tissue, including muscles, tendons, and ligaments. With the goal of stimulating, balancing, and realigning the body's energy flows, the Bowen technique is used by many health care professionals as an adjunct to their work; however, it is increasingly used as a stand-alone therapy, with many practitioners maintaining their own clinics.

History

The Bowen technique was developed in Australia by Thomas A. Bowen (1903–1982). He began his professional training with a year of medical school, followed by service in the Australian army during World War II. After the war, while working in an industrial plant, Bowen gained a reputation for being able to help his coworkers with their aches and pains. He decided to open a clinic using his method of muscle manipulation. By 1975 he was seeing 13,000 patients per year. After his death, Bowen's colleagues Oswald and Elaine Rentsch continued his work. The Rentsches had previously documented Bowen's technique, and since his death they have introduced it throughout Australia, North America, and Europe. More than 6,000 people worldwide have been trained to practice or administer the Bowen technique.

Practice

The Bowtech therapist uses two or four fingers to gently roll muscles from side to side. Known as the Golgi tendon reflex, this movement triggers muscles to relax. It appears to affect the body's autonomic nervous system and creates balance on a cellular level. Some believe that Bowtech sets up vibrational patterns that correspond to particular areas of the body. The body then attempts to alter its usual vibrations to match those ideal vibrational patterns, and in doing so, brings itself into harmony.

A typical treatment lasts between twenty and forty minutes. It is usually done on a massage table or bed, where a client will lie comfortably and fully clothed on his back or abdomen. The therapist relaxes a muscle, tendon, or ligament by gently rolling it back and forth with her fingers. Each session includes a series of waiting periods when the therapist will pause to allow the recipient's body to integrate the changes to the area being treated. Generally an increase in blood supply and lymphatic drainage results in the release of tension and reduced muscle spasms. Unlike traditional Swedish massage, the technique is gentle and contacts only muscles on the surface of the body, with no deep rubbing.

Benefits

The Bowen technique may be performed on anyone, from newborn infants to seniors. It may be incorporated into the treatment of the disabled or patients with chronic illnesses, including multiple sclerosis, cerebral palsy, muscular dystrophy, acute and chronic fatigue, and stress disorders. It has also been used to speed rehabilitation of sports injuries and accidents, regardless of how old or recent the injuries may be.

—*Oswald Rentsch*

Resources

Bowtech©
P.O. Box 733
Hamilton, Victoria 3300
Australia
Tel: 011-61-3-55-723000
e-mail: bowtech@h140.aone.net.au
Promotes the study and use of the Bowen technique.

Connective Tissue Therapy^{SM}

 Connective Tissue Therapy^{SM} is a form of bodywork, sometimes called binde or bindegewebs-massage, which stimulates the tissue between skin and muscle in order to relieve pain and promote mental, emotional, and physical well-being. Developed by a German physiotherapist, Elizabeth Dicke, it posits a powerful association between particular areas of connective tissue and specific paths of the nervous system and internal organs. Following Dicke's teachings, Connective Tissue Therapy plots treatment so as to activate relays between areas of tissue and different parts of the body. It can help restore balance to the neuromuscular and organ systems after illness and has a relaxing effect beneficial to self-healing and health maintenance.

History

Dicke discovered the basic principle of Connective Tissue Therapy in 1929, when she was incapacitated by toxemia of the right leg so severe that doctors recommended amputation. While touching an area of her lower back, she came across abnormally thick, tense layers of tissue and realized she felt sensations of warmth and tingling in her infected leg whenever she stroked the area of abnormal tissue in a pulling manner. Though recovery required three months and the help of a physiotherapist who followed Dicke's specific instructions, the transmission of energy from the lower back became the means by which Dicke saved her leg.

After returning to work, Dicke began to explore the ramifications of her discovery. She noticed, for example, correspondences between malfunction in various organs and changes in tension on specific areas of the body's surface, named "Head zones" after Henry Head, the nineteenth-century English neurologist who first studied them. According to Head, the nerves, organs, and their correlated Head zones of skin are rooted in the same segment of the spinal cord. Dicke built on Head's work, using the zones as a guide for locating pathways of connective tissue that could be manipulated to improve organ function.

By 1938 Dicke had formulated the system of bodywork she called bindegewebsmassage, literally connective tissue massage, and started to search out ways to introduce it to the medical community and the general public. She collaborated with a number of scientists in publishing the material in article and book form and became active as a teacher.

Theory

Connective Tissue Therapy concentrates on the subcutaneous sheaths of tissue, known as fascia, that are found throughout the body surrounding, supporting, and connecting the nerves, blood vessels, muscles, and organs. Distinct from muscles, fascia is an important determinant of strength and range of motion and in a healthy person is usually robust and flexible. Conversely, tension in the fascia, evident in a thickening of tissue and loss of ease in movement, is a sign of dysfunction caused by disease or by an imbalance likely to cause disease if it is not corrected.

Through massage, Connective Tissue Therapy attempts to restore suppleness and vitality to fascia that has tightened and become numbed or painful. It is postulated that the massage is effective because it activates the parasympathetic nervous system, which controls relaxation as well as pain relief and healing in the vital organs and all other parts of the body.

Practice

Length and frequency of sessions vary according to the needs of the receiver. Since the benefits increase with each additional session, a series of ten to twenty sessions may be recommended for a receiver with a severe problem or one interested in learning about the body's potential for health. During treatment, done without oils or lotions, the receiver sits on a chair or lies flat. The treatment starts at the pelvic area, then proceeds over the body, using a technique in which the therapist hooks his fingers into the skin and upper layer of fascia while performing a pulling stroke. The strokes cause temporary marks on the skin and sensations ranging from dull to sharp. As the treatment continues the receiver may experience a desire to sleep, excessive perspiration, deepened breathing, or a drop in body temperature. Benefits from the session may last for months following a series of treatments.

Benefits

Connective Tissue Therapy brings about a relaxation of the fascia that is particularly helpful in restoring function and range of motion and in stimulating bone and muscle repair of damage from injuries, arthritis, and other degenerative disorders. It has a tonic effect on the circulatory and nervous systems that can aid the elimination of toxins, promote the healing of wounds in a way that

The Elizabeth Dicke Society was founded in 1954 to preserve and expand her legacy. Bindegewebsmassage is a widely accepted physical therapy in Germany and in many countries is regarded as a medical treatment for organ and circulatory disease. In the United States, Connective Tissue Therapy remains less well known than other types of bodywork, but it is taught at various massage schools, and the technique is part of the repertoire of many massage therapists.

prevents the formation of scar tissue, promote recovery from kidney and other organ malfunction, and lessen stress and anxiety. It can also be an effective adjunct to other forms of treatment.

—JACKIE HAND

Resources

Theresa Lamb
2140 Lower Smith Gap Road
Kunkletown, PA 18058
Tel: (610) 826-5957
Provides training in CTT^{SM}.

Wholistic Pathway
152 N. Wellwood Ave., Suite 5
Lindenhurst, NY 11757
Tel: (516) 226-3898
Offers training in bindegewebsmassage.

Further Reading

Dicke, Elizabeth, et al. *A Manual of Reflexive Therapy of the Connective Tissue (Connective Tissue Massage) 'Bindegewebsmassage.'* Scarsdale, N.Y.: Sidney S. Simon, 1978.

Ebner, Maria. *Connective Tissue Massage: Theory and Therapeutic Application.* Huntington, N.Y.: Robert E. Krieger Publishing Co., 1980.

Tappan, Frances. *Healing Massage Techniques: Holistic, Classic, and Emerging Methods.* Norwalk, Conn.: Appleton & Lange, 1988.

CORE Structural Integrative Therapy

 CORE structural integrative therapy is a system of bodywork that seeks to improve the structure and function of the musculoskeletal system and connective tissues of the human body. CORE practitioners utilize client-assisted movement while applying massage techniques, which creates heightened awareness of the body and allows the client to participate in releasing tension and pain. This system was originated by George P. Kousaleos, founder of the CORE Institute School of Massage Therapy and Structural Bodywork.

Practice

A typical session includes an analysis of the client's structural alignment and movement patterns, the application of full-body or regional bodywork techniques that stretch and tone the body's myofascial network, and instruction of corrective and postural exercises. CORE bodywork techniques vary from moderate to deep pressure, and sessions can be organized for specific ailments or for general benefit.

CORE structural integrative therapy usually involves ten sessions of bodywork, but also includes introductory and maintenance sessions that support a lifelong system of improved alignment and optimal performance. The CORE system includes CORE myofascial therapy, a full-body session that introduces the client to the concepts and benefits of structural alignment; CORE ex-
trinsic therapy, a three-session series that aligns the superficial musculature, which allows for greater freedom of movement; CORE intrinsic therapy, a four-session series that aligns the deepest musculature, which supports the pelvis, spine, and cranium; and CORE integration therapy, the final three-session series, which provides integrated movement patterns throughout the body.

Benefits

A person will experience the physical benefits of CORE structural integrative therapy immediately. Clients may feel a lighter, longer, and looser relationship of muscles and joints. Some recipients often perceive that they are using less energy to produce all physical activities, and that they sleep and rest at a deeper level. Some clients will also experience a release of emotional memories and trauma, often resulting in a greater sense of self-reliance.

While CORE structural integrative therapy can be beneficial for every age group and activity level, the positive aspects are greater for those who are actively engaged in rigorous physical or mental endeavors. Many clients report immediate improvement in their physical and psychological stress levels, resulting in a higher state of clarity and focus. From 1994 to 1996 CORE practitioners worked with British Olympic athletes who were in training for the 1996 Atlanta Olympics. It is estimated that more than three hundred Olympic athletes and coaches have received CORE treatments.

—GEORGE KOUSALEOS AND GARY GENNA

Resources

The CORE Institute
    223 W. Carolina St.
    Tallahassee, FL 32308
    Tel: (904) 222-8673
    Fax: (904) 561-6160

Offers training for CORE practitioners. All CORE practitioners have been trained through the faculty of the CORE Institute and are nationally certified in therapeutic massage and bodywork. Training in CORE structural integrative therapy is offered throughout North America.

Infant Massage

Infant massage is an ancient tradition in many cultures throughout the world. Since the 1970s this art has been enjoying a renaissance in the West. Traditional infant massage strokes, like those practiced in India, are used in the United States as a way for parents and other caregivers to communicate their love, caring, and respect for their babies and children. Studies seem to indicate that the positive effects of practicing infant massage are just as profound on the parent's physical, mental, and emotional well-being as they are on the child's.

History

Vimala McClure was one of the first to bring the practice of massaging babies to the United States. While living in India in the early seventies, McClure observed the beneficial effects of daily massage on infants. She returned to the United States and put together a curriculum for parent-infant classes. McClure wrote a book on the subject, *Infant Massage: A Handbook for Loving Parents*, developed an instructor training program, and in 1981 founded the International Association for Infant Massage (IAIM). The purpose of IAIM is to integrate the art of infant massage into the parenting traditions of Western cultures. IAIM offers courses for parents and other caregivers and, according to its mission statement, works to "promote nurturing touch and communication through training, education, and research so that parents, caregivers, and children are loved, valued, and respected throughout the world community." There are presently more than 1,500 active certified infant massage instructors (CIMIs) throughout the world.

Theory

Infant massage includes the critical elements of bonding: eye-to-eye and skin-to-skin contact, smiling, soothing sounds, cuddling, and sound and smell reciprocity. "Touch communication" provides a common language for parent/child communication. Babies communicate through many types of nonverbal cues, such as rubbing their eyes when tired, sucking their hands when hungry, smiling when happy, and crying when hungry, wet, or in need of attention. By learning to read the nonverbal cues that babies use to express a full range of emotions in response to the massage, caregivers develop a tangible sense of their own powers to help soothe, comfort, and nurture their babies.

Renowned British anthropologist Ashley Montagu points out in his book *Touching* that all mammals except human beings lick their young. This licking process serves to stimulate the physiological systems and aids in the bonding process. Montagu postulates that the massage tradition, found in most countries of the world, is the human equivalent of mammals licking their young for health and well-being.

Clinical evidence shows that loving, touching, and nurturing contact between caregiver and infant has a positive impact on subsequent physical, mental, and emotional development of the child. Many studies suggest the benefits of positive, interactive contact as an integral part of early life. They also suggest that a lack of early interactive touch can have a negative impact on a child's development.

Research conducted over the years in regard to human touch has indicated that it is particularly beneficial for vulnerable babies. A landmark study by F. A. Scafidi shows that premature babies who were massaged daily developed more rapidly both physically, with greater weight gain, and neurologically. In 1987 researcher K. J. Ottenbacker analyzed nineteen separate infant stimulation studies and found that 72 percent of the infants receiving some form of tactile stimulation were positively affected. Most of the investigators in these nineteen studies reported greater weight gain and better outcomes on developmental assessments compared to those infants who did not receive as much stimulation.

Studies conducted at the Touch Research Institute (TRI) at the University of Miami Medical Center confirm the effectiveness of the techniques outlined in McClure's book. TRI studies have shown that massage improves cardiac and respiratory output, promotes longer and deeper sleeping patterns, and develops immunological factors. In one study conducted by Tiffany Field, babies of depressed adolescent mothers were massaged by their mothers. These babies fell asleep faster and became more vocal, mother-baby interactions improved, and the mothers perceived that the babies were easier to soothe. Field has also identified other positive effects that providing massage can have on the caregiver, including improved mood and a reduction in anxiety. In addition, caregivers' stress levels decreased and they reported improved self-esteem.

Practice

CIMIs conduct parent education classes in a variety of settings, usually in small groups to facilitate communication and support among the caregivers in the group. Instructors teach a series of classes over a four- to five-week period. It usually takes about a month for a healthy baby to learn to accept a full-body massage.

Parents are encouraged to massage their babies on a regular basis, every day if possible. Since the premise of the work is that parents are teachers of relaxation, parents are also encouraged to set up relaxed environments for themselves, so that they can pass on this sense of relaxation to their babies. Infant massage's precepts also encourage self-care for parents as a means of caring for one's child.

An important tenet of infant massage is learning to show respect for the baby. It is important that caregivers learn to use tactile, auditory, and visual cues to ask the baby's permission to massage. This can be done by rubbing small circles around the hairline, holding the baby's hands together, or placing the baby's hands on her chest and then waiting for a response from the baby. Learning to understand and respect the baby's answer, which is given with the same kinds of nonverbal cues, is part of learning to communicate through appropriate touch. By asking permission in this way, parents also teach their children to discern touch that is loving and appropriate. Asking permission is also a way of demonstrating respect for the baby. By showing the baby respect, the caregiver helps the baby develop self-respect.

Babies are massaged without clothing, using edible oils that are absorbed by the skin, such as sunflower or almond oil, so that the baby will not be harmed if she swallows any oil. A massage lasts as long as the baby gives permission and the caregiver is available. This can be as short as two minutes or as long as an hour. Most massages are twenty to twenty-five minutes long.

Massaging a baby is a tactile expression of love and security. Experience and clinical research show that babies enjoy and benefit from firm, confident touch as opposed to light, feathery touch. Babies typically move, kick, and talk throughout the massage. They are not quiet recipients like adults. Parents are encouraged to actively listen to their babies' responses to the touch of the massage. This type of interaction teaches parents to talk with their hands and listen with their hearts.

Massage is a dance between the parent and baby. The techniques taught in classes or learned from a book or video are the basic choreography. Once a parent is comfortable with the massage, improvisation begins. Parents use the same strokes that generations of parents all over the world have used, yet each parent and child develop a "duet" that is their own unique expression of love.

Benefits

The practice of infant massage enhances the parent-baby bond, helping to create loving and respectful relationships among family members. The massage time offers parents an opportunity to explore and develop their responses to the baby's sounds, movements, and facial expressions. Babies are taught that they are aware human beings who deserve respect, tenderness, warmth, and above all, a listening heart. This type of interaction serves as a model for the child as he grows and for the parent as well, encouraging both to develop respectful, loving relationships with an ever-widening circle of people.

—MINDY ZLOTNICK

Resources

International Association for Infant Massage
   1720 Willow Creek Circle, Suite 516
   Eugene, OR 97402
   Tel: 1-800-248-5432
   Fax: (541) 485-7372
   e-mail: iaimus@aol.com
   Organization that trains and certifies
   instructors.

The International Association for Infant Massage trains and certifies individuals to teach parents and caregivers to massage their babies. Many CIMIs are branching out to work with special-needs populations, such as physically challenged infants, infants who are drug-exposed, HIV-positive, or medically fragile infants, and teen mothers, incarcerated mothers, homeless families, and women recovering from drug and alcohol addiction.

Further Reading

Books

Kennel, J., and M. Klaus. *Parent-Infant Bonding.* 2nd ed. St. Louis, Mo.: C.V. Mosby, 1982.

McClure, Vimala. *Infant Massage: A Handbook for Loving Parents.* New York: Bantam Books, 1989.

Montagu, Ashley. *Touching.* New York: Harper and Row, 1978.

Journals

Field, Tiffany. "The Benefits of Infant Massage on Growth and Development." *Pediatric Basics,* vol. 71, 1996.

Ottenbacher, K. J., et al. "The Effectiveness of Tactile Stimulation as an Early Intervention: A Quantitative Evaluation." *Journal of Developmental Behavioral Pediatrics,* 8 (1987): 68–76.

Scafidi, F. A., T. Field, and S. M. Schanberg, et al. "Effects of Kinesthetic Stimulation on the Clinical Course and the Sleep/Wake Behaviors of Pre-term Neonates." *Infant Behavior and Development,* 9 (1986): 91–105.

Scafidi, F. A., et al. "Massage Stimulates Growth in Preterm Infants, a Replication." *Infant Behavior and Development,* 13 (1990): 167–68.

Muscular Therapy

 Muscular therapy, also referred to as the Benjamin system of muscular therapy, consists of a series of techniques and exercises designed to promote physical health and reduce muscular tension and stress caused by physical injury. It is also an educational process in which the client learns to understand the cause of his physical symptoms and what needs to be done to alleviate them.

History

Muscular therapy was developed by Ben Benjamin, Ph.D., from a synthesis of several approaches to working with the body. Benjamin's interest in the field began in 1958, when he sustained a serious injury. After several failed attempts to obtain relief, his injury was successfully treated by Alfred Kagan, a well-known French practitioner who had developed original techniques for the treatment of muscular tension and injury. During the course of his treatment, Benjamin became interested in Kagan's method and studied with him after his recovery. From his observations Benjamin created a series of more than seven hundred discrete muscular manipulations.

Following his work with Kagan, Benjamin spent several years studying the origins of physical tension and learning how people could care for themselves without requiring continual treatment from a physician or therapist. He became particularly interested in the work of Dr. Wilhelm Reich, F. M. Alexander, and Dr. James Cyriax and sought ways of incorporating some of their ideas into his approach to tension reduction. In Reich's work, Benjamin learned of the emotional component of muscular tension. This understanding of the physical manifestation of emotional distress could help the practitioner distinguish between emotional distress in the body and mechanical or injury-related tension. In his study of the Alexander technique, Benjamin discovered a method for establishing proper movement habits. By using these techniques, practitioners could learn to use their bodies more effectively and avoid movement habits that cause pain, tension, and injury. Benjamin also was influenced by Cyriax's injury evaluation and deep friction treatment.

These three approaches, combined with Benjamin's original treatment techniques, provide a comprehensive understanding of the nature and treatment of physical tension. They enable the practitioner to determine if an injury has been caused primarily by overuse, an alignment problem, or emotional stress. Using these techniques, Benjamin was able to distinguish between a serious injury, which requires a physician's attention, and one that is relatively minor and could be safely handled with muscular therapy techniques. His techniques are not designed to treat muscular tension caused by emotional stress.

Practice

A therapist works with the client by performing deep massage, including a variety of area-specific strokes, pressure, and rhythms to reduce chronic tension and pain. In a typical session, therapists may educate clients about the causes and effects of tension. Clients learn techniques designed to prevent the buildup of new tension. These may include basic exercises for warming up, stretching, and building strength.

—BEN BENJAMIN, PH.D., AND MARY ANN DI ROBERTS

Resources

Muscular Therapy Institute
   122 Rindge Ave.
   Cambridge, MA 02140
   Tel: (617) 576-1300

The Muscular Therapy Institute offers a two-year training program in massage therapy that emphasizes physical technique, clear professional boundaries, and good communication skills.

Further Reading

Benjamin, Ben E. *Are You Tense? The Benjamin System of Muscular Therapy*. New York: Pantheon, 1978.

———. *Exercise Without Injury*. New York: Summit Books, 1979.

———. *Listen to Your Pain: The Active Person's Guide to Understanding, Identifying, and Treating Pain and Injury*. New York: Viking/Penguin, 1984.

Myofascial Release

 A gentle, hands-on therapy that involves applying an extremely mild and gentle form of pressure to the body to relieve tension in the soft connective tissue, myofascial release is the release of this connective tissue, or fascia. The therapist applies a stretching technique to the body that exerts a small amount of pressure on the fascia. Myofascial release experts have shown that fascia softens and begins to release tension when the pressure is sustained over time. It is used to relieve chronic pain, especially in areas such as the neck, jaw, and back. With the release of physical pain, patients often report a release of emotions that were formerly buried deep in the subconscious. Myofascial release uncovers "secrets" stored in the body.

History

Myofascial release was developed by John F. Barnes, P. T. Barnes graduated from the University of Pennsylvania in 1960 with a degree in physical therapy and started his own practice in 1966.

Barnes's first experience with what we now know as myofascial release began at age seventeen, when he accidentally injured his back while lifting weights. He initially ignored the pain, but later, in his own work as a therapist, he came to the realization that he was in worse shape than most of his patients. The pain grew so bad that from ages twenty-five to thirty, he could not sit for more than two to three minutes at a time. Finally, Barnes consulted a neurologist and an orthopedist, who diagnosed him with a crushed disc. The removal of the disc took the intensity out of his pain and allowed him to function. However, he still had problems with his back, and through his frustration in trying to help himself before and after his surgery, he developed techniques that relieved the symptoms. The injury also gave Barnes an understanding of what it is like to be "trapped" in pain.

Despite the fact that he did not know why these techniques worked, Barnes began trying them on his patients. He noticed that patients were responding consistently. While attending a course on the connective tissue system, he realized his therapy dealt directly with the body's fascia. The soft tissue mobilization techniques he learned from this course were basically an old form of myofascial release. He had used these techniques to control his own pain, but he tended to hold each position for an extended period. This extended time factor turned out to be the key to releasing the total myofascial complex. Older forms of myofascial release were too superficial to give complete release.

Theory

Fascia extends from the head to the feet. In a normal, healthy state, the fascia is relaxed and wavy in configuration. It has the ability to stretch and move without restriction. When we experience physical trauma, such as inflammation, a fall, whiplash, surgery, or even just habitual poor posture over time, the fascia loses its flexibility. It becomes tight, restricted, and a source of tension to the rest of the body. The changes these traumas cause in the fascial system influence the skeletal framework for our posture, and the fascia can exert excessive pressure, producing pain, headaches, or restricted motion.

Fascia permeates all regions of the body and is interconnected. When it scars and hardens in one area following a trauma, it can create tension on adjacent pain-sensitive structures as well as on structures in faraway areas. Thus, a restriction in one region can theoretically put a "drag" on the fascia in any other direction. Because all muscle is enveloped by and ingrained with fascia, *myofascial release* is the term that has been given to the techniques used to relieve soft tissue from the abnormal grip of tight fascia.

Made of a fibrous, soft, gel-like substance, fascia can be softened when released. This release allows therapists to become sculptors with their fingers, hands, and elbows. By steadily releasing the fascia, they can remold the body back into a more healthful, functional, and comfortable position. This is because the pressure stretches the connective tissue and removes the tightness that causes the pain.

Practice

A myofascial release session usually lasts thirty to ninety minutes. The client undresses down to her underwear and lies on a massage table. Unlike massage, no oil is used. The therapist uses his fingers, palms, elbows, and forearms to warm and stretch the fascia. The pressure is gentle but firm and is used for at least 90 to 120 seconds with each therapeutic stroke. When an individual first begins this form of treatment, therapists recommend several sessions a week. As her condition gradually improves, the patient needs less treatment.

Benefits

Barnes has seen consistent, positive results using myofascial release to treat acute pain, chronic pain, fibromyalgia, headaches, scoliosis, chronic fatigue syndrome, birth injuries, cerebral palsy, geriatric problems, pediatric problems, and movement dysfunction.

Myofascial release experts say this form of therapy works especially well for individuals seeking long-term relief for chronic pain and immobility caused by extreme tightness of the muscles. Common areas of treatment include the neck, jaw, and back. Myofascial release can also reduce muscle tension and treat recurring injuries and other stress-related problems.

—TARA WELCH FOR MYOFASCIAL RELEASE TREATMENT CENTERS AND SEMINARS

Resources

Myofascial Release Treatment Centers and Seminars
    Routes 30 and 252
    10 S. Leopard Road, Suite 1
    Paoli, PA 19301
    Tel: (610) 644-0136 or 1-800-FASCIAL (327-2425)
    Web site: www.vll.com/mfr
    Provides information, organizes seminars and training programs, offers treatment programs, and refers patients to qualified practitioners.

Further Reading

Barnes, John F. *Myofascial Release: The Search for Excellence, a Comprehensive Evaluatory and Treatment Approach.* Paoli, Pa.: Rehabilitation Services Inc. T/A, Myofascial Release Seminars, 1990.

Myofascial Trigger-Point Therapy

 Myofascial trigger-point therapy (MTPT) is a physical, therapeutic discipline for treating myofascial, or muscular and connective tissue, pain in muscles and joints by focusing on trigger points, which are defined as sensitive areas in the muscle that are tender to the touch. MTPT therapists apply pressure, among other techniques, to trigger points in order to release these areas of constriction and pain. It is intended to provide the client with a greater awareness of his body, and to release stress and tension.

History

While many people contributed to the development and spread of MTPT, the person most responsible for its birth was Janet Travell, M.D. Born in New York City in 1901, Travell began practicing medicine in 1926. Her concentration was in the areas of internal medicine, cardiovascular disease, neurology, pharmacology, and musculoskeletal pain. In 1961 she was appointed physician to the president of the United States, serving both presidents John F. Kennedy and Lyndon B. Johnson. Her major interest over the last forty years was the mechanism and management of chronic pain syndromes, especially those related to myofascial trigger points.

She initially reported on the phenomenon of trigger points in 1942, determining that these points of tenderness could limit a person's range of motion and produce pain in other parts of the body. She also noted that sustained pressure applied directly to trigger points could be an efficient treatment technique. Over the next forty-seven years, Travell continued her research and mapped out the locations of common trigger points, their pain patterns, and methods of treating them.

She coauthored the textbook *Myofascial Pain and Dysfunction: The Trigger Point Manual* with David Simons, M.D. It is considered the most comprehensive work available on the subject of myofascial pain. Travell died in 1997.

In 1979 Bonnie Prudden founded the Bonnie Prudden School for Physical Fitness and Myotherapy, based on the trigger-point principles described by Travell. The school teaches the treatment of muscle pain through pressure applied to trigger points.

Theory

MTPT is a noninvasive therapeutic program for the relief and control of myofascial pain and dysfunction. The goal of treatment is the client's recovery to a normal or as near normal function as possible with either complete recovery from or significant reduction in pain. This is achieved through a systematized approach, which consists of ischemic compression (direct pressure) applied to trigger points, spray-and-stretch technique (spraying a vapocoolant along the muscle while simultaneously stretching it), passive stretch, and a specifically designed stretch and corrective exercise program. The exercise program requires the client to be very aware of his body to avoid future pain.

Factors that aggravate trigger points must be eliminated or modified to achieve lasting results. If a client is having neck and shoulder pain, and her job involves working at a computer, the therapist will make suggestions for ways of doing the activity with less stress on the muscles. Posture, sleep positions, daily activities, and nutrition may also be addressed. Success of therapy is measured by the level of pain reduction experienced by the client, as well as increased range of motion, strength, endurance, and other measures of improved function.

MTPT is part of an interdisciplinary approach to myofascial pain and dysfunction. Although myofascial trigger-point therapists are knowledgeable in the areas of myofascial pain and dysfunction, they are not diagnosticians. They must, therefore, rely on medical clearance (prescription) and support by a licensed doctor of medicine, chiropractic, or osteopathy, or a dentist before beginning a treatment plan. This protects the client from delayed diagnosis, delayed treatment, or treatment that might conflict with some other aspect of the healing process.

Practice

A session is usually an hour in length. At the initial visit a complete medical history is taken. Muscles are palpated or touched to determine the exact locations of trigger points. Range of motion, the distance the client can comfortably move a particular limb or joint, is also noted.

As patients are palpated, they are also treated. Treatment consists of the application of sustained direct pressure to the trigger point and/or the use of spray-and-stretch technique. The muscle is then passively stretched. Moist heat may be applied to further induce relaxation. The patient is given exercises, usually in the form of stretching, in order to maintain the effects of therapy and retrain the muscle to function at its normal resting length. Perpetuating factors may also be discussed at this time, such as eliminating or modifying certain activities that may aggravate the muscles, alternate sleeping positions, and correct posture. The therapist checks the patient's progress by monitoring pain levels and evaluating the range of motion periodically.

Benefits and Risks

The benefits of MTPT are as follows: the decrease or elimination of pain, increased movement and flexibility, and increased energy and activity levels. Common problems that are helped by this therapy are pain in the lower back, neck, shoulder, face, arm, hand, knee, leg, and foot; temporomandibu-

lar joint disorder; sciatica; carpal tunnel syndrome; whiplash; fibromyalgia; tennis elbow; plantar fascitis; and headaches.

People with any of the following conditions should not engage in MTPT: systemic or localized infection, acute circulatory condition, aneurysm, obstructive edema, acute healing fracture, advanced diabetes, and hypersensitivity of the skin.

—ELLIOT SHRATTER

Resources

Academy of Myofascial Trigger-Point Therapy
   Richard Finn, Director
   1312 E. Carson St.
   Pittsburgh, PA 15203
   Tel: (412) 481-2553
   Offers training in myofascial trigger-point therapy leading to national certification.

National Association of Myofascial Trigger-Point Therapists
   Web site:
   www.frontiernet/painrel/index.shtml

Further Reading

Travell, Janet, and David Simons. *Myofascial Pain and Dysfunction: The Trigger Point Manual.* Volumes I and II. New York: William & Wilkins Co., 1992.

Reflexology

Reflexology is both an ancient and modern hands-on therapeutic technique that activates and facilitates the natural healing powers of the body. This is accomplished by applying noninvasive, penetrating pressure to specific reflex points and areas on the feet, hands, and ears. In most instances this pressure work is focused on the feet because of the accessibility and larger size of the reflex points, the sensitivity of the feet, and their physical and energetic connection with the earth. Reflexology has been found to be most effective in stimulating and balancing the energy flow to specific organs, glands, and other physiological systems of the body that correspond to these reflex points, so that the body can utilize this energy to begin healing or to maintain optimal function.

History

Reflexology was practiced in many ancient cultures, including Asian, Egyptian, Greek, Japanese, and Native North American cultures. The rediscovery and promotion of this technique in the West is attributed largely to Eunice Ingham, an American masseuse, who formulated her own unique "pressure technique" for the feet after many years of working with patients who had various complaints and illnesses. She synthesized different popular theories with her own personal explorations and experiences to create what is recognized as modern reflexology.

Basic Principles

Reflexology works through the nervous system, through the circulatory system, and through correspondences of subtle energy currents. As in Fitzgerald's principles of zone therapy, the body is divided into ten vertical zones that run the entire length of the body from head to foot. The ten zones on the feet (five on each foot) contain the reflex points that are worked in a session. The theory is that the whole body is superimposed on a zone grid on the feet (also on the hands and ears). Therapeutically working a reflex point on the foot will result in the stimulation of all the body parts relating to that zone. In this way a practitioner can release blocked energy in any part of the body by applying systematic pressure to the corresponding reflex point on the feet.

Like acupuncture, reflexology is still not completely understood. The feet are extremely sensitive, with more than 7,200 nerves, and no doubt the stimulation of these nerve endings partially accounts for the beneficial results. However, there are also less easily discernible energy currents and relationships in the body that also contribute to the healing power of this technique. In addition, the skill of the practitioner, enhanced by his personal sensitivity, awareness, empathy, intention, and integrity, contributes to the effectiveness of reflexology.

Practice

How a client experiences a session depends on the style or method of reflexology being employed as well as the quality of resonance between the practitioner and client. Depending on the style of the practitioner, some clients may share thoughts and feelings—what is referred to as "verbally unwinding"—as the practitioner applies pressure to the reflex points. Others may maintain an interior focus, as in a meditative state, or may relax into a deep, restful sleep. It is important for the client to be in communication with the practitioner with regard to the degree of pressure being applied, which could be described as a "good hurt," but which still allows the client to feel relaxed. Many people express feelings and sensations of tingling, warmth, and expansiveness, as well as electrical currents, pleasant numbness in certain areas, and overall euphoria. The effects of reflexology are cumulative, producing subtle, long-term results, although dramatic and immediate results are also quite common.

Reflexology has been found to be most effective in stimulating and balancing energy flow to specific organs, glands, and other physiological systems of the body that correspond to these reflex points, so that the body can utilize this energy to begin healing or to maintain optimal function. Clients are fully clothed during sessions with only their feet exposed, and are usually most comfortable reclining on a padded bodywork table or bed. The practitioner applies pressure to the feet in a systematic fashion to induce deep relaxation (one of the hallmarks of reflexology), which facilitates the flow of energy.

Benefits and Risks

As with any type of therapeutic bodywork, personal health habits, genetic factors, emotional and mental attitudes, and amount of physical activity all play a part in one's personal health. Reflexology is not recommended for those suffering from the following conditions: hemorrhaging, intense pain of an unknown origin, any break in the skin, severe swelling characterized by red-hot pain with loss of motion, contagious or infectious disease of the foot (such as ulcerations), burns, chronic inflammation, neoplasms/tumors, varicose veins, severe sprain of the ankle or foot, severe bruises, hematomas, and in some instances, recent surgery. When the foot is too painful, the corresponding points on the hand can be worked instead.

Reflexology reduces and alleviates the debilitating effects of stress, the prime cause of many ailments. It provides a natural way of promoting balance within and between all the systems of the body by affecting all the organs, glands, and body parts. Added benefits include a deep feeling of groundedness. It also assists in detoxification by breaking up crystallized deposits of uric acid that lodge in the feet. It contributes to relief from nervous disorders, intestinal disorders, poor circulation, digestive problems, glandular disorders, headaches, fatigue, postmenstrual syndrome, back spasms, infertility disorders, sinusitis, eye problems, emotional shock and grief, and a great variety of sports injuries. In extreme chronic conditions, it is best used in conjunction with other therapies and under the supervision of a medical doctor.

—LAURA NORMAN

Resources

American Reflexology Certification Board
P.O. Box 620607
Littleton, CO 80162
Tel: (303) 933-6921
Web site: www.ns.net/quantum/arcb
Offers information regarding certification requirements and testing, and provides certification for qualified practitioners.

Laura Norman & Associates
Reflexology Center
41 Park Ave., Suite 8A
New York, NY 10016
Tel: (212) 532-4404
Offers services and certification training in reflexology.

Reflexology Association of America
4012 S. Rainbow Blvd.
Las Vegas, NV 89103-2059
Provides information about educational programs and recommends certified practitioners.

Further Reading

Grinberg, Avi. *Holistic Reflexology*. London: Thorsons Publishing, 1989.

Ingham, Eunice. *The Original Works of Eunice P. Ingham: Stories the Feet Can Tell Through Reflexology/Stories the Feet Have Told Through Reflexology*. With revisions by Dwight C. Byars. St. Petersburg, Fla.: Ingham Publishing, Inc., 1984.

Kunz, Kevin, and Barbara Kunz. *The Practitioner's Guide to Reflexology*. Englewood Cliffs, N.J.: Prentice Hall, Inc., 1985.

———. *Hand Reflexology Workbook*. Englewood Cliffs, N.J.: Prentice Hall, Inc., 1985.

Norman, Laura. *Feet First: A Guide to Foot Reflexology*. New York: Simon & Schuster, 1988.

Rolfing®

 Rolfing® is an original methodology of structural integration of the body through the use of fascial (also known as connective tissue) massage. Structural integration is a holistic approach that seeks to align a person's body in order to improve physiological and psychological functioning. It starts with the body's relationship to gravity; in fact, one of its primary objectives is to reeducate the body to move more efficiently and without tension and pain.

History

Dr. Ida P. Rolf, an American biochemist who studied the flexibility of proteins in connective tissue in the 1930s and 1940s, developed the technique of Rolfing. Rolf was a young research biochemist at the Rockefeller Institute in New York City studying connective tissue (a network of tissue beneath the skin that links other tissues and forms ligaments, tendons, and aponeuroses), particularly its plasticity, or capacity for being molded or altered. With other researchers, Rolf discovered that connective tissue is the organ of structure of the human body and that its shape, elasticity, even its length, can be altered with the application of appropriate pressure. She spent the next fifty or so years traveling widely—studying and eventually teaching a systematic way to go about organizing human structure. She called her method structural integration, and in the late 1960s it became more widely known as Rolfing.

Basic Principles

Rolfing is based on the following three ideas: First, the human body is affected by gravity, and when the body's major segments (head, shoulders, chest, pelvis, legs) are properly aligned, gravity works to lift the body rather than pull it down. Second, connective tissue, or the myofascial network of the body—a continuous bandage that forms a sheath around the whole body and all parts of the body, even individual muscle fibers—can be molded and changed. Third, the key to aligning the body in gravity is systematically releasing the connective tissue network. This will allow the muscles to return to a balanced relationship. It will also free the body of many chronic tensions and aches.

"When the body gets working appropriately," Rolf said, "the force of gravity can flow through. Rolfers make a life study of relating bodies and their fields to the earth and its gravity field, and we organize the body so that the gravity field can reinforce the body's energy field. This is our primary concept."

When a body is properly aligned, it can release the physical tensions and holding patterns resulting from years of compensation resulting in impaired balance and movement. It can also release the emotional stress that accompanies the physical symptoms.

After many years of searching, Rolf discovered that Rolfing works best in a ten-session format. The ten sessions are designed to slowly and methodically get the body—probably stuck from many years of poor compensation from accidents and injuries and from poor postural habits, along with a multitude of other possibilities—to lengthen, widen, deepen, or just let go.

Practice

The first session of Rolfing begins after a thorough interview and structural analysis, during which Polaroid pictures are usually taken. Rolfers attempt to identify the main structural issue in a person's body, or the reason a person remains stuck and unable to find the ease or support she needs.

Rolfing functions on three levels:

- Releasing the outer or superficial layer, relieving the body of accumulated stresses and strains (sessions 1–3);
- Freeing the body of its deeper core issues from which shortness, rotations, and imbalances emanate. This can be done successfully only if the way has been paved by the first level of sessions (sessions 4–7); and
- Integrating the body in gravity and assisting clients to use and enhance the changes that have occurred in Rolfing in their lives (sessions 8–10).

For example, in a person who has been slumping with the head forward for a number of years, the tissue of the upper chest has been responding by getting shorter; the muscles of the upper back (now assigned the task of holding the head on) have become more rigid. The person is unable to voluntarily get her head back over the shoulders where it belongs. The pelvis will very likely be tipped forward, unable to provide support for the shoulders and head. In turn the pelvis is probably not getting the support it needs from having the legs and feet under it. Rolfing examines the relationships among body parts—left and right, back and front, lower and upper, core and limb.

During the sessions the client either lies on a low table or, occasionally, sits or stands. Using the fingers and hands as primary tools, the Rolfer begins to release tension from the outer layers of the tissue with the application of pressure. The first session begins on the torso to release the outer wrapping (superficial fascia) and free up the breath. The work is done slowly and with the cooperation of the client, usually through specific feedback to help the Rolfer relax the fascial tissue. There is some pressure—the proper application of pressure is what makes the tissue release and change.

Although some clients find the degree of pressure painful, most clients find it acceptable, at times even pleasurable. Rolfers ask their clients to guide them and to participate in the process. At various times the client may be asked to stand and move about so that the results of the work can be felt and assessed by both the client and the Rolfer.

Sessions are cumulative and work progressively deeper into the body's structural issues. An important goal is not just to get the body to change, but to get the whole system to incorporate and use that change. Sessions generally last an hour and are usually spaced about a week apart.

Benefits and Risks

The primary objective is the release of the body's chronic and limiting holding patterns. After Rolfing sessions, people have reported freer movement and breathing, increased flexibility, release of chronic muscular tension and pain, psychological growth, and most important, continuous and progressive change.

Not everybody is an ideal candidate. Rolfing is designed to get at the underlying roots of chronic body issues or for people who want to feel and understand their bodies. In general, Rolfing deals with chronic rather than acute problems. People seeking immediate pain relief would be better served by a wide range of body therapies that would better address those issues.

—*ALLAN DAVIDSON*

Resources

The Rolf Institute
    205 Canyon Blvd.
    Boulder, CO 80302
    Tel: 1-800-530-8875 or (303) 449-5903
    Web site: www.rolfinst.com
    Founded in 1971, the institute trains Rolfers
    and Rolfing movement integration teachers,
    conducts research, and provides information
    to the public.

Further Reading

Anson, Briah. *Rolfing: Stories of Personal Empower-ment.* Kansas City, Mo.: Heartland Personal Growth Press, 1991.

Fahey, Brian. *The Power of Balance: A Rolfing View of Health.* Portland, Ore.: Metamorphous Press, 1989.

Feitus, Rosemary, ed. *Ida Rolf Talks About Rolfing and Physical Reality.* Rochester, Vt.: Healing Arts Press, 1990.

Rolf, Ida. *Rolfing: Reestablishing the Natural Align-ment.* Rochester, Vt.: Healing Arts Press, 1989.

Schultz, R. Louis, and Rosemary Feitus. *The Endless Web.* Berkeley, Calif.: North Atlantic Books, 1997.

Rosen Method

 The Rosen method is a form of therapeutic bodywork that uses gentle touch and supportive words to bring about a release of muscular and breathing constrictions, called "holdings," that limit our physical, emotional, and spiritual well-being. Developed by Marion Rosen, this method enables the mind and body to work together for optimal healing and growth, by facilitating awareness and integration of repressed emotional experiences that underlie and sustain physical holdings. The Rosen method is often used as an adjunct to psychotherapy and to physical therapy, for it is considered a preventive practice that enables people to alter their predispositions to psychological and physical illness.

History

Marion Rosen trained in Munich in the 1930s with Lucy Heyer, who had been a student of Elsa Gindler, the "grandmother" of today's breathing and relaxation techniques. She apprenticed with Heyer's group of therapists, giving breathwork instruction and massage to the psychoanalytic patients of Carl Jung. Rosen studied physical therapy further in Stockholm and at the Mayo Clinic in the United States. Since 1950 she has operated a private physical therapy practice in Oakland, California. During this time she developed the Rosen method of bodywork and the Rosen method of movement.

Over several years Rosen made two intriguing discoveries. The first was that some of her clients would improve, only to relapse, while other clients maintained their improvements. Rosen wondered: The body likes to feel well, but if the body feels better after treatments, why do the same problems recur?

Second, when she worked with some clients, they began to tell her deeply emotional things that they had never before told to anyone. Why, Rosen wondered, were they telling me these things? She observed that those clients who talked with such openness were the clients who made lasting changes. The intriguing question became, What is the link between a client's spontaneous verbalizations and his or her physical healing? Perhaps, thought Rosen, there is something behind recurring dysfunction and chronic pain that is revealing itself via these spontaneous verbalizations.

Following this line of inquiry, Rosen thus discovered a route to lasting physical improvements that involves touching the body in such a way that the mind, via memories, images, and emotions, becomes an active participant in the body's healing.

Basic Principles

Current memory research supports the theory that the sensory modalities (visual, emotional, kinesthetic, verbal, and so forth) store information in different parts of the brain, forming interactive networks throughout the brain. Rosen believes that memories can be accessed by the re-stimulation of any of these sensory areas. Rosen's touch stimulates the kinesthetic area to release memories, emotions, and associated images, also known as body-memory.

Body-memory includes emotional states because emotions are patterns of brief physiological responses whose function may be to move us to act. Every emotion has its own biological signature; for example, fear makes our sensory circuits more sensitive and activates the autonomic nervous system. Each emotional state has its own repertoire of physical reactions, thoughts, and memories.

We are mentally and physically equipped to suppress and override our emotions and their programs of action. This is called inhibition and takes place in the prefrontal cortex of the brain. The physical equivalent of this is muscular tightening. Rosen method practitioners believe that from infancy on, when events give rise to feelings that are overwhelming, threatening, or unacceptable, we inhibit them neurologically and physiologically. These responses, becoming automatic, may assume a life of their own over time. We forget, or we have never consciously known, their original purposes and meanings, yet they live on in our bodies as muscular holdings and affect our current physical and emotional well-being. We usually are not aware that we are restricting our muscles and our breath until these holdings create dysfunction and pain. When the body and the breath are chronically held, all of our emotions, whether happy or sad, are diminished, leaving us with the experience of inner deadness or emptiness.

When a Rosen method practitioner attends to these muscular holdings, she believes she is contacting the body's "barriers to self-awareness." As the practitioner's touch and verbal encouragement elicit memories from the body, information that had been unconscious moves into conscious awareness. This is of great importance, for now the traumatic memories—events, emotions—can be acknowledged and accepted.

Practitioners believe that as participants discover clues to the origin and meaning of their holdings, and as they experience their suppressed emotions, they come to a greater acceptance and appreciation of who they actually are. In finding these components of themselves that were forgotten, or never known, they gain a larger view of themselves in which living life more fully becomes possible.

Perhaps the greatest benefit of the Rosen method is its ability to bring people to the point of choosing different ways of expressing themselves and of being in the world: different ways of interacting, moving, looking, and feeling. The Rosen practitioner intends to be a midwife in the client's process of self-discovery. Rosen quotes Jesus from the Book of Thomas: "If you bring forth what is within you, what you bring forth will save you. If you do not bring forth what is in you, what you do not bring forth will destroy you."

Practice

A Rosen session lasts one hour. The participant lies on a massage table, removing as much outer clothing as he is comfortable with, always keeping on undergarments or wearing a swimsuit. Sessions are conducted with the client lying both faceup and facedown, so that the entire body can be contacted. No oils are used.

With gentle, noninvasive touch and supportive, encouraging words, the practitioner directs the client's awareness to shifts in muscle tension and breathing patterns. The Rosen touch is an open, soft, listening hand, but with the quality of curiosity. The practitioner asks through touch, "How is this person, really?" The practitioner's hands do not attempt to fix or change the client's body, for the intent is that the client experience what her body feels like, and what it is doing, in this moment. Through an open hand, the Rosen practitioner attempts to communicate acceptance, appreciation, and engagement. In this environment of safety and support, the participant's body seems to relax and open to healing itself.

The practitioner focuses on a muscular tightness until it relaxes. It is a basic premise of the Rosen method that these shifts in the quality of the breath indicate and mirror changes in the quality of the client's emotions and associated images, memories, and thoughts. The Rosen method aims to increase the client's awareness of these shifts by asking, "What just happened?" "Can you say more about that?" or by simply saying "Yes." Rosen method practitioners do not reinforce thoughts and emotions that are not echoed in the body and the breath. Marion Rosen calls this "one's body supporting the truth of one's words."

Benefits and Risks

Rosen method practitioners believe that the Rosen method's greatest contribution to health is preventive: enabling people to recognize tendencies or predispositions toward illness and then to reverse those tendencies. It can provide relief from symptoms caused by stress, injury, and fatigue. It has been shown to be an effective adjunct to psychotherapy, shortening the treatment process. People who are at appropriate stages of recovery from trauma, physical and sexual abuse, eating disorders, and addictions may benefit from adding the Rosen method to their treatment programs.

The Rosen method is not recommended for individuals suffering from severe emotional disturbance or acute physical pain.

—IVY GREEN

Resources

The Rosen Institute
    825 Bancroft Way
    Berkeley, CA 94710
    Tel: (510) 845-6606
    Web site: www.rosenmethod.org
    e-mail: info@rosenmethod.org.
    Organization that promotes the study and use of the Rosen Method.

Rosen Method Professional Association
    Tel: 1-800-893-2622
    Organization that makes worldwide referrals of Rosen Method practitioners.

Videotapes
Roziere, Gael. "Rosen Method Movement: Marion Rosen Teaches Movement." 45 minute class of Rosen Movement. Available from Gael Roziere, P.O. Box 372, Santa Cruz, CA 95061. Tel: (831) 479-8654

Further Reading

Rosen, Marion, with Sue Brenner. *The Rosen Method of Movement.* Berkeley, Calif.: North Atlantic Books, 1991.
Calvert, Robert, and Judi Calvert. "Exclusive Interview: Marion Rosen," *Massage,* Issue 32, July/August 1991.
Crawford, Bevalyn. "The Healing Touch of Rosenwork," *Yoga Journal,* March/April 1990.
Wooten, Sandra. "Rosen Method," *Massage,* Issue 44, July/August 1993.

St. John Method of Neuromuscular Therapy

 The St. John method of neuromuscular therapy combines bodywork and physical rehabilitation techniques to alleviate chronic pain related to stress or injury. Although recently developed, it rests on the assumption, formulated in a number of much earlier holistic therapies, that pain can be traced to a block or distortion in the flow of messages from the nervous system to the rest of the body's structures.

This hybrid approach to treatment distinguishes the St. John method from forerunners such as chiropractic. Through massage as well as analysis of a client's posture and gait, it seeks to free the transmission of nerve impulses and restore harmony to the entire organism.

History

Paul St. John, founder of the St. John method, began to study the phenomenon of pain in 1974 after he was involved in a devastating automobile accident. Noticing that firm pressure on his neck and shoulders brought temporary relief from the constant aches caused by his injuries, he undertook research that started with massage and led to the disciplines of chiropractic and neurology. By 1978 St. John had cured himself and put together a method of bodywork aimed specifically at the problem of persistent pain arising from trauma rather than disease. Convinced of its efficacy, he set up a clinical practice and eventually established an information and teaching center, the St. John Neuromuscular Pain Relief Institute.

Today his treatment is widely acclaimed as an important addition to the repertoire of physical and massage therapists specializing in pain management. They receive their training in a series of four seminars available only through the St. John Neuromuscular Pain Relief Institute.

Theory

While the St. John method incorporates Eastern and Scandinavian techniques of massage, its approach to the diagnosis of pain derives from the concept of homeostasis first popularized by American chiropractic teaching. Homeostasis (meaning human equilibrium) refers to the belief that the human organism functions perfectly so long as it exists in a state of ease and harmony, free from mental or physical disturbance. With this idea as its foundation, the St. John method views chronic pain as a symptom of a trauma that lingers on in the form of a block or imbalance in the organism's mechanisms of response.

Further, the St. John method posits that such old injuries are often neglected because they manifest themselves in an indirect fashion. They may appear healed yet be the cause of acute pain in another, apparently unrelated part of the body. Chronic pain is thus a systemic, not a localized, problem and cannot be understood or cured unless the totality of the organism's neuromuscular activity is examined.

Instead of X rays, the St. John method directly observes the nervous system's capacity to maintain the equilibrium of the body. These symptoms have been codified into the five so-called principles of pain: tissue with an insufficient blood supply; imbalance in the muscle and skeletal system; habitual distortion of posture and gait; "trigger points" of pain explicable only by reference to another region of the body; and "nerve compression" by soft tissue, cartilage, or bone.

By means of these five principles, the method charts chronic pain's pathway from the nervous system through the bones, muscles, and blood vessels to soft tissue and the experience of distress. Since the pain is habitual, successful treatment is believed to require bodywork that goes beyond relaxation to disruption of the unhealthy pathways and reeducation of the neuromuscular system. A type of therapeutic massage that exerts strong pressure on tissue is accordingly a standard feature of the St. John method.

Practice

Treatment is usually received from a physical or massage therapist who has completed the seminar program of the St. John Neuromuscular Pain Relief Institute. A first office visit will include a conversation about the patient's needs and a physical examination based on the five principles of pain.

The patient's posture, gait, and tone of body tissue are analyzed through visual observation. Additional information about trigger points and thickened, unhealthy areas of tissue is obtained by palpating the body. Once a diagnosis has been reached, the therapist and patient agree on a plan of treatment, which varies according to individual need but generally consists of a series of office visits for therapeutic bodywork.

The form of massage used is designed to interrupt dysfunctional responses in the neuromuscular system and stimulate healthy blood circulation. Manual pressure is exerted on selected portions of the patient's body in a rhythmic series of eight- to twelve-second applications.

Though the therapist will be sensitive to the patient's condition, the pressure is supposed to be strong enough to produce moderate discomfort. The discomfort is regarded as crucial evidence that the bodywork is affecting receptors in the nervous system and initiating the desired balancing of the body's structures.

Benefits

The St. John method has gained recognition for its success in relieving soft tissue pain without the use of drugs or costly laboratory tests. Advocates also claim that it can help rebuild injured tissue, eliminate spasms and hypercontractions, enhance the flow of blood and lymphatic fluids, restore alignment to posture, and free the individual from the aftermath of severe stress and trauma.

Resources

American Pain Association
    1615 L St., N.W., Suite 925
    Washington, DC 20036
    Tel: (202) 296-9200
    Provides information about techniques for the relief of chronic pain.

Swedish Massage

Swedish massage, also known as traditional massage, is characterized by its use of five distinct stroke techniques. Developed by Per Henrik Ling, these techniques are applied by Swedish massage therapists to improve blood flow to the heart. The combination of these strokes is believed to be extremely effective in bringing about relaxation, stress reduction, better circulation, and a general sense of well-being.

History

Swedish massage has its origins in the dedicated work of Swedish fencing master and gymnastics instructor Per Henrik Ling (1776–1839). Ling suffered from a form of rheumatism that affected his fencing arm. As a result, he began to use anatomical and physiological principles as a basis of a systematic method of massage to relieve his symptoms. His method became known as the Ling system. In 1813 the Royal Gymnastic

Central Institute of Stockholm added the Ling system of massage to its curriculum, where it became known as Swedish massage.

Basic Techniques

Five stroke techniques are used in Swedish massage: effleurage, petrissage, friction, tapotement, and vibration. As a general rule, the majority of strokes move toward the heart in order to facilitate blood flow back to the heart. For example, an effleurage stroke may begin at the foot and travel toward the pelvis.

The most often used technique is effleurage. These are long, gliding strokes that may be deep or superficial. Effleurage is used to initiate the massage in order to disperse a lubricant over the body part being massaged, to accustom the recipient to the touch of the therapist, and to allow the therapist to discover areas of spasm and tenderness. It is also used as a transitional stroke interspersed with other strokes. Deep effleurage may be used to passively stretch a muscle group.

Petrissage is a kneading stroke that gently lifts the muscle mass and rhythmically rolls, squeezes, or wrings it. This stroke has a stimulating effect on the muscles, deeper blood vessels, and lymphatics. It helps to break down adhesions in the soft tissues and relieves the muscles of metabolic wastes while increasing blood supply to the area.

Friction is most often performed in small circular motions with the tips of the fingers or the thumb. It is a deeper stroke used around the joints, bony prominences, or scar tissue. This stroke should be followed by effleurage to promote absorption of localized blockages or swelling.

Tapotement, or percussion, is the stereotyped, often misrepresented stroke commonly portrayed in motion pictures. This stroke is done with the hand rapidly alternating in hacking, clapping, or cupping movement. Tapotement has a stimulating effect on the muscles as well as on the nerves if done for brief periods, and a sedating effect on the nerves if prolonged. If, however, a stimulating effect is desired, tapotement renders a slight sense of stimulation and well-being.

Vibration is performed in a rhythmical, vibrating motion coming from the whole arm, with the elbow, wrist, and fingers kept stiff in a slightly flexed position. The pressure applied with this stroke should be very light, to impart a smoothing effect.

Practice

Swedish massage begins with the recipient lying on his back, fully draped with a sheet or towels so that only the part being massaged is exposed. A full-body massage follows a general order of right arm, left arm, right leg, left leg, chest, abdomen. The person then rolls over, and the massage continues with the back of the left leg, back of the right leg, and lastly the back. A typical massage ranges from thirty minutes to one hour depending on the person's needs.

For maximum comfort, the room should be warm but not stuffy. The person should be positioned in a comfortable, relaxed position, with the part of the body being massaged properly supported. Massage strokes should begin at a moderate intensity and increase in intensity based on the tolerance of the person being massaged. The massage should end as gently as it was begun.

Benefits and Risks

There are many beneficial effects of Swedish massage. The most discernible effect is its analgesic, soothing effect on sensory nerve endings in the skin. Depending on the type of strokes used and the length of the massage treatment, the massage may produce a sense of relaxation, stimulation, or even exhaustion on the nervous system. These effects are useful in eliminating many painful muscular, neurological, and arthritic conditions.

Swedish massage also improves circulation and increases nutrition to the joints and soft tissues while easing the demand on the heart by assisting the heart's ability to move blood through the circulatory system. Massage improves nutrition to the tissues of the body by facilitating a cellular exchange of oxygen and nutrients in the blood with carbon dioxide and cellular metabolic wastes as circulation is increased. This is essential for people who have been incapacitated by injury or disease.

It should be noted, however, that not everyone should be massaged. Massage enhances circulation; therefore any condition that can be spread via the circulatory system should not be massaged. These include cancer, acute febrile conditions, jaundice conditions, bacterial infections, pain associated with infections, and areas of acute inflammation. Massage should not be given to frac-ture sites, as it may cause a separation of bony fragments. Hemorrhages, acute phlebitis, thrombosis, and varicose veins should not be massaged due to the risk of dislodging a clot in the blood vessels. Persons with cardiovascular problems should be carefully screened and massaged only with a physician's recommendation.

Care should be taken in areas of abnormal or decreased sensation due to stroke, diabetes, or people using medications such as muscle relaxants. The person receiving the massage may have an abnormal vasomotor response to massage or may not be able to give accurate sensory feedback on the depth of the massage.

—*Janie McGee*

Further Reading

Tappan, F. M. *Healing Massage Techniques: Holistic, Classic, and Emerging Methods*. 2nd ed. Norwalk, Conn.: Appleton & Lange, 1988.

PART 8:

Acupuncture and Asian Bodywork

Acupuncture and Asian bodywork are holistic methods of healing, health maintenance, and human development based on the principles of traditional Chinese medicine (TCM). Many professionals in the field formally refer to Asian bodywork as Oriental bodywork, and in the United States the professional organization of Asian bodyworkers is the American Oriental Bodywork Therapy Association. All Asian bodywork practices are part of a larger group of methods that have come to be known collectively as *bodywork,* a general term describing a wide variety of methods that use touch to improve awareness of feelings and sensations in the body and improve physical functioning. They are also used to relieve pain and encourage relaxation. Many disciplines in this book are included in the bodywork category and can be found under Body-Oriented Psychotherapies, Massage, Movement Therapy Methods, Skeletal Manipulation Methods, Somatic Practices, and Subtle Energy Practices.

All acupuncture and Asian bodywork practices view the physical, mental, and emotional states of a person to be the result of *chi,* an invisible life energy. As water flows through canyons and riverbeds, *chi* travels through the body in channels called meridians. All the methods described in this section are based on observing and manipulating the flow of *chi* through twelve major meridians, each of which corresponds to organs and systems in the physical body.

According to TCM theory, when *chi* is flowing freely through the meridians, an individual will be healthy, well balanced, and able to adapt quickly and easily to changes in her internal and external environments. When the *chi* is blocked, it will produce uncomfortable physical and emotional conditions that will eventually produce debilitating diseases.

Manipulating *Chi*

Each of the methods included in this section employs different techniques to manipulate the flow of *chi* through the body. Acupunctur-

ACUPRESSURE

ACUPUNCTURE

JIN SHIN DO®
BODYMIND
ACUPRESSURE™

JIN SHIN JYUTSU®
PHYSIO-PHILOSOPHY

PROCESS
ACUPRESSURE

SHIATSU

TUI NA

ists insert thin, stainless-steel needles at specific points along the meridians known as acupoints. Acupressure and tui na, the ancient Chinese forms of massage, use many different techniques from gentle stroking to firm grasping and pinching of the acupoints. In shiatsu massage the practitioner uses his arms, elbows, knees, and feet to create the many different pressing, stroking, stretching, and percussive movements applied to the acupoints. Jin Shin Jyutsu®, revived in Japan in the early part of this century from ancient Chinese and Tibetan sources, is characterized by its technique of applying pressure to two points simultaneously. Contemporary methods such as Jin Shin Do® and process acupressure combine the ancient techniques with others developed by Western body-oriented psychotherapies in order to affect the flow of *chi*.

Although these methods work to alleviate physical pain, they all recognize the many different causes of illness and imbalance. Because every aspect of life, from inner emotions to external environment, is seen as interdependent with the others, an acupuncturist or Asian bodyworker may also suggest changes in diet, exercise, or lifestyle to help an individual find and maintain a harmonic relationship with the constant flux of the forces of nature.

Since TCM theory holds that no two people have exactly the same physical, mental, or emotional methods for coping with nature's flux, all changes will be recommended according to the particular needs of the individual and his symptoms and energy patterns. All methods stress the need for moderation to achieve balance and harmony with nature. Some methods of Oriental bodywork stress the importance of self-applied bodywork, as the responsibility associated with self-care is seen as a necessary part of the process of strengthening *chi*.

A Multitude of Benefits

Acupuncture and the various forms of Asian bodywork have been used by millions to heal hundreds of physical problems. They are useful for acute muscle and soft tissue problems such as sprains and strains as well as conditions resulting from overwork. These techniques have also been shown to effectively treat many chronic problems related to stress, such as headaches, insomnia, stomach disorders, asthma, and arthritis. Other complex chronic problems that combine emotional and physical attributes, such as addictions to alcohol, tobacco, and drugs, have been treated successfully with these methods. On a physical level, acupuncture and Asian bodywork aid circulation of all body fluids, removing harmful toxins from the system. By clearing blockages on the physical level, these practices tone and balance the interdependent organs and systems, opening neurochemical lines of communication in the body. But it is by clearing away blockages on the energetic level, and by treating every individual as a unique image of nature, that these methods teach awareness and respect for the inner and outer needs of each person at each stage of life, providing a means for living a long, healthy, happy, productive life.

—NANCY ALLISON, C.M.A.

Resources

American Association of Acupuncture and Oriental Medicine
    4101 Lake Boone Trail, Suite 201
    Raleigh, NC 27607
    Tel: (919) 787-5181
    Offers information about traditional Chinese medicine.

American Oriental Bodywork Therapy Association
    Glendale Executive Campus, Suite 510
    1000 White Horse Road
    Vorhees, NJ 08043
    Tel: (609) 782-1616
    Fax: (609) 782-1653
    A professional organization that has determined and enforces minimum entry-level standards (500 hours) for all types of Asian bodywork. Currently represents about 1,200 members.

Further Reading

Claire, Thomas. *Bodywork: What Type of Massage to Get—And How to Make the Most of It.* New York: William Morrow, 1995.
Knaster, Mirka. *Discovering the Body's Wisdom.* New York: Bantam Books, 1996.

Acupressure

 Acupressure is an ancient practice of applying hand and finger pressure to specific points on the body in order to control the flow of *chi*, or vital energy, which, according to traditional Chinese medical theory, courses through the body at all times. It is believed that doing this helps alleviate tension, pain, and other discomforting symptoms, and prevents harmful toxins and disease from spreading throughout the body. As a formal and defined therapeutic practice, acupressure originated in China more than 2,000 years ago. Oral tradition suggests that the practice is even older than that, up to 5,000 years old.

Acupressure is a part of traditional Chinese medicine, the system of holistic medicine that relates all of the parts of the body to one another through the flow of *chi*. Further, it relates the health of the human body to a person's genetic background and psychological conditions, and to exterior conditions of nature, such as climate and the changes of the seasons.

History

It is hard to pinpoint the exact date of acupressure's origin, since it is known to predate existing written records. The art is thought to derive from the instinctive practice of people rubbing, holding, or kneading painful places on the body for relief. Through experimentation and close observation, early healers developed an understanding of certain places on the body that could assist in the recovery from illness and promote wellness. Over many years of practice and experience, healers came to identify the points on the body, called acupoints, where stimulation produced maximum effects. Stimulation of these points cured numbness, stiffness, and chills in afflicted areas. The use of acupoints was refined and tested through study of the body, experience with patients, and contemplation over a period of at least 2,000 years. It is still practiced in Asia today.

Though traditional Chinese medicine was overshadowed somewhat during the last century by the introduction of Western medicine, it has now come back into widespread use. At present both Eastern and Western medical practices are often used together in order to provide maximum relief to patients. Since the "opening" of China in the 1960s, the principles and methods of traditional Chinese medicine are now being disseminated throughout the West in acupuncture, acupressure, and herbal medicine programs in which Westerners are able to study these ancient methods with traditional Eastern practitioners. Training for acupressure specialists begins with a basic 150-hour certification program and can range up to 850 hours for advanced training programs.

Various styles of acupressure were developed over time, although they all rely on the basic traditional model of energy flow through the meridians, acupoints, and whole person. Tui na is the Chinese massage method of using acupoints to regulate energy flow. Amma was the name used in Japan for a similar method. Shiatsu, meaning "finger pressure" in Japanese, is a vigorous form of acupressure that uses firm and rhythmic pressure on acupoints over the whole body for three to ten seconds each. Jin shin jyutsu® is the practice of holding two-point combinations at the same time until a release of energy and tension is felt. It was developed by Jiro Murai in Japan in the twentieth century and has been taught throughout the world. Contemporary American progressions from jin shin jyutsu are: Jin Shin Do®, developed by Iona Marsaa Teeguarden, which combines gentle yet deep finger pressure on acupoints with simple verbal techniques that heighten awareness of the connection between the body and the mind; and process acupressure, developed by Aminah Raheem, which combines psychological and spiritual work in consciousness with acupressure. In addition, self-acupressure techniques such as acu-yoga, developed by Michael Reed Gach in America, teach people how to find their acupoints and to release energy and relieve tension through self-massage.

Basic Principles

The Chinese holistic system is postulated on the premise that when the energy system and the internal organs of the body are functioning normally, a person will be in good health. Conversely, if either the energy or the organs are out of balance or distressed, illness will eventually occur. Therefore, the therapeutic approach is to locate any site of congestion, tension, or imbalance in either energy or organs, and then to apply the method that will release this obstruction, thereby returning the body to its own internal regulation processes and health.

The energy system of the body was mapped during ancient times. It is defined by explicit energy pathways (called meridians) that flow up and down the body from head to toe. Twelve of these pathways are linked to internal organs and are said to help regulate the health of these organs. The pathways are accessed by acupoints, or "windows," into the pathways, which can be stimulated to affect energy flow. Originally 361 acupoints were located on the surface of the body. These are still the primary acupoints today. Through the centuries more acupoints have been added to the map so that there are now some 2,000 points in the contemporary Chinese system.

Practice

In initial meetings with an acupressure therapist, open communication is established between patient and therapist. A therapist will determine a patient's total body symptoms and establish a thorough family and childhood history to uncover genetic or environmental reasons that could cause or contribute to a patient's disorder. Once the patient and therapist are satisfied that all significant issues have been discussed, the patient is encouraged to relax. Pressure is applied to the body using the hand, knuckle, finger, or a blunt-tipped instrument called a *tei shin*, which causes the body to release endorphins, an important neurochemical credited with effective pain relief. Various styles of acupressure have been developed over time, although they all rely on the use of acupoints to control energy flow through the meridians and regulate the whole person—body, mind, and spirit.

During the session, acupressure should result in lessened muscle tension, increased blood circulation, and a release of endorphins and subsequent pain relief. Toxins are also released and purged from the body. Length and frequency of the sessions are determined by the therapist and patient and depend on the severity of the problem.

Benefits and Risks

Acupressure is particularly beneficial for those who suffer with severe back pain, arthritis, nonarticular rheumatism, or chronic muscle aches. It can aid in relieving the pain of headaches. It is also credited with balancing the different systems of the body and eliminating harmful toxins. In this sense it is considered a powerful preventive tool against the onslaught of illness and disease as it purifies and strengthens the body's resistance, resulting in a healthy, vital existence.

As a caution, self-acupressure requires no special tools, but instruction is encouraged in order to effectively determine pressure points.

—*AMINAH RAHEEM, PH.D.*

Resources

Acupressure Institute
    1533 Shattuck Ave.
    Berkeley, CA 94709
    Tel: (510) 845-1059
    Offers certification programs from basic to advanced, including specialized classes and an 850-hour program.

American Oriental Bodywork Therapy Association
    Glendale Executive Campus, Suite 510
    1000 White Horse Road
    Vorhees, NJ 08043
    Tel: (609) 782-1616
    Fax: (609) 782-1653
    Web site: www.healthy.net/pan/pa/bodywork
    A professional organization that has determined and enforces minimum entry-level standards (500 hours) for all types of Oriental bodywork. Currently represents about 1,200 members.

Jin Shin Do Foundation for Bodymind Acupressure
    P.O. Box 1097
    Felton, CA 95018
    Tel: (831) 763-7702
    Fax: (831) 763-1551
    Provides information on Jin Shin Do® acupressure, including a list of registered practitioners, newsletters, books, videotapes, and training courses.

Further Reading

Academy of Traditional Chinese Medicine. *An Outline of Chinese Acupuncture.* Peking: Foreign Languages Press, 1975.

Raheem, Aminah. *Soul Return: Integrating Body, Psyche, and Spirit.* Santa Cruz, Calif.: Aslan, 1991. (Available from author at Process Acupressure Unlimited, P.O. Box 1096, Capitola, CA 95010.)

Serizawa, Katsusuke. *Tsubo: Vital Points for Oriental Therapy.* Tokyo: Japan Publications, Inc., 1976.

Steinfeld, Alan. *Careers in Alternative Medicine.* New York: Rosen Publishing, 1997.

Teeguarden, Iona Marsaa. *Acupressure Way of Health: Jin Shin Do.* Tokyo: Japan Publications, Inc., 1978.

———. *A Complete Guide to Acupressure.* Tokyo: Japan Publications, Inc., 1996.

Acupuncture

Acupuncture is one of the ancient healing practices recommended by traditional Chinese medicine to cure disease, relieve pain, and maintain health. A holistic medicine, acupuncture stresses the interconnectedness of one's body, mind, and spirit. An acupuncturist understands that physical ailments can affect one's emotional or psychological state and, equally, emotional, spiritual, or psychological difficulties can lead to disease. According to Chinese philosophy, energy—called *chi* or *qi*—circulates through all things, including our bodies. The proper flow of *chi* is essential to good health. The practice of acupuncture involves placing needles into specific points on the body to control the flow of this energy.

History

Evidence suggests that acupuncture has been practiced for more than five thousand years. It is mentioned in one of the first written records of traditional Chinese medicine practices, called the *Huang-ti Nei Ching* (*The Yellow Emperor's Classic of Internal Medicine*) This text was compiled sometime between 213 B.C.E. and 240 C.E., and is reputed to document practices used during the legendary reign of the Yellow Emperor in China (2697–2595 B.C.E.). Acupuncture started spreading throughout Asia around 1000 C.E. and reached Europe by around 1700 C.E.

Until recently in the United States, acupuncture was used mostly for anesthesia and for the treatment of alcohol, tobacco, and drug addictions. These are very limited uses that may be of help in some situations but do not embrace the underlying holistic philosophy of acupuncture. As more studies reinforce the benefits of acupuncture, its use as a method of health care and health maintenance seems to be increasing in the West.

Philosophy

Acupuncture is based on the belief that the body, mind, and spirit are fully integrated aspects of our being and cannot be separated from one another. They must be balanced in order for us to be healthy. *Chi* is the energy of our lives, what motivates us, our life essence—it affects our whole being. When the energy flows we feel generally well, and when it is impeded we feel out of balance and begin to develop the symptoms of disease. *Chi* is thought to travel in channels, called meridians, deep inside the body. Acupuncture points are the places where these meridians come close to the surface and where the *chi* can then be influenced.

Like all aspects of traditional Chinese medicine, acupuncture is firmly rooted in Chinese philosophy. The Tao, yin and yang, the five elements, and the twelve meridians provide the foundations for acupuncture's origin, development, and procedures.

Tao.
The principle of the Tao comes from the book *Tao te Ching (Book of the Way of Life)*, written by the philosopher Lao-tzu (604–531 B.C.E.). Like the Taoist principles that Lao-tzu described in this classic text, acupuncture emphasizes the importance of balance and harmony, change and growth, and ever-flowing energy of one's life.

Yin and Yang.
The terms *yin* and *yang* represent polar opposites that according to Taoism are continually merging into and creating balance with each other. Yin and yang create balance in the world and in ourselves. Yin is the cool, nighttime, reflective energy that takes things to completion; yang is the hot, daytime, active energy that puts things into motion. Yin is often considered representative of female energy and yang, male energy.

The Five Elements.
Chinese philosophy sees individuals as an integral part of nature, a microcosm reflecting the macrocosm. In nature we have elements such as fire, earth, metal, water, and wood. In acupuncture we envision these elements within us. We can feel all fired up or burned out; dry and stiff as dried wood or flexible and supple as a willow shoot; hard and cold as steel or hot and flowing as molten gold; fresh and pure as a freshwater stream or stagnant and dank like a polluted well. An acupuncturist uses these and many, many more images to conceptualize a person's state of well-being.

Meridians.
The twelve meridians, or officials, are seen as channels within our bodies that act as conduits for the *chi* to flow through, to animate and nourish us. The meridians have names akin to Western medical terms for organs but are much broader in scope. For example, the lung meridian is thought of as the receiver of *chi*. It takes energy in and lets it go. In addition to breathing, the lung meridian has the capacity for inspiration on an emotional and spiritual level. The small intestine meridian is in charge of "separation of pure from impure." On a physical level this determines which nutrients to absorb or discard. On an emotional and spiritual level it determines which aspects of ourselves we will keep and which we will let go.

Practice

Today a session with an acupuncturist is conducted in much the same way it was thousands of years ago. The acupuncturist talks to each patient individually, for hearing each person's description of the illness is particularly important. The practitioner wants to hear the patient describe the problem in her own words rather than recite a standard medical definition or diagnosis. The practitioner will want to know about the patient's background, including family history and childhood. According to traditional Chinese medicine, no two people ever have exactly the same illness, even if the Western diagnosis would be the same. A person's individuality affects how and why one becomes ill and must be taken into consideration when deciding on a treatment. Listening to the sound of the patient's voice, seeing subtle face color, palpating (touching), noticing any unusual breath or body odor, examining the tongue, and taking the pulse at the wrist are all very important methods of diagnosis and aid in formulating a treatment plan. There are several hundred acupuncture points, and the practitioner chooses which will be used in a session by using these diagnostic methods.

The goal, simply stated, is to restore the flow and balance of *chi*. The acupuncturist accomplishes this by inserting very thin, solid, sterile stainless-steel needles into acupuncture points in order to open blockages and manipulate the *chi*. Needles are placed and either taken out quickly or left to stay in for up to thirty to forty minutes, depending on what the acupuncturist wants to accomplish. On occasion the acupuncturist will warm or energize the *chi* by burning an herb called *Artemesia vulgaris* (mugwort, moxa) on the skin. This technique is called moxibustion. The practitioner may check the patient's pulse again and will decide whether or not to treat more points. An acupuncturist may also recommend herbal remedies, dietary and/or lifestyle changes, or exercises to assist in recovery.

Benefits

The World Health Organization accepts acupuncture as a treatment for more than a hundred health problems, including migraines, bronchitis, back pain, sinusitis, high blood pressure, ulcers, arthritis, premenstrual syndrome, hay fever, and the common cold. Various studies in China, Europe, and the United States have shown acupuncture to be useful in treating drug and alcohol addictions, mental disorders, depression, anxiety, insomnia, and stress.

Theories from the Western Perspective

From a Western perspective, two theories as to how acupuncture works have been put forth. One, proposed by researchers Ronald Melzack and Patrick Wall, is called the double-gate theory of pain. This theory suggests that acupuncture stimulates certain nerves that close a neurological "gate" in the spinal column, inhibiting pain fibers from ascending to higher cognitive levels. The other theory, suggested by the studies of several different researchers, suggests that acupuncture stimulates opiatelike substances called endorphins and enkephalins that account for its pain-relieving effects. These theories are enlightening but, acupuncturists contend, do not account fully for the far-reaching and long-lasting effects that acupuncture can have on a patient's body, mind, and spirit.

—DR. ROBERT J. ABRAMSON

Resources

American Association of Acupuncture and Oriental Medicine
  4101 Lake Boone Trail, Suite 201
  Raleigh, NC 27607
  Tel: (919) 787-5181

Works to improve awareness and acceptance of acupuncture as a form of complementary medicine.

National Acupuncture and Oriental Medicine Alliance
  638 Prospect Ave.
  Hartford, CT 06105-4298
  Professional organization with a membership of individual practitioners and medical colleges. The group lobbies to integrate acupuncture into American health care.

Worsley Institute of Classical Acupuncture, Inc.
  6175 N.W. 153rd St., Suite 324
  Miami Lakes, FL 33014
  Offers information, resources, and training in five-element acupuncture.

Further Reading

Mann, Felix. *Acupuncture: The Ancient Chinese Art of Healing*. Magnolia, Mass.: Peter Smith, 1990.
————. *Acupuncture: Cure of Many Diseases*. 2nd ed. Oxford, U.K.: Butterworth-Heinemann Ltd., 1992.
Melzack, Ronald. *The Puzzle of Pain*. New York: Basic Books, Inc., 1973.
Mitchell, Ellinor R. *Plain Talk About Acupuncture*. New York: Whalehall, Inc., 1987.
Worsley, J. R. *Traditional Acupuncture*, Vol. 2. Warwickshire, U.K.: College of Traditional Acupuncture, 1990.

Jin Shin Do® Bodymind Acupressure™

 Jin Shin Do® Bodymind Acupressure™ is a form of Asian bodywork developed by Iona Marsaa Teeguarden. It combines gentle yet deep finger pressure on specific points on the body (acupoints) with simple verbal techniques to release tension and heighten the connection between body and mind. Jin Shin Do is effective in helping to relieve muscular pain and stress-related problems such as headaches, backaches, anxiety, fatigue, insomnia, eye strain, menstrual and menopausal discomfort, digestive distress, joint pain, urogenital problems, sinus pain, and allergies.

History

Iona Marsaa Teeguarden was born in 1949 in Rugby, North Dakota. She studied piano performance and philosophy at the University of Michigan but was still in search of a profession when she met Mary Burmeister, who practiced Jin Shin Jyutsu®, a Japanese acupressure technique developed in the twentieth century by Jiro Murai. Teeguarden turned to Burmeister in 1971 for relief of back pain due to scoliosis. The improvement that Teeguarden experienced motivated her to study acupressure and, two years later, she began to treat clients in her home, working mainly with patients suffering from pain. She subsequently studied with Chinese, Korean, and Japanese acupuncture and acupressure specialists.

To better understand how to respond to emotions released by her patients during sessions, Teeguarden returned to school in 1979, receiving an M.A. in psychology from Antioch University in 1980 and a license to practice psychotherapy in 1982. Integrating Western and Eastern theories, she developed the emotional kaleidoscope, a detailed map of body-mind connections identifying acupoints that have an effect on specific emotions.

In 1982 Teeguarden began to develop a new teaching approach that included a color-coded system illustrating where the forty-five basic points are on the body and how to combine them in a simple way. She also established the Jin Shin Do Foundation and began offering teacher-training programs. There are now about eighty authorized Jin Shin Do teachers, and more than three hundred registered Jin Shin Do acupressurists throughout the world.

Basic Principles

In ancient times practitioners of traditional Chinese medicine mapped the energy system of the body. This system is defined by meridians, or energy pathways, that flow up and down the body from head to toe. These meridians help regulate the health of internal organs as well the physical and psychological processes that these organs control.

To develop Jin Shin Do, Teeguarden connected four main energy flows taught by Jiro Murai with the eight "strange flows," or "extraordinary meridians," of acupuncture. The strange flows are a primary self-regulating system that when functioning correctly, move energy around the body, continually adjusting and moderating the balance of the twelve organ meridians. They also store and release energy for the meridians. Teeguarden then added a Western component— Dr. Wilhelm Reich's view of the body as a series of segments that contain muscular tension related to specific emotional experiences. Reich stated that the health of human beings depends on proper flow of energy within the body. He believed that a stoppage of energy flow is unhealthy and results in both character armoring and muscular armoring.

Character armor is evident in the attitudes of people and the makeup of their personalities. For example, a common type of character armor is aloofness stemming from guilt and shame. Muscular armor is apparent in muscular tensions and contractions, which are physical barriers to the flow of energy. Both forms of armoring eventually lead to pain. Reich contended that they are unconscious techniques used by the bodymind complex to cope with early traumatic experiences and that character armoring and muscular armoring are just different aspects of the same defense.

Teeguarden related classic Chinese theories of the emotions and acupoints with Reichian theories of character and muscular armoring. She found that armoring could be released by holding "local points," or acupoints in the area of tension, with "distal points," which are far away from the area of tension but enhance the effectiveness of local-point pressure. At the same time she uses psychotherapeutic techniques, verbally encouraging the individual to remain open to emotions and thoughts that arise when muscular armor begins to dissolve.

Practice

A typical session lasts between sixty and ninety minutes, with the client clothed and lying on his back on a massage table. The practitioner evaluates the tension pattern in the body by asking questions and through pulse reading and inquiring touch, or "point palpation." After identifying main points of muscular contraction, the practitioner holds combinations of acupoints to release tensions and rebalance energy. The individual being treated will feel sensitivity at the point of pressure, but that is quickly replaced by a pleasurable feeling of tension being discharged. The general effect is a state of deep relaxation in which the individual achieves a peaceful mental state and a deeper awareness of his body. After a session, clients typically feel relaxed and rejuvenated. Over a series of sessions, armoring is progressively released in the head, neck, shoulders, arms, back, chest, diaphragm, abdomen, pelvis, and legs.

Like Reich, Teeguarden believes that when we are not allowed to express an emotion, we hold it back by tightening the muscles that would normally express it. This tension can become chronic, with the muscles involved becoming rigid and incapable of expression. Teeguarden believes that when we hold our emotions back with muscular tension, we also impede the flow of the Oriental energy pathways.

At its basic level, Jin Shin Do is a relaxation method that helps release physical and emotional tension, and so is named "The Way of the Compassionate Spirit." In the hands of a trained psychotherapist, it appears to help ease the effects of childhood abuse and other trauma trapped by the body in the form of physical tension. Treatment can have the intensity of catharsis but is generally characterized by gentleness. Jin Shin Do acupressurists avoid pressing on open sores and rashes, and pressing too hard in cases of phlebitis (inflammation of a vein), varicosities (swollen veins), broken blood vessels, or extensive bruising. Certain points are forbidden during pregnancy. Of course, clients should first consult their medical doctors, particularly in the case of chronic or acute conditions.

—*Iona Marsaa Teeguarden*

Resources

American Oriental Bodywork Therapy Association
   Glendale Executive Campus, Suite 510
   1000 White Horse Road
   Vorhees, NJ 08043
   Tel: (609) 782-1616
   Fax: (609) 782-1653
   Web site: www.healthy.net/pan/pa/bodywork
   Founded in 1984, this organization represents practitioners and teachers of all types of Oriental bodywork, including acupressure, shiatsu, and amma. The American Oriental Bodywork Therapy Association Council of Schools and Programs includes the Jin Shin Do Foundation among its members.

Jin Shin Do Foundation for Bodymind Acupressure
   P.O. Box 1097
   Felton, CA 95018
   Tel: (831) 763-7702
   Fax: (831) 763-1551
   Founded in 1982, the Jin Shin Do Foundation is a network of Jin Shin Do teachers and acupressurists throughout the United States,
Canada, Europe, and elsewhere. Write for a free newsletter, which includes a list of books, charts, and audio- and videotapes available as well as a description of the Jin Shin Do training program. An international directory is also available.

Further Reading

Teeguarden, Iona Marsaa. *The Acupressure Way of Health: Jin Shin Do.* New York: Japan Publications, Inc., 1978.
———. *Color-Coded Strange Flows Chart.* Watsonville, Calif.: Jin Shin Do Foundation, 1981.
———. *A Complete Guide to Acupressure.* New York: Japan Publications, Inc., 1996.
———. *Fundamentals of Self-Acupressure.* Watsonville, Calif.: Jin Shin Do Foundation, 1989.
———. *The Joy of Feeling: Bodymind Acupressure.* New York: Japan Publications, Inc., 1987.

*Jin Shin Jyutsu®
Physio-Philosophy*

 Jin Shin Jyutsu® Physio-Philosophy is an ancient art that uses the hands on specific areas of the body to harmonize the flow of life-giving energy throughout the body. Jin Shin Jyutsu provides an excellent opportunity to restore and maintain physical, mental, emotional, and spiritual well-being. It can be utilized either as a self-help tool or received from a practitioner.

History

According to records in the Imperial Archives of Japan, the principles of Jin Shin Jyutsu date back to ancient times. This understanding was passed down in the oral tradition from generation to generation until many of the principles became distorted and the art was nearly lost.

Near the turn of the twentieth century, Jiro Murai, the second son born into a family of medical professionals, rediscovered this art. Faced with a life-threatening illness considered terminal by traditional medicine, Murai turned to the wisdom of the great sages for his salvation. He healed himself through the application of hand mudras and through breathing exercises. Murai vowed to dedicate his life to the study and development of the art he eventually named Jin Shin Jyutsu, which translates as "the art of the Creator through man of compassion and knowing."

In the late 1940s Jiro met Mary Burmeister, an American-born Japanese working in the U.S. diplomatic corps. Murai asked if Burmeister would like to bring a gift from Japan back to America. Without knowing what he was referring to, she accepted his offer and became his first student. Burmeister studied with him for the next six years, then corresponded with him after she returned to the United States for another six years until Murai's death.

Burmeister spent the next several years deepening her understanding of the art of Jin Shin Jyutsu. In the early 1960s she was approached by the doctor of a neighbor she had been helping. Having noted positive change in the neighbor, this doctor wanted to learn more about what had helped so much and became Burmeister's first student. She continued to teach until 1990, sharing her awareness and understanding of this profound art with thousands of students across the United States and western Europe. Burmeister has since selected eight instructors whom she has certified to continue her teachings and those of Jiro Murai.

Basic Principles

Jin Shin Jyutsu employs twenty-six safety-energy locks throughout the body. These are found along the various pathways through which the universal energy travels. This energy flow creates and supports life and all the functions of the body. For many reasons—hereditary, character, stress, accidents, tension of daily lifestyle, and so forth—these pathways may become blocked, causing symptoms and illnesses. By placing the hands (jumper cables) on these safety-energy locks in specific sequences (flows), practitioners can unlock these areas to restore harmony, balance, and the proper functioning of the body. Many different sequences can be used, and these are determined by listening to the pulse and reading the conformation of the body.

To apply Jin Shin Jyutsu, the hands are placed on a clothed body. There is no massage or manipulation. Practitioners wait to feel the rhythmic pulsation in the safety-energy lock to know that area is in harmony with the universal energy. Then they move on to the next area of the sequence. Upon completion of this sequence, they will have become aware of the harmony restored to this particular flow of energy. Symptoms will disappear over time or, in some cases, immediately.

These sequences can be applied by a practitioner to another person, or by an individual utilizing them for self-help. This self-help is an important aspect of Jin Shin Jyutsu, as self-awareness, or "now know myself," helps us to maintain balance and harmony, or to simply feel relaxed and peaceful. In order to find the proper techniques and sequences for self-help, people can consult their practitioner or self-help books.

Jin Shin Jyutsu is not merely a technique but also an art. A technique is a mechanical application, whereas an art is a skillful creation. This art is supported strongly by its underlying philosophy, which emphasizes an awareness of ourselves and our connection to the universal energy. By maintaining this, we remain in harmony—happy and healthy. When we forget the philosophy, we can utilize our "jumper cables" to recharge our batteries and restore the proper functioning of our bodies. As Mary Burmeister has said, "Philosophy is the richness of Jin Shin Jyutsu, and the technique is for when we don't live the philosophy. It's a tool to get us out of trouble."

Practice

A Jin Shin Jyutsu session lasts about an hour. The recipient lies faceup on a table or any available comfortable surface. The practitioner will "listen" to the pulse not for diagnosis, but to determine which energy function flows might be utilized to bring the body to its natural state of harmony. At this point the practitioner uses the hands in specific sequences to restore energy flow. By the end of the session, the pulse should be even and balanced.

The practitioner often provides the client with information during or after the session. The actual experience and results may vary from person to person. The recipient may feel a sense of relaxation and deeper breathing as the energy flow is restored. The immediate effects of the session will continue for eight hours as the circulation pattern is completed.

—IAN KRAUT

Resource

Jin Shin Jyutsu®, Inc.
    8719 E. San Alberto
    Scottsdale, AZ 85257
    Tel: (602) 998-9331
    Fax: (602) 998-9335
    Web site: www.inficad.com/*.010jsjinc
    Offers information on seminars, books and materials, and practitioner referrals.

Further Reading

Burmeister, Alice. *The Touch of Healing: Energizing Body, Mind, and Spirit with the Art of Jin Shin Jyutsu.* New York: Bantam Books, 1997.

For those interested in studying Jin Shin Jyutsu, the basic five-day course is offered in the United States, Canada, Brazil, and Europe. The number of locations expands each year as interest grows. At this point only eight instructors are authorized by Jin Shin Jyutsu®, Inc., the sole organization offering instruction in this discipline. The class includes lecture, material, and hands-on experience. Instruction is broken down into two parts. Part 1 lasts for three days and covers the safety-energy locks. Over the remaining two days, Part 2 covers the seventeen "individualized" body function energy flows. Anyone is welcome to attend; there are no prerequisites.

Process Acupressure

Process acupressure (PA) was developed as a single modality for addressing and supporting all parts of an individual. According to PA, touch is able to release tension stored in a person's body, allowing her to develop more balance, strength, and clarity to understand and handle problems better. As in traditional acupressure, gentle pressure is applied to the body to strengthen, release, and balance the body's energy systems. PA also is concerned with revealing a person's soul, or inner wisdom. This deep inner knowing is accessed as a guiding influence over one's healing and development.

History

PA grew out of Dr. Aminah Raheem's search for ways to support a person's wellness and growth in body, mind, emotions, and soul simultaneously. In PA, she combined traditional acupressure methods with the unique touch of Zero Balancing®. It also uses skills developed from transpersonal psychology, which includes Carl Jung's analytical psychology, Roberto Assagioli's psychosynthesis, and Arnold Mindell's process-oriented psychotherapy. It took six years for Raheem to test and develop her theoretical framework into a hands-on application. PA premiered in Zurich, Switzerland, in 1986. Since then it has been continuously taught there and in the United States and England to bodyworkers, psychologists, and laypersons.

Basic Principles

According to PA, energy offers the most natural access to the whole person because it integrates the body, mind, emotions, and soul. Two energy systems—meridians and chakras—are referenced. While the meridians comprise the network of energy pathways used in Chinese acupuncture, chakras are an ancient Hindu system of energy vortices along the central midline of the body. Both of these systems are directly connected and intermingled, with the meridians feeding energy into and out of the chakras.

By allowing personal history to surface from the body during bodywork, PA is able to process directly the most relevant psychological material for the person's growth at the time. If memories or traumas from the past arise during the bodywork, the practitioner knows how to help a person bring feelings and images to consciousness, allowing him to reach a resolution. If feelings, images, or issues come to mind during the bodywork, they can be explored for the client's health and well-being.

Practice

Typically a PA session takes from one to one and one-half hours. The client lies on a massage table, fully clothed, and relaxes deeply while the practitioner applies custom-designed acupressure techniques. Physical, psychological, or spiritual issues are addressed in a team approach by both practitioner and client. In some cases a problem is clarified and resolved in one session. More commonly, several sessions are required to resolve a condition and prevent recurrence.

PA has been used to address a variety of physical symptoms, including back problems, headaches, respiratory, digestive, and systemic problems as well as colds, flu, allergies, and healing from injuries. Advocates also recommend PA to help relieve stress-related conditions, including post-traumatic stress. PA is promoted as a method of furthering and empowering development in the healthy person who wishes to grow toward his full potential.

PA should not be used to treat severe medical problems and does not supplant medical care. It should not be used for psychotics or people during severe psychotic episodes because it uncovers and releases unconscious material that may be overwhelming for a person in a weakened ego state.

—*Aminah Raheem*

Resources

Process Acupressure Unlimited
P.O. Box 1096
Capitola, CA 95010
Certifies health care professionals as PA practitioners after progressive levels of training, supervised experience, and examination. PA does not give licensure. Therefore, practitioners must be licensed in a professional health care modality, such as massage, medicine, or osteopathy; or in a psychological field, such as marriage and family counseling, psychology, or psychiatry, before they can be certified in PA.

Further Reading

Raheem, Aminah. *Process Acupressure I.* Palm Beach Gardens, Fla.: The Upledger Institute, Inc., 1994.

———. *Process Acupressure II: Releases for the Whole Being.* Palm Beach Gardens, Fla.: The Upledger Institute, Inc., 1994.

———. *Process Acupressure III: The Hologram.* Aptos, Calif.: Process Acupressure Association, 1996.

———. *Soul Return: Integrating Body, Psyche, and Spirit.* Santa Rosa, Calif.: Aslan Publishing, 1991.

Shiatsu

 Shiatsu is a method of Japanese bodywork derived from ancient healing practices. Practitioners apply pressure using the fingers, palms, elbows, forearms, knees, and even feet, to pressure points (called *tsubos* in Japanese) along a receiver's body. This practice encourages the proper flow of *qi*, or life energy, which, according to traditional Chinese medicine, is necessary for the optimum health of body and mind. Primarily, shiatsu is recommended as a preventive technique, that is, to be practiced even when one is healthy in order to maintain good health. It is also practiced for the relief of pain, to improve mental functioning, and to relieve a variety of ailments, including chronic stress, digestive problems, and lower back pain.

History

The use of bodywork and massage for curing disease and improving health has ancient origins in China. Massage is one of the treatment principles of traditional Chinese medicine, the basic tenets of which are thought to date back to the legendary reign of the Yellow Emperor in China from 2697 to 2595 B.C.E. Although the principles of traditional Chinese medicine were not recorded until sometime between 213 B.C.E. and 240 C.E., people believe that the practices had been passed from generation to generation for thousands of years before that.

The various practices of traditional Chinese medicine spread throughout Asia, making their way to Japan in about 500 to 600 C.E. In Japan massage became known as amma, which literally means "rubdown." By the early 1900s amma was still being practiced in Japan but had earned a reputation as folk medicine and became associated more with pleasure, relaxation, and sensuality than with medicine. As a result, some practitioners who wanted to continue practicing therapeutic massage began calling their practice shiatsu. These practitioners worked to raise public awareness of the healing aspects of massage. Today shiatsu is one of the most popular forms of massage in Japan.

Basic Principles

Shiatsu is a holistic form of bodywork in which the body and mind are viewed as connected to each other, as well as to the external environment. Practitioners believe that a vital life energy, called *qi*, surrounds and interpenetrates the physical body. *Qi* flows through the body through invisible channels called meridians. Practitioners of shiatsu are trained to manipulate pressure points that lie along these channels of energy in order to balance a receiver's energy. According to the traditional Asian worldview, illness or disease (including emotional and psychological problems) is the result of an imbalance in the flow of *qi*. By balancing and fortifying vital life energy, the shiatsu therapist can help a client maintain and improve her health. Shiatsu is thought to help prevent the onset of illness. If illness or disease has already set in, shiatsu is used to encourage the body's healing process.

Shiatsu therapy is widely available. Anyone interested in experiencing this rejuvenating form of treatment should have no trouble finding an experienced practitioner. Many spas, health clubs, and resorts offer shiatsu as one of their treatments. As the training of practitioners can vary widely, you should check the educational background and experience of any practitioner you are considering visiting.

Practice

Shiatsu emphasizes the physical manipulation of the body. It aims to work with both the physical body and the energy that surrounds and interpenetrates it. As the number of practitioners grows, the variety of styles of shiatsu also grows. A shiatsu session may be a vigorous massage or it may employ only gentle touch, depending on the practitioner. Some people find the more vigorous method painful. One should seek a shiatsu therapist that best meets his own personal needs. Increasingly, Western shiatsu practice is gentle and less invasive than the traditional Japanese approach. The most well known and representative form of this style of shiatsu is Ohashiatsu®. Ohashiatsu was developed by Wataru Ohashi, who probably did more than any other person to introduce and popularize shiatsu in the West. Ohashi's style of shiatsu is taught and practiced at the Ohashi Institute.

Traditionally, the recipient dresses in loose, comfortable clothing and lies on a comfortable futon—a kind of Japanese mattress—or cushioned space on the floor. The practitioner kneels and crawls around the person she is massaging. Because there are different approaches to shiatsu, however, some practitioners have receivers disrobe to their level of comfort and lie on a padded massage table rather than on the floor. A typical shiatsu session lasts from half an hour to

an hour and a half. Pressure can be light or deep depending on the style practiced and what is best for the recipient.

Practitioners may also gently stretch the client's body. They may also act as a kind of coach or teacher in order to help the client achieve better energy balance. A shiatsu therapist might recommend a more nutritious diet, getting additional exercise, or other helpful suggestions regarding lifestyle.

Benefits and Risks

People who receive shiatsu often say they feel both energized and relaxed at the same time. They may also feel calm and peaceful, and lighter in spirit, and physical aches and pains may diminish. Shiatsu is considered by many to be a wonderful healing practice for individuals seeking physical relief of muscle aches and soft tissue pains. It is also useful for exploring the energetic aspects of bodywork.

Shiatsu can be an important part of an ongoing health maintenance program. By taking time to be more aware of our bodies, we may be able to spot physical and emotional problems before they have a chance to make us sick. In addition to helping relieve aches and pains, shiatsu can fortify the functioning of the immune system, which protects us from illness; stimulate circulation, which is vital to life; provide massage to the internal organs; and encourage proper functioning of the nervous and endocrine systems. Those who receive shiatsu often report relief from a variety of complaints, including low back pain, sinus problems, constipation, and premenstrual syndrome.

The therapy can be used by nearly anyone. However, there are some instances in which it should be avoided, or caution should be exercised in its use. You should not receive shiatsu if you have cancer. It should also be avoided if you suffer from brittle bones or are on cortisone treatment, which weakens the bones. Shiatsu should not be practiced under the influence of alcohol or by anyone with a fever or contagious disease. If you have high blood pressure, you should not receive shiatsu to the abdomen; pregnant women should consult with their doctors before treatment.

—THOMAS CLAIRE

Resources

American Oriental Bodywork Therapy Association
> Glendale Executive Campus, Suite 510
> 1000 White Horse Road
> Vorhees, NJ 08043
> Tel: (609) 782-1616
> Fax: (609) 782-1653
> Web site: www.healthy.net/pan/pa/bodywork
> The AOBTA is a professional organization that represents practitioners of a number of different styles of Asian bodywork, including shiatsu.

The Ohashi Institute
> P.O. Box 505
> Wallace Road
> Kinderhook, NY 12106
> Tel: 1-800-810-4190
> Fax: (518) 758-6809
> The Ohashi Institute has twelve locations in the United States and Europe. It is the leading worldwide educational institute devoted to the teaching and practice of shiatsu, and serves as a bridge between Western and Eastern healing arts.

Further Reading

Bienfield, Harriet, and Efrem Korngold. *Between Heaven and Earth: A Guide to Chinese Medicine.* New York: Ballantine Books, 1991.

Claire, Thomas. *Bodywork: What Type of Massage to Get—and How to Make the Most of It.* New York: William Morrow, 1995.

Connelly, Dianne M. *Traditional Acupuncture: The Law of the Five Elements.* Columbia, Md.: The Centre for Traditional Acupuncture, 1989.

Haas, Elson M. *Staying Healthy with the Seasons.* Berkeley, Calif.: Celestial Arts, 1981.

Ohashi, Wataru. *Do-It-Yourself Shiatsu: How to Perform the Ancient Japanese Art of "Acupuncture Without Needles."* New York: E. P. Dutton, 1976.

Ohashi, Wataru, with Tom Monte. *Reading the Body: Ohashi's Book of Oriental Diagnosis.* New York: Arkana, 1991.

Tui Na

 Tui na is an ancient form of massage used to maintain and improve health, cure disease, and relieve pain. It is one of several methods recommended by traditional Chinese medicine. The philosophy of traditional Chinese medicine and the methods that it recommends are holistic in nature, viewing the health of an individual as affected by three equally important and interconnected aspects of our being: body, mind, and spirit. Practitioners of tui na manipulate the physical body by pushing, pulling, pinching, and tapping on it. The goal is to affect the flow and balance of the vital energy called *qi*, which, according to Chinese philosophy, flows through our bodies and affects the health of mind, body, and spirit.

History

Chinese massage can be traced as far back as 4,000 years. Archaeologists have discovered an early form of Chinese writing dating to this time that looks more like pictograms than the sophisticated characters used today. In this early form of writing they have found what they believe are mentions of massage. Some experts have concluded that massage had developed to such an extent that it was used and discussed at the court of the emperor, where all writing took place.

Massage is also mentioned in the oldest existing medical text, *Huang-ti Nei Ching*

(*The Yellow Emperor's Classic of Internal Medicine*). This text was compiled during the Han dynasty in China, which spanned 206 B.C.E. to 240 C.E. Some experts believe that the *Huang-ti Nei Ching* documents practices that had been handed down verbally for thousands of years, from the time of the legendary reign of the Yellow Emperor in China (2697–2595 B.C.E.), suggesting that medical massage may be up to 5,000 years old.

Massage evolved to such a point that in the fifth century C.E., a doctoral degree was created for it at the Imperial College of Medicine in Xian, the ancient capital of the Tang dynasty. Originally called *moshou*, which means "hand rubbing," massage later became known as *anmo*, which means "press and rub." By the Ming dynasty (1368–1644) the name *tui na*, meaning "push and grasp," was used.

During the Republican period (1911–1949) in China, all forms of traditional medicine were overshadowed by Western allopathic medicine. Traditional medical practices gained a reputation as folk medicine, and more and more young people began to study and practice Western medicine. With the establishment of the People's Republic in 1949, the government made an effort to gather and systematize traditional medical practices under the heading Traditional Chinese Medicine and to integrate Chinese and Western healing methods. Today in China, clinics are available for both styles of healing, and patients can choose where they want to go. In addition, many hospitals use a combination of Western allopathic and traditional practices to create the most effective treatment.

Basic Principles

All of the treatment methods of traditional Chinese medicine, including tui na, take a holistic view of humans as composed of inseparable components of body, mind, and spirit. The principles of traditional Chinese medicine are influenced by the naturalist school of Taoism, which emphasizes a lifestyle based on moderation and harmony with natural cycles. According to Taoism, the highest ideals of human attainment—wisdom, serenity, and compassion—come with age. This medical system seeks to maintain health and vitality into old age, with a strong focus on preventing disease.

According to traditional Chinese medical theory, a major component of life is called *qi*, a vital life energy that is in constant motion through channels in our bodies. If *qi* is deficient, excessive, or stagnant, we feel disease, which can eventually lead to disease. Tui na uses a variety of hand techniques—massaging the body, applying pressure to specific points that affect the *qi*, and holding the body in certain poses. These techniques act on the *qi* to move and invigorate it and restore balance in the individual's whole self.

Practice

In a typical session, a practitioner will use traditional Chinese medicine's five methods of evaluation—looking, listening, smelling, asking, and touching—to gather information about the patient. Practitioners believe that interior disharmonies can appear in the exterior of the self and that exterior stresses can affect the interior of the self. Since each aspect of life and behavior reflects the other, all are important to the therapist, including specific complaints, pain, movement patterns, sleep and dietary patterns, and lifestyle. The massage therapist will weave all the data together to see the entire tapestry of the patient's energetic landscape to determine how the *qi* is flowing, where it may be blocked or stagnant, and how this is affecting the individual as a whole.

After the assessment, the therapist will choose specific points, pathways, and hand techniques to create a massage specifically helpful for that patient on that day. Hand techniques can vary from gentle stroking to firm grasping and pinching with innumerable combinations and possibilities. The session can last for thirty to sixty minutes. The therapist's intention is to see some immediate change and lay the groundwork for long-term progress.

Benefits and Risks

In China tui na is used as a health maintenance program to treat chronic stress-related problems such as headaches, insomnia, and stomach disorders; illnesses such as asthma and arthritis; and injuries such as sprains. Patients often feel an increase in energy, relief from pain, diminished fevers, improvements in digestion and sleep, and a regulation of the processes of the internal organs. Tui na is not recommended for fractures, in the case of infections, or when there are open wounds or lesions on the body.

Tui na is a quickly growing therapy in the United States, with licensed practitioners available throughout the country. Because tui na is considered a complementary therapy to Western scientific medicine, each state regulates it differently. Always check to see if your practitioner is state licensed and/or nationally certified. This will ensure that he is adequately trained and familiar with pathologies and conditions that make this treatment inadvisable.

—GINA MARTIN

Resources

The American Oriental Bodywork Therapy Association
   Glendale Executive Campus, Suite 510
   1000 White Horse Road
   Vorhees, NJ 08043
   Tel: (609) 782-1616
   Fax: (609) 782-1653
   Web site: www.healthy.net/pan/pa/
   bodywork

Physicians in traditional Chinese medicine have always been required to demonstrate a mastery of bodywork to increase their digital sensitivity for competent palpatory and assessment skills. Today in China, massage is a doctoral study that takes five to six years to complete.

A national organization of bodyworkers in eleven different styles. Certifies practitioners, teachers, and schools throughout the United States. The organization enforces minimum entry-level standards (500 hours) for all types of Oriental bodyworkers. Currently represents about 1,200 members.

Swedish Institute of Massage Therapy and Allied Health Sciences
   226 W. 26th St.
   New York, NY 10010
   Tel: (212) 924-5900
   Master Jeffrey Yuen and licensed massage therapists Reggie Crosan, Alix Kasat, Paula Chin, Tom Banaciak, and Gina Martin offer classes and sessions.

Further Reading

Chengnan, S., ed. *Chinese Bodywork: A Complete Manual of Chinese Therapeutic Massage*. Berkeley, Calif.: Pacific View Press, 1990.

Eisenberg, D., and T. L. Wright. *Encounters with Qi: Exploring Chinese Medicine*. Rev. ed. New York: W. W. Norton, 1995.

PART 9:

Movement Therapy Methods

Movement therapy methods are disciplines that seek to relieve pain, improve physical performance, and increase the potential for emotional and creative expression by developing awareness of body movement and repatterning it. These methods are part of a larger group of methods that have come to be known collectively as *bodywork*, a general term describing a wide variety of methods that use touch and movement to improve awareness of feelings and sensations in the body and improve physical functioning. Bodywork methods are also used to relieve pain and encourage relaxation.

Many disciplines in this book are included in the bodywork category (see under: Acupuncture and Asian Bodywork, Body-Oriented Psychotherapies, Massage, Skeletal Manipulation Methods, Somatic Practices, and Subtle Energy Practices). Movement therapy methods are distinguished from other bodywork methods by their use of the process of movement itself as their primary diagnostic and therapeutic tool. These disciplines share certain common origins. All were developed in the West in the twentieth century. Many of the originators of these disciplines were driven by the urgent need to solve their own physical health problems. In doing so they each recognized a lack of mental awareness of body movement patterns as a root cause of their symptoms. Eventually each found a way to teach his or her unique path of discovery to others.

Pioneers in Movement Therapy

No single figure can be credited with the start of the field of movement therapy. Like the invention of the television, movement therapy is an idea that was developed simultaneously by several people working separately in different parts of the world. At the turn of the century F. M. Alexander (1869–1955), an Australian actor, while searching for a cure for his own recurring loss of voice, developed a

ALEXANDER
TECHNIQUE

ASTON-
PATTERNING®

BARTENIEFF
FUNDAMENTALS℠

BODY-MIND
CENTERING®

FELDENKRAIS
METHOD®

HANNA SOMATIC
EDUCATION®

HELLERWORK

IDEOKINESIS

KINETIC AWARENESS

MEIR SCHNEIDER
SELF-HEALING
METHOD

SENSORY
AWARENESS

SOMA
NEUROMUSCULAR
INTEGRATION

SOMATO
RESPIRATORY
INTEGRATION

TRAGER
PSYCHOPHYSICAL
INTEGRATION

method for freeing the body of excess tension and changing inefficient movement patterns. He named his method the Alexander technique.

Working several continents away, a young German woman, Elsa Gindler (1885–1961), developed her method of "restorative observation" as a cure for her own life-threatening bout with tuberculosis. Later, while working as a young movement educator, Gindler met the musician and teacher Heinrich Jacoby (1889–1964), who was exploring teaching methods that addressed the effects of mental attitudes on performance. They combined their ideas and methods to create sensory awareness, a practice designed to "free people from conditioned habits, fears, and tensions."

At about the same time that Gindler was curing herself of tuberculosis, an American teenager, Mable Elsworth Todd (n.d.–1956), was teaching herself to walk and move after a severe back injury. The methods she discovered became the basis of her private dance education practice, and eventually the method known as ideokinesis.

A second wave of movement therapy methods occurred in the 1940s and 1950s. At this time performing artists such as Irmgard Bartenieff (1900–1981) were exploring the ways in which body and mind interact in the process of movement. But people from other fields, such as Milton Trager, an athlete, and Moshe Feldenkrais, a physicist and engineer, also turned their attention to the connection between movement and health. While some of these pioneers continued to be driven by self-healing needs, others were responding to mass healing crises, such as the polio epidemic of the 1940s. This helped take movement therapy beyond the performing arts and directly into the world of health care.

In the 1960s and 1970s a third wave of movement therapy methods was developed by performing artists, engineers, philosophers, healers, and people from the established medical profession. Most of these explorers were students of second-wave founders, and the new disciplines they created were firmly rooted in the principles and theories of their teachers. Many individuals developing new methods were deeply influenced by Dr. Ida Rolf, making use of Rolf's method of physically manipulating the tissue covering the muscles (see the entry on Rolfing for more information on this discipline). Joseph Heller, founder of Hellerwork, and Drs. Bill and Ellen Williams, founders of soma neuromuscular integration, combined Rolf's methods with movement exercises and psychological processing techniques to bring greater levels of body-mind integration to the process of healing and maintaining health through movement.

In the late 1990s many of the organizations that support the teaching and professional activities of the various methods described in this section banded together under the umbrella of the International Somatic Movement and Education Therapy Association (ISMETA). ISMETA aims to increase public awareness of the value of movement therapy in health and education and to ensure quality among movement therapists. Recently ISMETA petitioned and won the right from the U.S. government to include the title Registered Movement Therapist® among the official U.S. Department of Labor occupational titles. This step integrates movement therapy methods further into the mainstream of American health care practices.

The Unifying Principles of Movement Therapy

Movement therapists stress the fact that the living body is in constant motion. From the subtle expanding and contracting motions of breathing to the more obvious exertion of muscles during strenuous activity, efficient movement is believed to be crucial for human health. Since movement therapists view the human being as an integrated combination of physical, mental, and emotional aspects, all body movement is seen as related to the emotional life of the mover.

Inefficient and painful movement patterns are seen as creative coping mechanisms that our bodies and minds develop to deal with traumatic experiences or chronically stressful physical or emotional situations. Learning to move painlessly or more freely and expressively is often an "unlearning" process by which our individual, intuitive coping strategies can be relinquished in favor of patterns that work more harmoniously with natural forces such as gravity and with the physical realities of our bodies.

The first step in this educational process is to become aware of habitual movement patterns that are restrictive and counterproductive. Some of these may be very deep and subtle, such as holding our breath when we want to exert our strength. Since oxygen is essential to the functioning of our muscles, holding our breath will only frustrate our efforts. Most methods use some form of touch to help develop awareness of counterproductive patterns. Many employ forms of manipulation that have grown out of specific bodywork, or massage practices.

The second step is described by ISMETA as "gaining increased awareness and control over basic psychophysiological processes which can begin to correct restrictive habit patterns and can lead toward optimal body-mind performance." For instance, as you continue to explore your ability to exert force in a powerful tennis serve, you may become aware of a buried psychological reason that causes you to hold your breath and prevents you from releasing all your power into the serve.

While all the methods described in this section support the belief that human beings have all the internal self-healing mechanisms they need to develop the increased awareness of the second stage of the movement therapy education process, different methods approach this stage of movement education in different ways. Some, like sensory awareness, hold that solely developing consciousness of your physical sensations without taking any subsequent action will stimulate the self-correcting mechanisms. Most methods, however, teach that conscious control over movement patterns is necessary to achieve a complete change and healing. In most methods it is believed that this conscious control will eventually function on an unconscious level. This occurs through a repatterning of the messages your brain sends to your muscles via your nervous system.

The third step in the movement therapy model is to be able to express these new movement patterns in all your daily activities. To help you do this, movement therapists might recommend certain exercises to practice at home, and might help you find visual images that will enable you to perform particular movements more efficiently. Therapists might help you evaluate lifestyle practices, such as the kind of shoes you wear or the arrangement of your study area, which could also be negatively affecting your performance.

Finally, it is the goal of all movement therapists to help you learn to be self-reliant so that you can continue developing without their help. Mastering the three levels of learning can help you develop new physical and mental awareness, along with newly ingrained neuromuscular reflex patterns that allow you greater freedom, ease, and pleasure living in your moving body.

—*NANCY ALLISON, CMA*

Resources

International Somatic Movement and Education Therapy Association (ISMETA)
    148 W. 23rd St., No. 1H
    New York, NY 10011
    Tel: (212) 229-7666

The Somatics Society
    1516 Grant Ave., Suite 212
    Novato, CA 94945
    Tel: (415) 892-0617
    Fax: (415) 892-4388
    Organization offering seminars and information for all movement therapy educators. Publishes the biannual magazine-journal *Somatics*.

Further Reading

Claire, Thomas. *Bodywork: What Type of Massage to Get—And How to Make the Most of It.* New York: William Morrow, 1995.
Knaster, Mirka. *Discovering the Body's Wisdom.* New York: Bantam Books, 1996.

Alexander Technique

The Alexander technique is a method used to help people illuminate their unconscious patterns of body tension and correct habits that cause physical and emotional problems. It allows a person to pattern his body's movement, inhibiting habits that cause tension or pain and replacing them with those that help the body to function more efficiently. Teachers of the Alexander technique believe that greater control over the body can be gained once these habitual movements are brought to consciousness. An individual may then apply new and healthier ways of using his body to improve the performance of activities in his life. For almost a century this technique has been used to help people find relief from many chronic painful conditions and to help performing artists and athletes expand their potential.

History

Development of the Alexander technique is credited to Frederick Matthias Alexander (1869–1955), an Australian actor who experienced a recurring loss of his voice. Through ten years of self-observation and experimentation with the aid of a three-way mirror, he observed that the manner in which he was breathing and holding his head was the source of his difficulties. He was able to correct his voice problems by altering his posture, muscular reaction patterns, and behavior. In addition, he observed that these changes improved his physical health, emotional outlook, and balance. Pursuing his findings further, Alexander began to study the way the body functioned during various activities, looking for signs of misalignment or misuse of his own muscular-skeletal system. He discerned that mental and physical habits, acquired early in life, often control one's everyday movements. Over time Alexander developed a technique for breaking inefficient and counterproductive habits and replacing them with conscious, constructive control. Throughout the rest of his life, Alexander taught his technique in England. Today there are more than 3,000 certified Alexander teachers worldwide, teaching privately or in schools, institutions, and corporations.

Theory

Alexander believed that the alignment of the head, neck, and spine was the most important relationship within the body, affecting the functioning of the entire body and mind. He called the relationship between head and neck the "primary control" and found it to be the integrating force for all movement. Alexander believed that from an early age constant stress and accommodation to both physical and emotional environments caused people to distrust the natural alignment and integration of the head and neck. According to Alexander's theories, by the time a person is fully grown he or she establishes patterns of postural and muscular-skeletal distortion that reveal uniquely identifiable movement characteristics, but also contribute greatly to individual physical and emotional problems.

Through his extensive self-examination process, Alexander found that proper positioning of the head creates a reflexive lengthening of the spine, which stimulates a gentle upward release, relieving forces of compression throughout the entire body. Compression can cause tight muscles, poor breathing, tightness or constriction around the joints, and poor communication throughout the nervous system. Because the nervous system, which consists of the brain, the spinal cord, and the nerves, is the communication system for the whole self, poor communication can lead to disorders including headaches, backaches, stomachaches, and even low self-esteem.

Alexander believed that all people could develop conscious awareness of their distorted muscular-skeletal patterns. By developing that awareness, people could learn to resist or inhibit old, restrictive, or dysfunctional patterns and thereby allow the body to function and develop effectively and effortlessly.

Practice

Experts in the Alexander technique are called teachers, since the process of therapy is considered a re-education of the body. A teacher seeks to equip students with the skills to recognize and modify movement patterns used in basic activities. During a session the student is led through a sequence of simple exercises such as sitting, walking, bending, or even crawling to help raise awareness of the body's movement. The student receives both verbal and hands-on instruction. A teacher may use touch to place a student's body in proper alignment. At the same time a teacher may verbally reinforce a student and direct her toward better posture and movement. These activities are gentle and painless. The teacher's goal is to familiarize a student with proper body alignment and patterns of motion, allowing her to use the lessons independently. The specific exercises in a session will be designed according to the activities the student wants to improve. For example, athletes, actors, singers, or musicians will want to focus on motions and parts of the body that are used in each activity. The emphasis throughout is on self-awareness and improved control.

A session generally lasts from thirty minutes to an hour. A series of twenty to thirty sessions, conducted once or twice a week, is typically recommended. People who have a poorly developed kinesthetic sense, or sense of movement, may take longer to become aware of their body movement.

Benefits

The result of lessons in the Alexander technique is often a sense of greater lightness, vitality, and well-being. Participants commonly report greater ease of motion, greater flexibility, and relief of pain. The technique is frequently used by people with chronic neck and spinal injuries and disorders, including scoliosis. Athletes, dancers, and other performing artists have found that it enhances physical functioning and creativity.

—DIANE YOUNG

Resources

The American Center for the Alexander Technique, Inc.
129 W. 67th St.
New York, NY 10023
Tel: (212) 799-0468
The oldest Alexander technique training center in the United States.

North American Society of Teachers of the Alexander Technique
3010 Hennepin Ave. S., Suite 10
Minneapolis, MN 55408
Tel: 1-800-473-0620
Fax: (612) 822-7224
e-mail: nastat@ix.netcom.com
Offers information on practitioners, training programs, reading lists, and other materials.

Further Reading

Alexander, F. M. Constructive Conscious Control of the Individual. 1923. Reprint, Long Beach, Calif.: Centerline Press, 1985.
———. The Alexander Technique: The Essential Writings of F. Matthias Alexander. Edited by Edward Maisel. New York: Lyle Stuart, 1990.
Barlow, Wilfred. The Alexander Technique: How to Use Your Body Without Stress. Rochester, Vt.: Healing Arts Press, 1990.
Caplan, Deborah. Back Trouble: A New Approach to Prevention and Recovery. Gainesville, Fla.: Triad Publishing. 1987.

Gray, John. *Your Guide to the Alexander Technique.* New York: St. Martin's Press, 1990.

Aston-Patterning®

 Aston-Patterning® (A-P) is an educational system developed by Judith Aston and based on more than thirty years of teaching and life experience. The Aston process combines bodywork, movement education, fitness, and ergonomics. Ergonomics is a method of arranging living and work areas so that they are used most efficiently and safely. A-P may be used as a rehabilitative process for those seeking relief from acute or chronic pain, and it is also used to help improve posture, athletic performance, or overall efficiency in daily living activities.

History

Judith Aston earned a bachelor's degree in fine arts at UCLA, with a specialization in dance therapy. She completed her master's degree at UCLA in 1965, with emphasis in theater, psychology, and dance. Aston also earned a lifetime teaching credential in secondary education. Her teachings focused on the relationship between dance movement and the movements encountered in everyday life.

Aston believed there was a better way to teach movement. One of her students, a track athlete, had reluctantly enrolled in her ballroom dancing course to meet college requirements. Though the young man was consistently able to post record times on the track, he had two left feet on the dance floor. When traditional teaching methods failed, Aston tried a different approach. She took the student out to the track, where she carefully observed his running style and movement patterns. Aston asked him to sprint, then jog, and also requested that he run forward, then backward, and to run left, then right. She used her creative skills to integrate the young man's individual running patterns into dance patterns. Before long, they were dancing the fox-trot right on the running track. This and similar success stories led Aston to focus on the "how-to's" of teaching. By understanding that what you teach is not as important as how you teach it, Aston achieved incredible results.

In 1966 Aston was in a car accident that caused severe whiplash and significant tissue injuries to her neck and back. Another accident the following year made her condition worse. Doctors recommended surgery but Aston looked for an alternative solution. One doctor suggested Aston get in touch with Dr. Ida Rolf at the Esalen Institute in Big Sur, California. Rolf, founder of the Rolfing system, was a respected expert in the field of soft tissue mobilization. Rolf was interested in Aston's educational background, and at Rolf's request Aston developed the first movement education system to be used at the Rolf Institute.

In the late 1960s Aston expanded her knowledge of movement therapy by completing massage training and Rolfing studies. As she continued to practice her own theories, she began to move away from traditional Rolfing principles, especially in regard to her perception of the body and movement as asymmetrical rather than symmetrical. By 1977 Aston had developed her own basic classes in movement and bodywork and trademarked the title "Aston-Patterning."

Theory

Aston-Patterning practitioners look at the alignment of your body, the ways that you move, and areas of tension and discomfort in your movements. It is believed that everyday activities—at work, school, and home—athletics, injuries, and emotional history all work together to develop patterns of movement in your body. Some of these patterns are easy on the body and some are not. They may be caused by reactions to injuries, by physical reactions to emotional distress, or by physical environments that are improperly designed. By understanding individual patterns, practitioners provide sessions that are highly individualized and produce positive changes in posture and movement habits that are long lasting.

Traditionally, medical understanding of body alignment has been based on a linear model. Lines are drawn up and down or side to side to define alignment. Movement is traditionally perceived as symmetrical—that is, balanced equally on each side. In contrast, Aston models of the body have volume—they are three-dimensional. When looking at alignment and movement, consideration is given to the unique length, width, and depth of each body. Aston concepts also consider the bodies' internal structure, which is naturally asymmetrical: the heart is on the left, the liver is on the right, and although there are paired organs (kidneys, lungs), each has its own shape and size. Therefore, A-P practitioners believe that since we are naturally asymmetrical, movement needs to be slightly asymmetrical in response to this internal design. This information helps individuals find their body's natural alignment along with efficient, tension-free ways to move.

Practice

Sessions are customized to individuals' interests, taking into account their own unique patterns created by their histories. Each client is required to take an active role in his process of change. Throughout a session, one wears comfortable clothing and may be asked to perform a variety of movements—sitting, standing, or lying down—as the practitioner assesses his three-dimensional body shape, movement, and muscular tensions. This information is used to design a program of therapy to release the muscular tension and re-educate the body for a new,

efficient movement pattern. These new patterns are practiced and, once learned, are applied to the person's goals and interests.

Each well-rounded session includes a blend of pain-free bodywork, movement coaching, fitness training, and ergonomics. Massage tables, padded stools, and lotions are used for releasing patterns of muscle tension. Stools, stretch cords, toning platforms, and exercise and ergonomic equipment are used to help clients be more aware of where their bodies are in space. This equipment also helps improve alignment and body mechanics and increase overall fitness. Mirrors and skeleton models are used for visual education and explanation. Special foam wedges designed by Aston help clients modify their environments (car seat backs, office chairs, and so forth) to support the new, more efficient alignment.

Private A-P sessions are normally one and a half to two hours long. Though sessions are most effective when offered as a series, they may also be beneficial on a onetime basis. Group lessons or clinics are also available for a wide variety of applications from athletics to daily activities.

Benefits

Aston-Patterning can help individuals use their bodies more efficiently and become aware of stressful movements that can be harmful to the body. Because it focuses on relearning how to use the body more efficiently, it has been offered as a rehabilitative therapy for those seeking relief from acute or chronic pain. It is also used to assist people who wish to improve posture, athletic performance, or overall efficiency of movement in activities of daily living. Many participants report that sessions help them to better understand their own bodies. As a result, these people seem to enjoy long-lasting benefits.

—ALLISON FUNK, CERTIFIED ASTON-PATTERNING
PRACTITIONER

Resources

The Aston Training Center
    P.O. Box 3568
    Incline Village, NV 89450-3568
    Tel: (702) 831-8228
    Fax: (702) 831-8955
    Provides printed material and course descriptions on request. Courses include two- to five-day options. A twenty-one-week practitioner training program is offered every two years. Also offers information about A-P practitioners or classes in specific areas of the country.

Further Reading

Aston, Judith. "Your Ideal Body." *Physical Therapy Today,* summer 1991, vol. 14, no. 2, pp. 30, 32, 34, 36.

Aston, Judith, and Jeff Low. "Your Three-Dimensional Body: The Aston System of Body Usage, Movement, and Fitness." *Physical Therapy Today,* fall 1993, vol. 16, no. 3, pp. 50–59.

Brody, Liz. "Axling: A New Spin on Fitness." *Shape,* April 1993, vol. 12, no. 8, pp. 80–84.

Calvert, Robert. "Exclusive Interview with Judith Aston, Developer of Aston-Patterning Bodywork." *Massage,* October–November 1988, Issue 16, pp. 12–13, 15, 17–19.

Cook, Jennifer. "Body Ease." *Self.* December 1985, p. 146.

Low, Jeffrey. "The Modern Body Therapies." *Massage,* October–November 1988, Issue 16, pp. 48–50, 52, 54–55.

Richardson, Nancy. "Aston-Patterning," *Physical Therapy Forum,* October 28, 1987, vol. 6, no. 43, pp. 1, 3.

Servid, Laura. "Aston-Patterning: Accessing the Power of the Ground." *P.T. and O.T. Today,* July 21, 1997, pp. 18–22.

Woods, Jenna. "Forces of Nature in the Aston Paradigm: Key Concepts of Aston-Patterning." *Massage and Bodywork,* spring 1997, pp. 123–125.

———. "A Patterns Tale: Moving into Aston-Patterning." *Massage and Bodywork,* fall 1996, pp. 95–97.

Bartenieff Fundamentals[SM]

Developed by Irmgard Bartenieff, a German dancer, choreographer, and physical therapist, Bartenieff Fundamentals[SM] are a set of movements that reinforce efficient communication between the mind and body as the body moves. A person trained in Bartenieff Fundamentals is able to observe an individual's movement style and diagnose what makes that individual struggle or succeed with certain movements. People who are recovering from injuries or coping with physical limitations caused by illness generally use the Fundamentals. Athletes, dancers, and people involved in fitness training use the Fundamentals to improve their coordination and overall performance.

History

Irmgard Bartenieff (1900–1981) studied biology, art, and dance before beginning her diploma studies in Berlin with Rudolf Laban in 1925. Laban was a Hungarian movement theorist, choreographer, and teacher who had introduced several influential theories about the nature of movement. Laban created a system to observe, record, and analyze all types of movement, including dance, the martial arts, and everyday actions. Bartenieff emigrated to America in 1936 and began applying her knowledge of human movement to help the ill and the injured. She studied physical therapy at New York University and began working in that field. She also explored the therapeutic possibilities of dance, helping to found the field of dance therapy.

Bartenieff is known for the innovations in physical therapy she developed in the 1940s and 1950s while chief physical therapist for the Polio Service of New York City at Willard

Parker Hospital and later at an orthopedic hospital for children. An epidemic of polio had swept America, crippling many children and adults. To help these individuals, Bartenieff drew from her knowledge of physical therapy and what she had learned from Laban about the dynamics of movement and how the mover can interact with the full circumference of space that surrounds him. She developed the Fundamentals to help polio patients regain their full range of movement. In traditional physical therapy, the therapist manipulates the limbs of a patient who remains, for the most part, passive. Bartenieff insisted that her patients take an active role mentally, physically, and emotionally in the movement sequences she designed to increase their mobility. Her methods were successful, and her patients progressed more rapidly than those treated with traditional physical therapy.

At first Bartenieff called her method "Correctives," a term doctors used to describe orthopedic exercises for correcting posture and the alignment of the spine. But the movement sequences she perfected were more than isolated exercises. She renamed them Bartenieff Fundamentals because she saw them as the building blocks of all human movement. She referred to the movements as "sequences" rather than "exercises" because she wanted to emphasize that a mover should always be thinking about each movement and its connection to the next; never should a mover simply count the number of repetitions. Doing the Fundamentals properly, she believed, helps the mover restore efficient neuromuscular pathways, the communication channels among muscle, nerve, bone, and breath within the body.

To promote her method and the theories of Laban, Bartenieff founded the Laban Institute of Movement Studies in New York City. Since the 1960s, Bartenieff and other Laban movement analysts, who are the only certified Bartenieff Fundamentals practitioners, have helped children and adults, among them athletes, actors, dancers, and musicians.

Some use the Fundamentals to recover from injuries, others to improve or polish their performance in a sport or specialized movement skill. Today there are more than eight hundred certified Laban movement analysts (CMAs) practicing throughout the world.

Theory

Like Laban, Bartenieff approached movement as requiring a person's commitment on a physical, emotional, and mental level. Through his observation of people engaged in such varied activities as t'ai chi ch'üan, folk dancing, and factory assembly-line work, Laban developed a system for analyzing movement known as Laban movement analysis (LMA). Laban's system breaks movement into four primary components: body, space, effort (dynamics), and shape. Although Bartenieff Fundamentals promote awareness of all four components, the Fundamentals primarily emphasize the body.

The Fundamentals are developmentally based; that is, they mirror the stages of development of the brain and motor skills through which babies and toddlers progress on their way to mastering mature movement patterns. Practicing the Fundamentals strengthens the body's internal support for both everyday and highly skilled movement. The Fundamentals require the use of deep muscles close to the core of the body, and the use of breath support to increase the power and flow of movement. They also require a clear spatial intent: an understanding of where movement initiates in the body and how it sequences through the body from one part to another. Practicing Bartenieff Fundamentals helps a mover understand how to initiate and complete a movement efficiently.

By watching a mover perform the Fundamentals, a certified movement analyst (CMA) can identify which body parts do or do not function together smoothly and where movement does or does not flow in the body. Astute observation skills allow a CMA to tailor movement sequences specifically for an individual who wants to address problem areas and meet goals for improvement.

Practice

Fundamentals are taught in groups or in one-on-one sessions that usually take place in a studio with a wooden floor. Participants should wear clothing that allows freedom of movement. The Fundamentals are usually done lying on the floor. There the individual more easily becomes aware of the body's parts, the center of weight, and how it relates to the initiation of action. Without the struggle against gravity or interaction with the environment or other people, the individual can focus mentally on what is going on in the body. In addition to demonstrating the movement sequences clearly, CMAs often use imagery to help students understand movement qualities or to sense more readily how the movement should flow through the body. Using a hands-on technique, CMAs also guide students in performing the movement sequences correctly, drawing attention to where in the body the movement begins.

Although there are many variations of Bartenieff Fundamentals, the most commonly known are the basic six: thigh lift (hip flexion), pelvic forward shift, pelvic lateral shift, vertical body half, knee drop, and arm circle. All practitioners use these six sequences to analyze movement. They also develop variations based on the principles of Bartenieff Fundamentals to address specific problems. Because the Fundamentals provide the foundation for so many other actions, they look simple. Once people begin to study them, however, they find that moving from the core of the body without excess tension is not easy. Most people tend to move inefficiently. Often they don't notice their inefficient habits until a teacher, a coach, or an injury brings it to their attention.

Benefits

Studying Bartenieff Fundamentals helps an individual learn to move more easily and more expressively. Athletes from many sports have improved their performance and reduced the risk of injury after incorporating the Fundamentals into their training. Dancers, actors, and musicians have found that practice of the Fundamentals brings greater clarity and expression to their performances. People rehabilitating from injuries and other conditions that limit mobility have used the Fundamentals to regain functional and expressive movements. Others practice simply for the joy they experience from moving more fluidly and with greater ease.

—*Janet Hamburg, CMA*

Resources

Laban/Bartenieff Institute of Movement Studies
234 Fifth Ave.
New York, NY 10001
Tel: (212) 477-4299
Offers classes in Bartenieff Fundamentals and certification programs in Laban movement analysis.

Further Reading

Bartenieff, Irmgard, and Dori Lewis. *Body Movement: Coping with the Environment.* New York: Gordon and Breach Science Publishers, Inc., 1980.

Laban, Rudolf. *The Mastery of Movement.* Revised and enlarged by Lisa Ullman. Boston: Plays, Inc., 1971.

———. *The Language of Movement: A Guidebook to Choreutics.* Lisa Ullman, ed. Boston: Plays, Inc., 1974.

Videotapes

Discovering Your Expressive Body. Directed by Peggy Hackney and Diane Ramsey. 60 min. Dance Horizons Video, 1981.

Body-Mind Centering®

 Body-Mind Centering® is a therapeutic and educational system combining movement, vocal, perceptual, and hands-on work with the study of life's physiological, psychological, and developmental processes. It can help one to balance one's inner and outer experience in the context of one's environment. While the work itself does not directly treat symptoms, by creating new options for listening and responding to one's own body and the external environment, Body-Mind Centering promotes self-healing and enhances one's quality of life.

History

Body-Mind Centering was developed during the 1960s by Bonnie Bainbridge Cohen, who studied occupational therapy at Ohio State University. She continued her studies in England, where she was certified as a neurodevelopmental therapist. She was also certified as a Laban movement analyst and as a Kestenberg movement profiler. Bainbridge Cohen's professional background and her interests in dance, martial arts, and yoga are reflected in her work, which combines Eastern and Western approaches to relating mind and body. By the late 1960s her work had begun to influence the fields of dance and body and movement therapies. In 1973 she founded the School for Body-Mind Centering to train and certify practitioners and teachers.

Basic Principles

Bainbridge Cohen has compared the relationship of mind and body to wind blowing sand. She has said, "The mind is like the wind and the body is like the sand. If you want to know how the wind is blowing, look at the sand." This kind of interrelationship is at the heart of Body-Mind Centering. Relationship is a key and multilayered principle in this work, where the mind and body are engaged in a dynamic, interactive process that shapes the development of the organism. Fundamental to this process is the interaction among the systems of the body and one's movement development.

Body-Mind Centering identifies seven body systems (skeletal, ligamentous, muscular, organ, endocrine, fluids, and nervous). Each contributes independently to the expression of the body-mind, and at the same time balances and interacts with all the other systems, creating a unique expressive quality for each individual. Although a Body-Mind Centering approach to study of the systems of the body may entail lessons in anatomy through pictures, models, and movement, it does not view the body as an object to be brought under the control of the intellect. This approach is based on the premise that the body has a wisdom of its own, and Body-Mind Centering seeks to mobilize and support this wisdom. This inner knowing is manifested in both a new awareness of the body-mind and a greater vitality and coherence among its various parts. The resonance of the voice, for example, is used to reach down into the torso to arouse the visceral organs and to promote integration of the inner and outer structures of the body—a key for gaining awareness of and healing the body.

The bones of the skeletal system are studied by means of illustrations and models and by tracing, or palpating, their forms through the skin with the hands. The learning process interweaves abstract and sensory knowledge of the body's structure, moving toward the goal of enhancing the body's functioning and range of expression.

Body-Mind Centering considers movement the expression of "inner learning" accumulated since infancy, as basic skills (such as breathing, nursing, rolling, crawling, and walking) are acquired and the structure of the organism takes form. How a person moves or even holds her body is a reflection of a process of personal evolution. Further, Body-Mind Centering assumes that each stage in human growth underlies and supports the next and must be fully realized if the individual is to achieve the balance and ease needed to withstand stress and interact with the world in satisfying ways. Conversely, skipped or unintegrated patterns can lead to alignment/movement problems, systems imbalance, and problems in perception, organization, memory, and creativity.

Body-Mind Centering strives to give the individual access to the totality of her development by enabling her to explore the body's structure through movement, sensory awareness, and imagery. First the cells, then the systems of the body, then movement and action in the world are examined as elements in a progressive formation of self. Participation in this review enables the individual to bring consciousness to bear on strengthening and focusing her own body-mind interaction.

Practice

Sessions in Body-Mind Centering can help identify developmental gaps and facilitate the learning of any absent patterns in infants, children, or adults, and allow them to realize new potential. These "repatterning" sequences involve exploring the anatomical and psychological ramifications of basic movements, such as breathing, pushing the hands against a surface, or reaching out for what one desires.

Group classes or private sessions are directed toward the individual's self-discovery and transformation. They may be organized around the specific concerns and goals of the participants, or they may present principles of the work for exploration. A typical class may involve movement or hands-on bodywork to heighten the student's awareness of a specific system or area of his body.

The class may also include repatterning exercises, study of anatomical illustrations and models, and experiential explorations to increase sensory awareness and integrate that awareness with one's intention and action. The number and frequency of private sessions are determined by the client in consultation with the practitioner. The work is designed to supply insights and skills that can be incorporated into daily experiences.

Benefits

By creating new options for how one senses, feels, and acts in the world, Body-Mind Centering can help individuals change limiting patterns or attitudes. It can be used to address problems such as headaches, chronic pain, sports injuries, hypertension, eating disorders, and perceptual and learning difficulties. It can also improve flexibility, coordination, creative expression, communication, and sense of self-identity and well-being.

—VERA ORLOCK

Resource

The Body-Mind Centering® Association
   16 Center St., Suite 530
   Northampton, MA 01060
   Tel: (413) 582-3617
   Organization that promotes the study and use of Body-Mind Centering.

Further Reading

Bainbridge Cohen, Bonnie. *Sensing, Feeling and Action: The Experiential Anatomy of Body-Mind Centering®.* Northampton, Mass.: Contact Editions, 1993.

Grossinger, Richard. *Planet Medicine.* 2 vols. Berkeley, Calif.: North Atlantic Books, 1995.

Hartley, Linda. *The Wisdom of the Body Moving: An Introduction to Body-Mind Centering®*. Barrytown, N.Y.: Station Hill Press, 1993.

Johnson, Don Hanlon. *Body, Spirit, and Democracy*. Berkeley, Calif.: North Atlantic Books, 1993.

———. *Bone, Breath, and Gesture: Practices of Embodiment*. D. H. Jonson, ed. Berkeley, Calif.: North Atlantic Books, 1995.

———. *Groundworks: Narratives of Embodiment*. D. H. Jonson, ed. Berkeley, Calif.: North Atlantic Books, 1997.

Olsen, Andrea, in collaboration with Caryn McHose. *Body Stories: A Guide to Experiential Anatomy*. Barrytown, N.Y.: Station Hill Press, 1991.

Videotapes

Bainbridge Cohen, Bonnie. *Experiential Anatomy in the Training of Young Dancers*. 1996. (Set of two videos on the foot and the pelvis with an accompanying text. Available from SBMC, 189 Pondview Dr., Amherst, MA 01002.)

Stokes, Beverly. *Amazing Babies: Moving in the First Year*. 1995. (Available from Beverly Stokes, 418 St. Claire Ave. E., Toronto, Ontario, Canada M47 1P5.)

Feldenkrais Method®

 The Feldenkrais Method® is an approach for improving physical and mental functioning through the exploration of body movement patterns and the use of attention. It is based on the brain's innate capacity for learning and the potential for lifelong development and growth. Movement is used as the medium toward understanding our habits and identifying, learning, and acquiring alternatives that promote ease and well-being. Applications range from pain reduction, improvement of neurologically based difficulties and learning disabilities, and increasing mobility to enhancing performance of professional athletes, dancers, musicians, and actors. Those who engage in Feldenkrais are referred to as students rather than patients, because learning underlies the basis of the method.

History

The Feldenkrais Method was developed by Dr. Moshe Feldenkrais. Born in Russia, Feldenkrais emigrated to Israel at the age of thirteen. After receiving degrees in mechanical and electrical engineering, he earned his D.Sc. in physics at the Sorbonne in Paris. He subsequently worked for a number of years in the French nuclear research program. Physically active, Feldenkrais played soccer and practiced the martial arts. He studied with Kano Jigoro, the originator of judo, and in 1936 became one of the first Europeans to earn a black belt in that discipline. A chronic knee injury prompted him to apply his knowledge of physics, body mechanics, neurology, learning theory, and psychology to the body and mind. His investigations resulted in the formulation of a unique synthesis of science and aesthetics known as the Feldenkrais Method.

Practice

A Feldenkrais lesson might begin with a practitioner saying, "As you're sitting, what are you aware of about your sitting? Perhaps it's your back against the chair, or your feet on the floor, or your buttocks on the seat. Now bring your attention to what the back of your neck is doing; to what your chest is doing; to what your shins are doing."

A student's reply might be, "My neck is scrunched" or "My chest is tight." Yet most often, it is "I have no idea what those parts are doing," which indicates that we give little or no attention to certain parts of ourselves or we tend to notice the same parts habitually. The fact is, our whole self is involved in everything we do, but we sense only certain parts of ourselves in our actions, and they generally tend to be the same parts. Through a more complete self-image in our actions and a more even distribution of effort and force throughout our whole selves, an overall enhancement of movement, action, and thought results.

The practitioner might continue, "While seated, without changing the placement of your feet, notice where you have placed your feet. Slowly come to a standing position. [You may find that it is impossible to get up without changing where your feet are placed.] Sit again, move your feet an inch closer together, and come to a standing position. Move your feet back to where you started, then move them an inch farther apart and come to standing. Do you observe that a different placement of your feet influences your ability to stand? You may notice the effects of this in your breathing, your jaw, your neck, your balance, or the amount of effort required in each action. Slowly start to stand as you look down. As you slowly get up, look up. Then get up looking right. Next get up looking left. Can you sense that the different placement of your eyes affects how you come to stand?" This process continues with more variations in order to help the student clarify, inform, and understand how one goes from sitting to standing.

This foundation of learning is not the kind based solely on information; rather, it involves learning that can lead to a change in action, a change in thinking and feeling. The introduction of new variations awakens curiosity and teaches adaptation for continually altering circumstances. Rather than attempting to learn the "right way" of doing something, or "correcting" or "fixing," a student can explore choices, options, and different ways of using himself. Thus, he can act more effectively and efficiently depending on the context and the intention in that moment.

The Feldenkrais Method utilizes attention in a learning environment that is safe, easy, and geared toward an appropriate degree of challenge. In this context, a student can dis-cover and shift habitual patterns that interfere with functioning. He becomes his own laboratory for developing understanding and awareness of his daily actions.

There are two main modalities of learning in the Feldenkrais Method: Awareness Through Movement® and Functional Integration®. Awareness Through Movement lessons are group sessions. Participants are verbally led through a series of structured movement sequences that utilize attention, perception, and imagination. Designed to evoke a more synergistic use of oneself, the lessons establish new patterns of movement. As the lessons progress, participants become more aware of their movement habits, affording new patterns of behavior. More than a thousand different lessons are possible, with movements ranging from developmentally based patterns to innovative configurations. The movements are usually done lying down or sitting, and in a manner that recognizes each participant's own pace and range of motion. Comfort, ease, and the quality of movement are the main criteria used as one is developing greater inner authority.

The other modality, Functional Integration, is a one-to-one, hands-on interaction specifically designed to meet the needs of an individual. Practitioners, primarily through the use of their hands, guide students to a new and more varied use of themselves. The quality of touch is noninvasive, informative, and interactive in nature. Students usually lie or sit and are comfortably dressed. As with Awareness Through Movement group lessons, these individualized sessions use movement as the means to promote changes in patterns of thinking, sensing, feeling, and interacting with others.

Benefits

The Feldenkrais Method aims to improve physical and mental functioning. It is applicable to anyone wanting to enhance the quality of her everyday life and activities. People from many different walks of life do

Each individual, Dr. Feldenkrais believed, possesses an inner body wisdom that when allowed will choose the most comfortable and efficient movement patterns for itself. As the individual develops greater awareness of movement patterns and feels the ease and comfort of new choices, a stronger self-image is formed. This in turn creates healthy new modes of thinking, feeling, and acting.

Feldenkrais. They report results of increased vitality, enhancement of self-image, better breathing and posture, greater flexibility and range of motion, and reduction of pain. By bringing attention to the process of movement, students usually feel lighter and more graceful, and have greater ease and effectiveness in turning their intentions into actions.

—ALAN S. QUESTEL

Resources

The Feldenkrais Guild of North America
P.O. Box 489
Albany, OR 97321
Tel: 1-800-775-2118
Fax: (503) 926-0572
e-mail: fldgld@aol.com
Offers information regarding practitioners in your area, training programs, and other services.

Feldenkrais Recordings
467 Cahill Lane
Santa Rosa, CA 95401
Tel: 1-800-722-7349 or (707) 577-8282
A source of tapes.

Feldenkrais Resources
830 Bancroft Way, Suite 112
Berkeley, CA 94710
Tel: 1-800-765-1907
Fax: (510) 540-7683
e-mail: feldenres@aol.com
Provides information regarding books, tapes, and materials related to the Feldenkrais Method.

Further Reading

Feldenkrais, Moshe. *Body and Mature Behavior: A Study of Anxiety, Sex, Gravitation, and Learning.* Capitola, Calif.: International Universe Press, 1970.
———. *Elusive Obvious.* Capitola, Calif.: META Publications, 1985.
———. *The Master Moves.* Capitola, Calif.: META Publications, 1985.
———. *Awareness Through Movement: Easy-to-Do Health Exercises to Improve Your Posture, Vision, Imagination, and Personal Awareness.* San Francisco: Harper, 1991.
———. *The Potent Self: A Guide to Spontaneity.* San Francisco: Harper, 1992.

Hanna Somatic Education®

Hanna Somatic Education® is a method in which people learn to relax chronically tensed muscles and regain control of various muscle groups and movement patterns. It seeks to change the body by working with a person's "soma," or internal first-person view of herself. A soma includes a person's internal feelings, movements, and intentions. Hanna Somatic Education seeks to bring all these internal aspects to conscious awareness and combine them with scientific knowledge of how muscles work, thereby helping patients to re-educate their bodies to move freely and without pain.

History

Hanna Somatic Education (HSE), also called Hanna Somatics, was developed by Thomas Hanna. A philosopher and former chair of the philosophy department at the University of Florida, Hanna wrote about the philosophy of the body in his book *Bodies in Revolt: A Primer in Somatic Thinking*. He first coined the term *somatics* in 1976 to describe a kind of training that addresses the unification of mind and body. Hanna began with the concept of the soma, which is the body experienced from within, *soma* being the Greek word for "body." Historically, somatology referred to the field that eventually divided into anatomy and physiology. This division separated the study of the structure of the body from the study of its functions.

Hanna perceived no division between body and mind. He used soma to describe a first-person view of the body in which a person is fully aware of his own internal feelings, behaviors, and intentions. This first-person perspective is an integral part of HSE.

In the early 1970s Hanna met Moshe Feldenkrais, an Israeli (Russian born) physicist and body educator, whose Feldenkrais Method was compatible with Hanna's somatic philosophy. Hanna created the first Feldenkrais training program in the United States under the sponsorship of the Humanistic Psychology Institute (now the Saybrook Institute), where he was a director. He continued his study with Feldenkrais for many years at the Novato Institute for Somatic Research and Training, an institution that Hanna founded in 1975.

As he practiced the Feldenkrais Method, Hanna observed characteristic postural difficulties in people of all ages and walks of life. He also noticed that certain techniques were extremely effective in helping clients regain control of the muscles that were holding them in these postures and restricting their movements. These techniques became known as HSE.

Basic Principles

Hanna Somatic educators believe that people stand in characteristic postures because they are being held by chronically contracted muscles. When muscles are balanced in their tonicity—front, back, and sides—people stand up against gravity in a comfortable, upright posture. When the muscles are more contracted on one side or another, people are pulled in that direction.

Muscles become contracted because the nervous system sends messages instructing them to shorten their muscle fibers. When this message is sent continually, the muscle becomes chronically contracted. The message to contract has become a habitual pattern that the person doesn't control consciously.

In his work Hanna identified three reflexes: the red light reflex, green light reflex, and trauma reflex. The red light reflex is also referred to as the startle response or the escape response. It is a set of changes that happen rapidly when there is a sudden change in environmental stimulation. This might be a loud noise nearby, or someone saying, "Boo!" The reflex includes a set of responses such as eyes widening, muscles contracting, and respiration stopping. It takes a while to release these responses and return to normal. With repeated triggering of the startle reflex, there will be some chronic muscle holdings. The muscular holdings contribute to a posture in which the person is bent forward, knees bent and pulled together, arms bent, with the head forward. The muscles on the opposite side of the body also become contracted, which may become painful.

The green light reflex refers to the postural reflex that an infant first experiences at six months of age, when she first contracts the back extensor muscles, arches the back, and extends the neck, arms, and legs. This movement enables the infant to sit up and eventually to stand in preparation for walking. The green light reflex, sometimes called the Landau reflex, activates our antigravity muscles.

The trauma reflex includes motor contractions, which surround any physical or severe emotional trauma—accident, surgery, long-term stress, and so on. This may result in the person being tilted to one side, or the trunk being tilted to one side, while the head tilts to the opposite side. There may be various rotations: head, shoulders, or pelvis rotated to one side or the other. The rotations may be slight or very noticeable.

Hanna put forth the concept of sensory-motor amnesia to describe the tendency of humans to forget certain movements or ways of relating to muscles or muscle groups, leaving them chronically contracted. This occurs when muscles are contracted from being constantly subjected to different kinds of stress responses or injuries over an extended period of time. Hanna believes the contraction is the result of ongoing brain stem–level impulses sent to the motor units, causing contractions of muscle fibers.

Practice

There are two approaches to HSE: hands-on table lessons, guided by the Hanna Somatic educator, and Somatic Exercises™, developed by Hanna and done by the individual. In the hands-on lessons, a typical session is one on one and lasts fifty minutes to one hour. The person is dressed and positioned on a low table. The practitioner guides the person to perform certain movements, evaluating and emphasizing them according to the person's needs. People can learn the exercises immediately. It is estimated that participants average only three visits with a Hanna Somatic educator before they become comfortable and able to move freely.

In the second approach, individuals do the Somatic Exercises on their own. These basic maintenance exercises, also called the "cat stretch," were developed by Hanna and are done once or twice daily. They take ten minutes to perform. There are many more specific exercises for specific purposes. In fact, these are not considered exercises, but are reminders to the brain about how to efficiently use the muscles of the body. They are done slowly and gently, with few repetitions.

Benefits and Risks

HSE provides significant postural improvements. It is especially effective with conditions that are characterized by chronic muscle contractions. HSE is recommended for the following conditions: accident trauma, whiplash, long-term stress, repeated-use stress, difficulties in moving, back pain, and headaches.

Great care must be taken with patients suffering from osteoporosis or other conditions that would be aggravated by movement.

—*Eleanor Criswell Hanna, Ed.D.*

The Novato Institute for Somatic Research and Training offers the only training in Hanna Somatics. It is a certified training program that began in 1990. The institute also provides seminars, books, audiotapes, and videotapes through Somatics Educational Resources. Practitioners can also join the Somatics Society, an organization for bodywork professionals.

Resources

Novato Institute for Somatic Research and Training
   1516 Grant Ave., Suite 212
   Novato, CA 94945
   Tel: (415) 892-0617
   Fax: (415) 892-4388
   Provides certification training programs to qualified students. Also conducts individual sessions and workshops.

The Somatics Society
   1516 Grant Ave., Suite 212
   Novato, CA 94945
   Tel: (415) 892-0617
   Organization for somatics educators and
   bodyworkers. Provides information on the
   practice of somatics and publishes newsletters as well as *Somatics: Magazine-Journal of
   the Bodily Arts and Sciences*. This membership
   organization is run by the Novato Institute
   for Somatic Research and Training, also at
   the same address.

Further Reading

Criswell, Eleanor. *An Introduction to Somatic Yoga.*
   Novato, Calif.: Freeperson Press, 1987.
Hanna, Thomas. *Bodies in Revolt: A Primer in So-
   matic Thinking.* Novato, Calif.: Freeperson
   Press, 1985.
————. *The Body of Life: Creating New Pathways for
   Sensory Awareness and Fluid Movement.*
   Rochester, Vt.: Healing Arts Press, 1993.
————. *Somatics: Reawakening the Mind's Control
   of Movement, Flexibility, and Health.* Reading,
   Mass.: Addison-Wesley, 1988.

Hellerwork

 Hellerwork combines hands-on bodywork, movement educa-tion, and dialogue to release the accumulated stress and trauma that cause people to become rigid in their bodies, in their movements, and in their thinking. The client experiences the insepa-rability of body, mind, and spirit by releas-ing the aches and pains stored in a type of connective tissue called fascia, thereby free-ing up movement patterns and mental pat-terns that waste energy. Its techniques, developed from those of Rolfing, differ in that Hellerwork emphasizes movement edu-cation over hands-on bodywork. The aim is to teach its clients how to live without pain.

History

Joseph Heller, founder of Hellerwork, was born in Poland in 1940 and received his early education in Paris. He emigrated to the United States at the age of sixteen, settling in Los Angeles. In 1962 he began working as an aerospace engineer for NASA and later be-came intensely involved in the field of hu-manistic psychology.

Heller left NASA in 1972 to train with Dr. Ida Rolf and learn her method of structural integration (techniques to rid the body of ha-bitual patterns of storing stress) for the body, called Rolfing. In 1973 he became a Struc-tural Patterner after studying with Judith Aston, creator of the discipline known as Aston-Patterning®. A few years later, while maintaining a successful Rolfing practice, Heller received advanced training from Dr. Rolf and from Dr. Brugh Joy, a noted physi-cian, author, and innovator in the field of preventive medicine and the use of energy as a means of healing. In 1976 Heller became the first president of the Rolf Institute.

As a result of his unique combination of expertise and training in structural integra-tion, movement education, and body energy awareness, Heller began to synthesize a new form of bodywork that emphasized move-ment re-education. In 1978 he left the Rolf Institute and moved to the San Francisco Bay area, where he founded Hellerwork and began training certified practitioners.

Principles

Although Hellerwork is effective for tempo-rary pain or tension relief, practitioners rec-ognize that pain and tension are usually the result of an overall pattern of imbalance oc-curring in the body. Rather than treating the pain or tension "symptom," Hellerwork fo-cuses on rebalancing the entire body, return-ing it to a more aligned, relaxed, and youthful state. To fully understand how the therapy works, one must learn about con-nective tissue and gravity.

According to Heller, any tissue in the body that has a connecting function is considered to be connective tissue. The form of connective tissue that Hellerwork primarily affects is called fascia. Fascia is a plasticlike tissue that wraps all muscles and all of the individual fibers and bundles of fibers that make up muscles. Fascia comes together at the end of the muscle and becomes the tendon, which attaches the muscle to the bone. The fascial system of the body can be seen as one multilayered body stocking, with fascial sheaths wrapping the muscles and organs throughout the body. Because of this, stress in any one area of the body has an effect on every other part of the body.

In its optimal condition, fascia is loose and moist. In a balanced body, the fascial stocking stays loose and mobile, facilitating movement. Under continual stress or lack of movement, however, fascia becomes rigid and layers begin to stick to one another, creating the "knots" people experience in their backs or necks. The sheaths of fascia stick in a systematic way based on our habitual patterns of holding and movement. Holding patterns are often created by emotional memories stored in the tissue of the body; movement patterns are often a result of genetic predisposition or unconsciously learned behaviors from parents and primary caregivers. Although people associate tension and stiffness with their muscles, it is actually the connective tissue around the muscles that accumulates most of this stress.

In Hellerwork, the practitioner uses concentrated deep tissue bodywork on fascial areas in order to release and alleviate tensions. Only then can the body attain its optimum alignment. Also, by eliminating stress and pain, practitioners believe the body should be able to rid itself of repressed mental memories and physical and emotional traumas that function as an obstacle to good physical and mental health.

Practice

During a session a practitioner interacts with a client in three major ways: working with his soft tissues while the client rests on a table; leading him through movement experiences; and discussing the relationship among body sensations, emotions, and thought.

At the start of the first session, the practitioner takes a health history and establishes with the client the goals for the series. The client then undresses to his underclothing and has "before" pictures taken as the practitioner observes the client's body for structural imbalance and restrictions in movement. The client then lies down on a bodywork table and the practitioner proceeds to work with her hands on the rigid parts of the client's soft tissues. Through pressure, movement, and stretching, the practitioner restores fluidity to those tissues and rearranges the parts so that they fit better in their alignment with gravity. When the structural work is done, the practitioner works with the client in establishing a new movement pattern that supports the new alignment. During the session, the practitioner talks with the client, highlighting the more common attitudes and emotions associated with the areas of the body that have been worked with in that session. As the client becomes aware of these emotions, he has the opportunity to become more responsive to them and is less likely to limit self-expression. When the client has integrated the changes in his structure with new movement patterns and attitudes, the series is complete.

Benefits and Risks

Reported benefits include increased flexibility and adaptability, increased energy levels, and a sense of wholeness and well-being. Although not a treatment for any specific condition, Hellerwork is said to reduce and even eliminate musculoskeletal pain from trauma and stress.

Hellerwork is particularly effective as first aid after trauma to the musculoskeletal tissues. It is not a treatment for any disease, conditions of organs, or symptoms of the nervous system. Use of Hellerwork is not advisable when pressure on the soft tissues cannot be tolerated.

All certified practitioners have completed the training program offered by Hellerwork International, LLC. In addition to being trained to deliver the Hellerwork series, they have received extensive training in anatomy, movement, psychology, and energy systems.

—SANDY SULLIVAN FOR HELLERWORK INTERNATIONAL

Resource

Hellerwork International, LLC
   406 Berry St.
   Mount Shasta, CA 96067
   Phone: (916) 926-2500 or 1-800-392-3900
   Fax: (916) 926-6839
   e-mail: Hellerwork@aol.com
   Web site: www.hellerwork.com
   Offers a list of Hellerwork practitioners. Also provides information about the discipline, as well as training opportunities.

Further Reading

Heller, Joseph, and William Henkin. *Bodywise: Regaining Your Natural Flexibility and Vitality for Maximum Well-Being.* Oakland, Conn.: Wingbow Press, 1986.

In Hellerwork practitioners use verbal dialogue with their clients to discuss the relationship among the client's body sensations, emotions, and thinking. During the bodywork session, the practitioner highlights the more common attitudes and emotions associated with the affected area of the body. As the client becomes aware of these emotions, they become easier to recognize and deal with, resulting in a discernible change in movement and mental outlook. When the client has integrated the changes in her structure with new movement patterns and attitudes, the session is complete.

Ideokinesis

Ideokinesis is a method of movement therapy that utilizes the capacity of the nervous system to correct awkward or inefficient movement. The term *ideokinesis* derives from two Greek words, *ideo*, meaning "idea," and *kinesis*, meaning "movement." Ideokinesis views the neurological system as the messenger of ideas or patterns of movement that stimulate and organize muscular and skeletal activity. Through anatomy lessons, exercises, and guided imagery, ideokinesis imparts healthy patterns of movement to the nerves and ultimately to the whole muscular and skeletal structure of the body. Either on its own or combined with other movement training, ideokinesis can aid in overcoming physical impairment caused by illness or injury. It is also considered a means of learning patterns of movement that enhance coordination, reduce tension, and promote a general sense of well-being.

History

Ideokinesis is an outgrowth of techniques Mabel Elsworth Todd discovered when, as a teenager in upstate New York, she struggled to cure herself after suffering a back injury. Once she had completely recovered, Todd developed her techniques into a form of movement therapy that she practiced first in Boston, then in New York City. By the late 1920s she was attracting a steady stream of patients to her private clinic and lecturing on her method at Columbia University and the New School for Social Research. Todd's books, *The Thinking Body* (1937) and *The Hidden You* (1953), remain essential to the study of ideokinesis. But Todd's method might have been forgotten without the efforts of a former student, Lulu Sweigard, and a former patient, Barbara Clark. They introduced her method into the curriculum of New York University and the Juilliard School of Dance, ensuring that her legacy would be passed on. *Human Movement Potential,* published shortly after Sweigard's death in 1974, is an important updating of Todd's original practice, which it dubbed ideokinesis. While ideokinesis is not well known to the general public and has no national professional organization or certification procedure, it is studied and used by a network of private practitioners throughout the United States. Many practitioners combine it with dance, Rolfing, or physical therapy.

Theory

Movement is an event in which each of three systems of the organism—neurological, muscular, and skeletal—plays a specific and integrated role. This event starts when the neurological system acts as a messenger and transmits impulses from the brain to the muscular system. In turn, the muscular system acts as a motor, responding to the impulses. It moves the third component in the event, the skeletal system or framework. This is the basis of ideokinesis.

The particular focus of ideokinesis is the subcortical level of nervous activity. Todd described the delicate subcortical nerves as "the hidden you," since it is through these nerves that ideas and images about the totality of the body are realized. If thoughts about the body are habitually faulty or weak, then the subcortical nerves will transmit debilitating messages to the rest of the body and movement will be impaired. To improve movement, ideokinesis accordingly concentrates not on increasing flexibility or muscular strength, though these often occur, but on changing the nervous system's coding of movement. This is accomplished through exercises and guided imagery, which modify both conscious and unconscious thought about body movements and positions.

Practice

A class in ideokinesis generally opens with a discussion of anatomy, physiology, and body mechanics, which furnishes some of the mental images used in the positions and movements to follow. Beginning-level work often centers on the constructive rest position, a recumbent position in which the arms are folded softly over the body and the legs are flexed at the knees and kept together. As the participants assume the constructive rest position, they are instructed to conceive of their bodies as empty suits of clothes. The ideokinesis teacher then uses suggestive language to evoke a process of gentle pressing that simultaneously removes wrinkles from the imagined suit of clothes and tension from the real body of the participant.

In a comparable fashion, work on sitting, standing, walking, and other basic movements makes use of exercises, mental images, and suggestive language. Participants attempt to perform various movement patterns while calling to mind the biomechanical and metaphorical images the teacher has introduced. Participants work in pairs, with one participant executing the movement while the other touches him lightly to clarify the initiation point and pathway of the movement.

By contrast, the experience of ideokinesis done on a one-to-one basis will vary from person to person, depending on the specific methods of the practitioner and the needs of the client. Instruction in the biomechanics of movement might be omitted and attention given over to diagnosis of difficulties and the establishment of a regimen of remedial exercises.

Benefits

When practiced consistently, ideokinesis can help restore range of motion and improve the integration of sensory and motor skills. Further, it is credited with producing or restoring homeostasis, a condition in which all the systems and subsystems of the organism function harmoniously. In a state of homeostasis, the individual experiences enhanced freedom of movement, release from tension and fatigue, increased vitality, and a sense of well-being that often leads to the discovery of unexpected inner potential.

—*ANDRE BERNARD*

Further Reading

Matt, Pamela. *A Kinesthetic Legacy: The Life and Works of Barbara Clark.* Tempe, Ariz.: CMT Press, 1993.

Sweigard, Lulu. *Human Movement Potential: Its Ideokinetic Facilitation.* Lanham, Md.: University Press of America, 1988.

Todd, Mabel E. *The Thinking Body: A Study of Balancing Forces of Dynamic Man.* Pennington, N.J.: A Dance Horizons Book, 1968. (Originally published 1937.)

Kinetic Awareness

 Kinetic awareness is a discipline that aims to increase knowledge of the human body on both physical and emotional levels. It aims to improve the individual's mental image of her body while also revealing ways that physical tension affects health, attitude, and emotional well-being. Practitioners of kinetic awareness believe that through the careful exploration of the body's responses to concentrated physical pressure, people can gain a heightened sensitivity to posture and movement, both in daily life and in specialized activities such as sports, dance, and martial arts.

History

Dancer/choreographer Elaine Summers developed kinetic awareness in the 1960s. Her career was interrupted at an early age when she began to experience symptoms of osteoarthritis, a potentially crippling disease of the joints. Doctors told her that within five years she would be unable to walk. Eventually, through her own determination, she was able to resume dancing. During her recovery she studied with Carola Speads, whose system of physical re-education evolved from the work of Elsa Gindler, a bodywork innovator. Summers's method of bodywork grew out of these studies and her own search for treatment of her physical condition. Upon experiencing positive results, she began to teach the technique to others.

Basic Principles

Through experimentation, Summers developed an extensive system of techniques to increase physical awareness and release muscular tension. A special feature of this

Kinetic awareness encourages the individual to experience the pleasure of movement for its own sake. Practitioners maintain that a strong link exists between a person's mental state and the level of muscular tension in the body. This discipline seeks not only to relieve muscular tension resulting from daily stress and agitated emotional states but also to achieve a corresponding enhancement of psychological well-being through holistic treatment of the human being.

method is the use of rubber balls of various sizes to highlight body parts in isolation.

When an individual rests his body on a ball, the ball provides a focal point of attention; the individual naturally concentrates on the muscles and body part directly above the ball, where pressure on the body is greatest. This both supports and stretches the body. Muscular tension dissipates because of the pressure of the ball and the intentional movement of the body as the individual slowly shifts his position over the ball.

As an individual moves, the ball tests the elasticity and responsiveness of the muscles and joints. The intensity of the pressure created by the ball is a direct result of the size and firmness of the ball and, therefore, can be controlled. People often feel a pleasurable ease and warmth in the part of the body where the ball has been and an alert quietness in the mind from the focused attention and overall relaxation that occurs from this.

As practitioners work, they release the unnecessary tension that causes many individual aches and pains. The work helps to prevent future injuries by revealing the body's warning signs. Practitioners also see how the mind and emotions manifest themselves in the body. For example, anger, sadness, or joy can each create a particular physical response in the body. Similarly,

how people feel physically can create a certain mood, which then affects behavior. Through kinetic awareness, individuals discover that they have choices about how they move, and that it is possible to let go of habits and images of the body that are restrictive. Moving with awareness is a profound way to reconnect the mind and the body.

Practice

Kinetic awareness can be taught both in classes and private sessions. People will often experience benefits such as relief of pain or greater range of movement after one or two sessions, but the method can be practiced on an ongoing basis—many dancers and performers incorporate it into their training.

A typical class begins with an evaluation of body sensations while the participant lies quietly on the floor. Close attention is paid to breathing and slow movement explorations with or without rubber balls. The individual focuses on one body part at a time, moving slowly through its full range of motion while noting any sensations. A person might become aware that certain parts of the body are dull and have little sensation while others are hypersensitive. He also begins to discover that tension can exist in very specific, concentrated locations in the body. Practitioners assert that each person has preferred ways of moving, and that these favored modes naturally exclude other possibilities for movement. Summers believes that moving every part of the body through its potential range, often and without pain, encourages the body to attain physiological balance.

After the initial warm-up is complete, the teacher will suggest an exercise that enables the students to work at their own pace on the part of the body that is chosen as a focus. Throughout the session, the teacher will invite the students to share their feelings and observations. The process may include some explanation of anatomy to further an understanding of the musculoskeletal system and how it works. After the first phase of kinetic awareness, people can then choose to explore more advanced phases that employ multiple simultaneous movements and a full range of speed. The technique is adaptable; there is ample room for creativity and experimentation.

Benefits

Those who practice kinetic awareness gain a deeper understanding of their bodies. They are able to release the unnecessary tension that causes many bodily aches and pains, and they can prevent future injuries by becoming familiar with the body's warning signs. Furthermore, advocates of this discipline emphasize that the mind and emotions are expressed in the body. By improving physical condition and relieving stress through kinetic awareness, a person is able to create a feeling of well-being that will affect behavior. Through this practice, then, individuals reportedly discover they have the capacity to choose how they move, and can enjoy more freedom and self-expression through movement.

—ELLEN SALTONSTALL; J. ROBIN POWELL, PH.D;
AND MICHELLE BERNE

Resources

The Kinetic Awareness Center
    1622 Laurel St.
    Sarasota, FL 34236
    or
    P.O. Box 1050
    Cooper Station
    New York, NY 10276
    Provides information about kinetic awareness as well as referrals to qualified teachers.

Further Reading

Saltonstall, Ellen. *Kinetic Awareness: Discovering Your Bodymind.* New York: Kinetic Awareness Center, 1988. (Available through the Kinetic Awareness Center.)

Meir Schneider Self-Healing Method

The Meir Schneider self-healing method combines massage, movement exercise, and other methods, including vision improvement exercises, into a comprehensive rehabilitation system. It focuses on establishing communication between the mind and the body, and on understanding the needs of the body as it strives to heal itself.

History

Meir Schneider, Ph.D., L.M.T., was born in Ukraine in 1954. Blind at birth, he suffered from cataracts and other serious vision problems. The family emigrated to Israel, and by the time the young Schneider was six years old, five unsuccessful surgeries had left his lenses shattered, which resulted in admitting less than 1 percent of light in one eye and 5 percent in the other. Doctors said that nothing further could be done. Schneider was given a certificate of legal blindness and taught to do his schoolwork in Braille. He refused to use a cane or guide dog, and insisted on doing everything a sighted child could do, even ride a bicycle, although he sometimes ran into walls. He was confident that he would gain functional eyesight one day.

At age sixteen, he learned about the Bates method of vision improvement, as well as massage. He began to develop his own theories and insights about movement and the body. He practiced eye exercises, self-massage, and movement exercises up to thirteen hours a day. His family and friends told him he was wasting his time. At first Schneider saw only blurry lights and shadows, but soon he began to distinguish some of the shapes as windows. Within eighteen months he could read print without glasses. After years of effort, he learned to see well enough to earn an unrestricted driver's license.

With the Bates exercises, he relaxed his eyes, adjusted them to varying levels of light, and trained his brain to use his eyes in different, more effective ways. But he also needed self-massage to improve circulation and relieve the underlying strain of his face and upper body. Movement exercises helped to balance his vision. Through all of this Schneider discovered how deeply the function of any one organ or area of the body is related to that of the whole body.

While still working to gain his own functional vision, he began to see clients who experienced chronic pain, multiple sclerosis, and other problems. The massage and movement techniques he had developed from his own experience resulted in improvement in his early clients. He opened his first clinic with two of these clients, a youth with muscular dystrophy and a young woman with polio. His clinic and work gained national attention in Israel. In 1977 he founded the Center for Self-Healing in San Francisco. A few years later he opened the School for Self-Healing.

Today Schneider's work with muscular dystrophy is the subject of scientific studies. An internationally known therapist and educator, he is the author of *Self-Healing: My Life and Vision* and coauthor of *The Handbook of Self-Healing*. A seminar, *Meir Schneider's Miracle Eyesight Method*, is available on tape.

Philosophy

Schneider believes the body has a powerful, innate ability to heal itself. Because we use the body only as a tool to accomplish our everyday goals, most of us lose touch with this ability.

For many people, the body is unexplored territory. Only a fraction of the total capacity of muscles, lungs, and brain are regularly called upon. We overuse about fifty of the body's approximately six hundred muscles, and underuse the rest. Stress-related tension is a major cause of this problem. It creates "frozen" areas where muscular tension restricts movement, feeling, and circulation. People respond to stress with shallow breathing, eventually impairing lung and heart function. Chronic stress exacerbates disease. For people with serious health problems, it aggravates the course of the disease and inhibits the body's natural tendency to repair itself.

According to Schneider, these problems stem from a lack of communication between the body and mind. So much of our attention is directed away from ourselves—toward other people, our work, and the constant barrage of external stimulation—that sensations within go unnoticed. In our culture we tend to listen to our bodies only in times of extreme crisis. By developing an intuitive sense of the body's needs, we can overcome serious health problems and increase health and vitality. This is the goal of self-healing therapy.

The School for Self-Healing offers training in the Meir Schneider self-healing method. Level 1 graduates are eligible in some places for massage therapy certification. Graduates of the full 760-hour program are recognized as self-healing practitioner/educators. Many students enroll in the beginning and intermediate stages of training in order to work with their own health problem or that of a family member. Some students are already health care professionals or bodyworkers, while others are newly entering the massage-bodywork field.

Practice

A self-healing therapy session usually lasts about one and a half hours. The client wears underwear or a swimsuit. With the therapist's guidance, the client explores the body-mind link by experiencing a combination of many different kinds of movement—massage, self-massage, visualizations of movement, breathing, coordination exercises, and eye exercises when appropriate. The session often begins with a movement that is problematic, difficult, stiff, or uneven. It is repeated at times as a checkpoint to see if there is any improvement. The methods that prove most successful during the session are incorporated into a home exercise program. In this way, deeply ingrained, harmful movement patterns, such as the habit of tensing up in order to move, can be reprogrammed.

One client, a bodybuilding champion, came to Schneider with constant pain in her shoulders, neck, and knees, which resulted in diminished performance. "Many bodybuilders have such tight muscles and joints, they can't pull a T-shirt on, and they're in constant pain," she told him. Athletes often exhibit this kind of harmful use of the body, which eventually jeopardizes their performance. He taught her to isolate specific movements, to use only the correct muscles for a specific action without compensating with the others, to stay soft, and to move through a sense of relaxation. Her muscles became longer and fuller, the pain disappeared, and her weight-lifting performance improved.

Benefits

The Meir Schneider self-healing method has helped athletes and musicians improve their performance. It prevents and alleviates the occupational health hazards of computer work and other detailed eye-hand tasks. It has been successfully used to treat problems with breathing, digestion, posture, the spine, and neuromuscular, joint, and heart/circulatory systems; injuries; chronic pain syndromes; poor vision from nearsightedness, farsightedness, astigmatism, and lazy eye; a wide variety of eye diseases; and many other health problems.

—CAROL GALLUP

Self-healing is unusual among the bodyworks because:
- It combines massage and movement equally.
- It includes vision improvement work.
- It offers detailed programs, carefully tailored to the needs of the individual at a given time, to nurture specific organs or organ systems that are fragile or damaged.
- It emphasizes client motivation and empowerment. Self-healing is above all an educational process, and the client becomes an active, inventive partner of the therapist.

Resources

School for Self Healing
2218 48th Ave.
San Francisco, CA 94116
Tel: (415) 665-9574
Fax: (415) 665-1318
Web site: www.self-healing.org
e-mail: info@self-healing.org
Organization that promotes the study and use of the Meir Schneider Self-Healing Method.

Videotapes

Schneider, Meir. *Yoga for Your Eyes*, 1997. (Available from Sounds True, P.O. Box 8010, Boulder, CO 80306.)

Audiotapes

Schneider, Meir. *Meir's Miracle Eyesight Method.* (Available from Sounds True, P.O. Box 8010, Boulder, CO 80306.)

Further Reading

Schneider, Meir, with Maureen Larkin and Dror Schneider. *The Handbook of Self-Healing.* Penguin/Arkana, 1994 (Foreign language editions available in Portuguese, Russian, and Hungarian.)

Schneider, Meir. *Self-Healing: My Life and Vision.* Penguin, Arkana, 1989 (Foreign language editions available in French, Portuguese, Hungarian, and Hebrew.)

Sensory Awareness

 Sensory awareness is a practice in freeing ourselves from conditioned habits, fears, and tensions that keep us from being what we really want to be and doing what we really want to do. The process promotes direct awareness of our sensations: sight, hearing, touch, taste, smell, and especially the subtle kinesthetic sense of body movement. In practicing this kind of awareness, we experience how we relate to ourselves, other people, and the world around us. We become present for what is happening from moment to moment—to be here, now—with greater interest and joy, and more creative responsiveness to things as they are.

History

In Germany at the beginning of the twentieth century, a young woman named Elsa Gindler contracted tuberculosis, for which there was no known cure at that time. Her doctor asked, "What have you done to yourself?" and she took this question literally.

From that moment on she began giving full attention to how she behaved and what happened inside her body, from the time she awoke in the morning until going to sleep at night. In doing so, her lungs began to function normally and she recovered.

Sensory awareness is the name now given to such "restorative observation"—this interested, nonjudgmental attention to the sensations of tension and release felt throughout the body as one moves in response to life's continually changing events. Through such attention, Gindler became aware of natural processes and learned to work with them instead of against them, particularly in regard to breathing and interaction with the pull of gravity, which attracts us to the earth at every moment.

Gindler not only cured herself of tuberculosis, but also discovered that being aware of what is happening in the physical body can bring about liberation from mental anxiety. This practice brought about a state where she was no longer disturbed by her own thoughts and worries. She came to understand that calm in the physical field is equivalent to trust in the psychic field.

At about the same time, a young musician named Heinrich Jacoby was asking himself why some of the singers on the operatic stage had beautiful voices but were blocked musically, whereas others could master the music but not move with it. He came to see how "talent" and "lack of talent" were mainly results of conditioning. A person was talented or untalented depending on the ideas imposed by family, teachers, society, and culture, rather than on inherent capacities.

Jacoby's thesis was that every human being born without physical defects has the biological equipment for every natural function, and that these include all possibilities of living, moving, experiencing, and creating. He demonstrated with thousands of people that there is an unrealized human potential for receiving impressions and allowing expression in every mode that can continue to unfold throughout our lives—if we are not blocked by our own limiting mental attitudes.

When Gindler and Jacoby came together, they found in each other's discoveries the missing pieces of their own work. Jacoby was a highly educated "intellectual," while Gindler had no formal education beyond public school and taught a bodywork called *gymnastik*—through which she had already recognized that one's attitudes are not just abstract thoughts, but tensions embedded in the physical tissue. When Gindler and Jacoby became colleagues, "mind" and "body" came together. In their classes students strove to consciously experience a state of balance that was not "physical" or "mental," but both—not only new ways of moving, but new ways of seeing and hearing, of thinking and relating, of being creative in many ways.

Students of Gindler and Jacoby have carried their work around the world: to Germany, Switzerland, England, Israel, Spain, the United States, Mexico, Canada, and Japan. Sometimes it is the practice as such that is offered; sometimes it is a transforming approach that is taught to various professions such as musical performance, dance, child care, or psychotherapy. Dr. Lily Ehrenfried took the work of Gindler and Jacoby to France, where she established a new kind of physical therapy called *gymnastique holistique*. The AEDE (Association des Eleves de Dr. Ehrenfried et des Practiciens en Gymnastique Holistique) was formed in 1986 and now has practitioners in ten countries in Europe and the Americas.

The Gindler/Jacoby theories and practice were brought to the United States in the 1930s by several of their students, including Else Henscke Durham, Clare Fenichel, Carola Speads (who called the work physical reeducation), and Charlotte Selver. Each offered the practice in her own way. Selver coined the name *sensory awareness*, presenting the first classes in "body awareness" and "nonverbal experience" ever given at the New School for Social Research in New York and the Esalen Institute in California. The Charlotte Selver Foundation, now the Sensory Awareness Foundation, was established in 1971 to support her work. The psychologist Erich Fromm studied extensively with Selver and found the work "of great significance for the full unfolding of the personality." Fritz Perls incorporated much of what he learned from her into his gestalt therapy, while Alan Watts, who presented many joint seminars with Selver, called this practice "the living Zen."

Practice

Sensory awareness sessions are simply an inquiry into what it feels like to be a living human being, when you are aware of what you are feeling and how you are living. There are no set "exercises." Experiments inspired by the felt needs of the student or students at that moment are outlined by the leader. Afterward, there is reporting as to what a student might have discovered. There are no preconceptions as to what ought to happen or what students ought to feel; feelings are neither "right" nor "wrong," they simply *are*.

All living is movement, and these experiments are not only large movements, such as walking, running, dancing, and stretching, but also the most subtle: inhalation and exhalation, the pulsing in a wrist, the vibration of the vocal cords in the throat as a person speaks or sings, the resting of a hand on a cheek or on a shoulder, the lifting of a partner's arm or having one's arm lifted. In noticing how these movements feel as they take place, the habitual tensional patterns that produce inappropriate and painful movements of the body can change.

Sensory awareness is offered privately, in regular group sessions, and in workshops. There are no formal training courses for leaders; leaders and students come to a mutual understanding as to when the student is ready to become a leader, usually after many years of practice.

> This work makes possible a way of being that is full of life, more security, and more courage to dare [to do] something new. The wonder is the blessed feeling that comes when I can be more fully, as if each cell in me were happy to exist.
>
> —RUTH VESELKO, LONGTIME GINDLER/JACOBY STUDENT AND SENSORY AWARENESS TEACHER IN SWITZERLAND

Benefits

As sensory awareness experiments continue over a period of time, muscles may become more elastic, aches and pains fade, illnesses subside. Fear may be replaced by self-confidence. Movement and thinking may become more spontaneous and creative. There may be less effort and greater joy in relating to others and taking part in private or professional activities. The fundamental aim is simply to wake up—to experience life in every bit of us and be happy to exist at this moment.

It is recommended that you study with an experienced sensory awareness leader, to help you begin to explore this unique practice of making friends with your body and of discovering all of the possibilities that can unfold when you learn to trust in the innate wisdom of the body-mind.

—MARY ALICE ROCHE

Resources

Sensory Awareness Foundation
    c/o Sara Gordon
    955 Vernal Ave.
    Mill Valley, CA 94941
    Tel: (707) 794-8496
    Distributes various publications concerning the practice of sensory awareness.

Sensory Awareness Leaders Guild
    c/o Louise Boedeker
    411 W. 22nd St.
    New York, NY 10011
    Tel: (212) 675-5730
    Recommends qualified sensory awareness leaders in the United States and abroad.

Further Reading

Brooks, Charles V. W. *Sensory Awareness: Rediscovery of Experiencing Through the Workshops of Charlotte Selver*. New York: Viking Press, 1974.

Soma Neuromuscular Integration

 Soma neuromuscular integration, or soma bodywork, utilizes ten individual sessions that address particular and progressive soft tissue manipulation, primarily through working with the fascia, or connective tissue. Founded in 1978, soma is a way of enabling people to function more optimally by providing greater access to the body-mind. People who inhabit their whole and integrated body-mind frequently experience greater levels of emotional openness, creativity, and self-reliance.

History

Soma neuromuscular integration was developed by Bill M. Williams, Ph.D., and Ellen Gregory Williams, Ph.D. Bill Williams taught and collaborated with Ida Rolf in the early development of her well-known ten-session work in fascia manipulation. He was a member of the founding board of directors that established the teaching institute for Dr. Rolf's methods. Ellen Williams is a psychologist who, after many years as a talk therapist, realized there must be an involvement with the body to effect deep and lasting psychological change. In his early years as a Rolfer, Bill continued to be aware of the interaction of the body and the mind and wanted to develop a training program that would more effectively address and work with integrating the whole person. He was one of the first to develop a hands-on training program that combined the physiological and psychological approaches to healing.

Basic Principles

Fascia is the tissue that wraps around muscles and gives them their shape. Ideally, muscles should be able to move independently and slide over one another, but often as a result of age, injury, or physical or emotional stress, the fascia glues together, causing the fascia and muscles to lose functional and structural differentiation. Someone who has experienced a serious neck injury may attempt to turn his head from side to side, but instead of using only the muscles necessary to accomplish the rotation, the muscles of the neck and shoulders act as one, and turning the head ends up requiring rotation of the entire upper torso. Such gluing is a restriction in movement that is expensive in terms of energy output and general vitality.

By working directly on the fascia, the soma practitioner frees the musculature, allowing it to assume a more effective structural relationship with the fascia. As a result, one stands taller with less effort and moves with greater ease and comfort. In addition, chronic muscle or joint pain is almost always reduced or eliminated as muscles have the opportunity to lengthen and assume optimal relationships with surrounding fascia.

Neural tissue is embedded within the myofascial system. In the process of freeing restricted and adhered fascia, practitioners work directly with the nervous system, sending sensory information to the brain that allows the body new options to organize itself in more comfortable, more energy-efficient, more satisfying ways. Practitioners believe that soma bodywork teaches the body to self-correct and continuously reprogram itself to greater levels of ease and freedom.

According to Marcia Nolte, codirector of the Soma Institute, "Life is change and change is movement, movement in our bodies, our feelings, our thoughts. It is the loss of the ability to move and change our bodies and our thinking that continues over time to diminish our ability to experience life. Soma bodywork focuses on accessing more somatic options. Soma therapists are not working toward the evolution of a 'perfect person' by replacing old patterns with new, 'right' ones, but rather toward a less rigid, more authentic individual who responds creatively rather than reacts to his or her environment."

To help accomplish this, therapists work with the three-brain model developed by Bill Williams. The three-brain model is a way of understanding human consciousness and the activity of the nervous system. It is based in part on neuropsychiatric research, which has clearly outlined specific differences between the roles and functions of the left and right sides of the brain. In simplified terms, the left half of the brain is more logical and the right side is more creative. The "third brain" in the model is the corebrain, which consists of nerve plexi located in the abdomen. According to Williams, it is the source of bodily energy and the means by which the left and right hemispheres translate cognition into activity.

Soma therapists believe that being stuck or dominant in any one "brain" prevents optimal functioning. They endeavor to educate people as to how to integrate all "three brains." The structural organization resulting from the soma bodywork, the integrative exercises, and somatic education are all designed to improve access to the "three brains."

Soma training is designed to be a unique, experiential, nonlinear training using Dr. Bill Williams's three-brain model as the underlying principle of integrating the body and mind. Training was first held in 1978 in Gainesville, Florida. In 1986 Marcia W. Nolte, LMP, and Karen L. Bolesky, M.A., CMHC, LPM, became codirectors of the Soma Institute. The following year the institute moved to Washington State, where it continues to expand and develop.

Practice

There are ten sessions in soma bodywork treatment. These sessions last for approximately ninety minutes to two hours and progress layer by layer, working progressively deeper. The practitioner and client work together to slowly release and rebalance layers of tissue until reaching the deepest layers of the core.

Unresolved feelings can surface in the rebalancing process. Past trauma that may have been understood intellectually will continue to remain buried in restricted tissues until it is addressed, released, and repatterned. The repatterning part of the work is accomplished through journaling with special goals, the three-brain model of body-mind functioning, a notebook of integrative movement, and individual somatic learning.

Results

The results of soma bodywork are not limited to the relief of symptoms, although relief occurs consistently. Participants may experience increased levels of energy and performance, fewer stress-related symptoms, increased flexibility, increased align-

ment and freedom of movement, heightened emotional and physical awareness, greater self-reliance, and creativity.

—*Karen Bolesky and Marcia W. Nolte*

Resources

Soma Institute
730 Klink
Buckley, WA 98321
Tel: (360) 829-1025
Fax: (360) 829-2805
Web: www.soma-institute.com
Provides the professional licensing program and the certification program in soma neuromuscular integration and somassage. Trainings are held in Washington State. The Soma Institute is licensed by the Washington Workforce Training and Education Coordinating Board, and the Washington State Board of Massage. It also lists soma bodywork practitioners.

Somatorespiratory Integration

 Somatorespiratory integration (SRI) is a system of breathing and touch that is used to allow a person to heal herself. It is not used to remedy a specific ailment; rather, SRI invites participants to access the body's inner rhythms and experience the present moment more fully. The body's rhythms are charted in a twelve-stage process through which a person experiencing SRI will progress.

History and Practice

Over nearly two decades Dr. Donald Epstein developed network chiropractic and network spinal analysis. He noticed specific patterns of breath, movement, and self-touch that spontaneously occurred in his clients after they received network care. Eventually he categorized these expressions into twelve stages of consciousness, each with its own pattern of breath, touch, and movement. The stages are suffering, polarities and rhythms, being stuck in a single perspective, reclaiming power, merging with an illusion, preparing for resolution, resolution, readiness in emptiness, light beyond form, ascent, descent, and community.

Most of the exercises are performed while lying down or seated. At the start of an SRI session, the participant is instructed to breathe gently while using her hand to feel the rise and fall of her chest and abdomen. The breathing patterns may involve various combinations of nose and mouth breathing. This exercise is used to transfer a peaceful rhythm to the person's hand, equipping it to heal other regions of the body. The individual then places her hands on various areas of the body to allow them to move in alignment with the rhythms. The exercises are used to find the most peaceful areas of the body and spread these areas of peace to other regions. These tools help individuals pay attention to themselves in a meaningful way.

A practitioner intends to educate the client in each of the twelve possible rhythms of healing. An entire session may involve connecting with up to four rhythms. The time it takes to transfer a rhythm will vary with a person's experience. This technique is valued for being simple and effortless. The body becomes increasingly able to dissipate stored tension or energy. The benefits of SRI will occur progressively over the twelve distinct stages of the healing process. With each session, the natural movement of the body overtakes the thinking mind.

SRI does not attempt to force any particular outcome or catharsis. The intent is to acknowledge and accept the body's rhythms without changing them. By observing the way a person moves, touches, and breathes, SRI is used to increase a person's self-awareness and respect for her own healing process.

The exercises are best learned under the guidance of a trained facilitator. SRI is not meant to be a replacement for any form of therapy, nor as a treatment for specific health conditions. It is ultimately intended as a self-care system that may be used in conjunction with other healing modalities.

—DONALD EPSTEIN

Resources

Innate Intelligence, Inc.
    444 N. Main St.
    Longmont, CO 80501
    Tel: (303) 678-8086
    Provides information about SRI workshops and a list of those who have taken the SRI programs.

Further Reading

Epstein, Donald, and Nathaniel Altman. *The Twelve Stages of Healing.* Novato, Calif.: New World Library, 1994.

Trager Psychophysical Integration

 Trager psychophysical integration is a type of bodywork that uses the human ability to feel pleasure and other sensations as the basis for developing and maintaining a healthy body. According to Trager theory, a healthy body is both a container for and a reflection of a healthy mind and spirit. Practicing the Trager approach can result in relief from pain and greater freedom of motion. It can also assist in correcting long-standing patterns of posture and movement that cause discomfort, unhappiness, and unfulfilled life potential.

History

Trager psychophysical integration was developed by Milton Trager, M.D. As a young man Trager was an aspiring boxer. At the gym, trainers and boxers used bodywork to alleviate muscular pain after rough workouts. One day, while giving his trainer a rubdown, Trager discovered he had a gift for bodywork. Shortly thereafter Trager quit boxing and began to practice his own intuitive form of bodywork on family, friends, and clients in his Miami neighborhood. He experienced success in cases of sciatica, polio, and many other conditions from which people had found no relief through conventional medicine.

After eight years of private informal practice, Trager sought out more formal training and certification. At age forty-one he entered the Universite Autonoma de Guadalajara in Mexico, where he studied medicine. While there he impressed the doctors, professors, and Catholic nuns with his treatment of a four-year-old polio victim. After working with Trager for just forty minutes, the girl, who had been paralyzed from the waist down for two years, could move her foot in four directions. The university organized a clinic for Trager, where he continued to treat polio victims throughout his years of study.

In 1959 Trager opened a private practice in general medicine and physical rehabilitation in Waikiki, Hawaii. While visiting Los Angeles in 1974, he worked on a patient with muscular dystrophy. At the patient's request Trager agreed to try to teach his approach to the patient's regular therapist. Such attempts in the past had been unsuccessful, but this time Trager first had the therapist place his hands over Trager's own as he worked. Then he had the therapist place his hands on the patient while Trager worked on top of them. Finally, he let the therapist work alone. Trager knew he was successful when the patient exclaimed, "That's it, Doctor, he's got it! It almost feels like you are doing it!"

Trager gave the first public demonstrations of his approach in 1973 at the Esalen Institute in California. There he met Betty Fuller and found he could teach her in the same fashion that he had taught the therapist. Fuller immediately recognized the significance of Trager's work and persuaded him to let her establish an organization that would allow others to study it. The Trager Institute was founded in 1980 with Fuller as director.

By 1977 Trager had closed his private practice in Hawaii to devote all of his time to his growing number of students. At present there are more than nine hundred students throughout the world, more than one thousand certified practitioners, and fifteen certified instructors.

Basic Principles

Trager believes that human beings are the sum total of all the experiences of their lives. These experiences are ingrained in both the body and the mind. Changes in reflex responses, tissue condition, and behavior are possible, he believes, because of the deep neurological associations between sensory stimulations, emotional feelings, attitudes, and concepts, as well as the body's motor response to all of them. He believes that clients should come to him ready to learn more about their bodies and minds rather than simply to receive treatment.

Trager's method of manipulating the body is actually a form of movement reeducation. The Trager practitioner is not concerned with moving particular muscles or joints. Instead, he uses motion in muscles and joints to produce pleasurable feelings. These enter the central nervous system and begin to trigger tissue changes by means of the many motor-sensory feedback loops between the mind and the muscles. The practitioner does not change the condition of tissue with his hands. He uses the hands to remind the nervous system how it can feel.

This feeling elicits tissue response within the client to achieve this relief and pleasure again. Over the course of many sessions a client learns how to move and hold her body in a healthier, more beneficial manner.

Practice

A Trager psychophysical integration session takes from one to one and a half hours. No oils or lotions are used. The client wears a bathing suit or underclothing and lies on a well-padded table in a warm, comfortable environment. The practitioner gently and rhythmically moves the body of the client, first as a whole and then by moving individual limbs and parts, in such a way that the client feels the sensation of free, effortless, and graceful movement.

In order to facilitate a successful bodywork session, the practitioner enters a relaxed state of consciousness known as "hook-up," in which she physically remembers pleasurable sensations. The practitioner transmits these pleasurable sensations through her hands directly to the client's body tissue, encouraging the tissue to release into a lighter and freer physical state. When the Trager practitioner encounters stiffened limbs or hardened muscles, her response is to apply gentle pressure to release tight, painful tissue and restore it to a deeply relaxed physical state. After getting up from the table, the client is given some instruction in the use of mentastics, a system of simple, effortless movement sequences developed by Trager to maintain and enhance the feeling of balance, freedom, and flexibility that was instilled by the table work. Clients can also take workshops focusing on the exercise of mentastics.

Benefits and Risks

For most clients, the effects of a Trager session appear to penetrate below the level of conscious awareness and continue to pro-

Mentastics is a program of do-it-yourself exercises, often given as a kind of homework after a psychophysical integration session. Instruction in mentastic exercise can be given by the practitioner at the end of the bodywork session or in a class. A mentastics class is taught in a workshop format and usually lasts thirty to ninety minutes. The exercises consist of simple, dancelike movements. Students stretch and rock gently and lightly. The objective is to relax and increase range of motion. The exercises are meant to allow the body to feel free and agile, and to release pain or tension.

duce results long after the session itself is over. Benefits include the disappearance of specific symptoms, such as discomfort or pain; heightened levels of energy and vitality; better posture and carriage with less effort; greater joint mobility; a deep relaxation of the body and mind; and a new ease in daily activities.

Although the session involves gentle and light movement and bodywork, it is not advisable for those suffering from joint, bone, and disk disorders; complicated or high-risk pregnancies; broken bones; or blood clots.

—NANCY ALLISON, CMA; WITH DEANE JUHAN

Resources

Trager Institute
21 Locust Ave.
Mill Valley, CA 94941-2806
Tel: (415) 388-2688
Fax: (415) 388-2710
e-mail: TragerD@trager.com
Manages the certification program in Trager psychophysical integration and mentastics movement education. Training is conducted

throughout North America and Europe. The Trager Institute is accredited by the California Nursing Continuing Education Board and the Florida State Massage Board.

Further Reading

Trager, Milton, and Cathy Guadagno. *Trager Mentastics: Movement as a Way to Agelessness.* Barrytown, N.Y.: Station Hill Press, 1987.

PART 10:

Somatic Practices

Somatic practices are movement practices that develop one's mental, emotional, and spiritual experience of life by awakening greater awareness of the sensations of one's physical body as it moves through space. The term *somatics* was coined by the American philosopher Thomas Hanna (1928–1990) in the 1970s. Derived from *soma*, the Greek word for "body," somatics describes "the field of study of the human being as experienced by him- or herself from the inside," according to Hanna. His definition includes many disciplines described in other sections of this encyclopedia. However, part 10 focuses on disciplines that were devised not for relief from a particular ailment or pain, but for those seeking to enhance understanding and awareness of what it means to be fully alive in a human body.

The Development of Movement Practices

Throughout history, various cultures have used movement to impart mental, emotional, or spiritual lessons. T'ai chi ch'üan, one of the oldest extant methods, was developed in China between the years 2205 B.C.E. and 1100 C.E., although its sources can be found in the even more ancient practices of qigong. Called "great dances" by Emperor Yü, one of its earliest developers, t'ai chi's sequence of movements was developed collectively by many generations of philosophers, healers, and artists. All were influenced by Taoism, an ancient Chinese religion that encourages a keen observation of the patterns of movement and change in nature as a means to help human beings understand the physical, mental, and emotional changes that occur during the course of human existence.

Many ancient Western educational and spiritual traditions also developed movement practices. Most of these, including those believed to have been developed by the Greek philosopher and father of geometry, Pythagoras, and those developed by Jewish and Christian esoteric sects, have been lost to us. They were often practiced in

BRAIN GYM®

CONTACT
IMPROVISATION

CONTINUUM

EURYTHMY

GURDJIEFF
MOVEMENTS

PILATES METHOD
OF BODY
CONDITIONING®

ROM DANCE

SKINNER RELEASING
TECHNIQUE

SPATIAL
DYNAMICS℠

T'AI CHI CH'ÜAN

secret and generally frowned upon by the dominant sects of the Judeo-Christian tradition, which condemned the body and its sensations.

For hundreds of years most of Western culture, including its educational methods and spiritual practices, maintained a separation of spirit and flesh, mind and body. In the latter part of the nineteenth century, however, some philosophers began to reexamine the possibility of using physical exercises to promote healthy mental and emotional functioning. One of the best-known explorers of this period was the philosopher George Ivanovitch Gurdjieff (1872–1949), whose "movements for educating the whole person" were inspired by "sacred dances" he observed in a remote part of Central Asia.

As the twentieth century dawned, the concept of learning mental, emotional, and spiritual lessons through body movements began to echo in many quarters. In 1919 the Austrian philosopher Rudolf Steiner (1861–1925) opened the Waldorf Schools to teach eurythmy, his movement practice to promote spiritual growth based on sound vibrations. Working from a different perspective, the German physical culturist Joseph Pilates (1880–1965) developed contrology, now known as the Pilates Method of Body Conditioning®, to free people from the stress and mechanization of living in the industrialized world. Pilates's sequence of exercises borrows heavily from the physical postures and concepts of the practice of hatha yoga.

In recent times the concept of enhancing one's experience of life through movement practices has been embraced by innovators in many other professions. Educational theorists Paul and Gail Dennison developed Brain Gym® as a corollary to contemporary educational practices. Dancer-choreographers Steve Paxton, Emilie Conrad-Da'oud, and Joan Skinner developed contact improvisation, continuum, and Skinner release technique, respectively, from their own creative explorations of movement. Occupational therapists such as Diane Harlowe—one of the originators of ROM dance—and clinical psychologists, such as Jaimen McMillan—the originator of Spatial Dynamics℠—have created new movement sequences that have become popular in many contexts outside their original healing work.

The Laws of Movement

The primary theoretical construct that ties these practices together was first elucidated by the ancient cultures of China, India, and the Middle East and has been given voice in our own time by physicists studying the physical laws governing the universe. This ancient construct holds that the entire universe is in constant motion. As parts of the universe, humans are subject to the same laws of movement. By learning to experience how those laws of movement are reflected in our own bodies, we improve our physical condition. We also develop an intuitive understanding of how these physical principles affect our everyday experience. These physical laws become metaphors for ways of thinking, feeling, and living.

Somatic practices help participants focus on the messages they receive from their bodies and become more aware of their physical sensations in the present moment. Each method begins by teaching a person a physical skill. In some practices, such as t'ai chi ch'üan, Pilates Method, or Spatial Dynamics, the movement patterns are extremely specific and must be precisely replicated. In others, such as contact improvisation, continuum, or Skinner release technique, the form of the movement is spontaneously created by exploring a particular concept of movement. Whether the form is set, like an ancient spatial architecture, or improvised, like a free jazz tune, the process used develops one's sensitivity to subtle changes in the body and its relation to its spatial environment. By developing heightened physical sensitivity, a person can experience freer, more graceful, original, or daring movements, creating a sense of pleasure, accomplishment, or calm.

Experiencing a Somatic Practice

Somatic practices are taught in almost every part of the world today. They may be experienced in public and private schools, at recreation and growth centers, at business seminars, or in private studios. Classes are generally taught in groups, although private instruction is sometimes available. Classes may be geared toward any age level or special needs group. In addition to conditioning the physical body and offering a pleasurable social interaction, these practices seem to imprint themselves on both the body and the imagination of the mover, empowering and freeing him to face the challenges of life. Many participants claim these practices have expanded their sense of connection to the rest of the universe and awareness of what it means to be a human being.

—*Nancy Allison, CMA*

Resources

International Somatic Movement and Education Therapy Association
    148 W. 23rd St., Suite 1H
    New York, NY 10011
    Tel: (212) 229-7666

The Somatics Society
    1516 Grant Ave., Suite 212
    Novato, CA 94945
    Tel: (415) 892-0617
    Fax: (415) 892-4388
    Organization offering seminars and information on many somatic practices. Publishes the biannual magazine-journal *Somatics*.

Further Reading

Arnheim, Rudolf. *Visual Thinking*. Berkeley: University of California Press, 1969.
Gardner, Howard. *Frames of Mind: The Theory of Multiple Intelligences*. New York: Basic Books, 1985.
Hall, Edward T. *The Hidden Dimension*. New York: Doubleday & Co., 1966.
Schneider, Michael S. *A Beginner's Guide to Constructing the Universe*. New York: HarperCollins, 1994.

Brain Gym®

 Brain Gym® is a system of exercises that joins physical and mental development in ways designed to improve a person's ability to learn and perform in all areas of endeavor. The training focuses on linked brain and motor skills but also includes exercises for the release of stress, now considered a major factor in children and adults with learning difficulties. Practice in Brain Gym has been shown to accelerate progress at school for students of all ages and skill levels, and to enhance success at work and in recreational pursuits.

History

Brain Gym was developed by Paul E. Dennison, Ph.D., in the late 1960s. The director of several learning clinics in the Los Angeles area, Dennison was discouraged by inconsistent results in some of his patients. He researched techniques and information from early childhood developmental theory, brain research, developmental optometry, applied kinesiology, language acquisition theory, dance and movement therapy, and his own field of learning theory to formulate a way to improve the skills of his patients. Dennison coined the name "Brain Gym" to describe the movement activities he developed, which were simple enough for anyone to do and effective enough that anyone could benefit.

After the initial success of Brain Gym, Dennison collaborated with his wife, Gail, in exploring its potential as a self-help tool of broad application in business, sports, and the arts. In 1987 they established a research-and-information center on body-mind development, the Educational Kinesiology Foundation, that oversees the training of Brain Gym instructors and coordinates the international network of foundation faculty and Brain Gym instructors.

In 1991 Brain Gym was recognized by the National Learning Foundation (NLF) as one of twelve "successful learning innovations." Established in response to the White House Task Force on Innovative Learning's 1989 Action Plan, the NLF's mission is to make the most effective innovations in education available nationwide.

Theory

Brain Gym is based on theories about the connection of mind and body in the formation of dynamic, balanced intelligence. The human brain has two hemispheres, each in control of one half of the body and a distinct type of mental function. The left hemisphere is in charge of the body's right side and carries out analytic processes, while the right hemisphere activates the left side and works with visual and spatial perception. Though the right "gestalt" hemisphere can absorb large amounts of sensory information simultaneously, it cannot easily express the material without the participation of the left "analytic" hemisphere. According to the Dennisons, modern educational systems are themselves imbalanced since they emphasize left-brain, logic-oriented skills at the expense of the comprehension and creativity of whole-brain learning.

Stress impedes whole-brain learning by stimulating the fight-or-flight reaction in which the body experiences profound physical changes. These changes include elevated pulse and blood pressure, increased breathing rate, slowed digestion, and unfocused vision—all normal, healthy responses to threat, and useful to mobilize energy to escape from or overcome the threat. However, these responses can make learning difficult at best and, if prolonged, can lead to illness. Using movement to activate the parts of the brain where logical, rational thinking takes place, Brain Gym helps the brain to recover from the fight-or-flight response, evaluate the nature of the threat, and respond appropriately. As the brain responds, the overall stress level drops and competence increases. In children, this is crucial to their entire process of growth and change, since stress disturbs the organism at every level of its relationship to the world.

Practice

There are several ways to use Brain Gym. A series of individual sessions with a certified instructor usually gets the quickest results. Each sixty- to ninety-minute session is focused on a specific goal and starts with PACE (positive, active, clear, and energetic), a series of steps that prepares the participant for the work ahead.

The instructor and the student then go through a process called a balance. Together they identify where the brain is working smoothly, and where it is responding less efficiently. The instructor guides the student through basic Brain Gym or in-depth edu-kinesthetics movements, to help the brain make those connections more effectively. Whole-body activities, exercises to activate eye-hand coordination, movements for fine motor coordination, and others may be used depending on each individual's needs.

By the end of the balance, the student notices positive changes in attitude, posture, and skills, and is assigned exercises to do daily at home. These exercises, called homeplay, support and stabilize the cumulative benefits of the balance. Parents are encouraged to do exercises at home with their children, and often the whole family will do Brain Gym together.

Benefits

Today Brain Gym is used in thousands of schools in the United States, Canada, Europe, Australia, New Zealand, Africa, and Russia. Improvements are reported in all areas of academic skills, including self-

In 1991 the White House Task Force on Innovative Learning praised Brain Gym for its effectiveness in improving basic math, reading, and writing skills. Its reputation is now international, and schools in countries such as New Zealand have incorporated Brain Gym into their curricula.

esteem, memory, recall, test-taking, listening and attention, technical and creative writing, reading speed and comprehension, and oral reading and self-expression. People with learning difficulties such as dyslexia, attention deficit disorder, and attention deficit hyperactivity disorder report improved focus, comprehension, and physical coordination with Brain Gym. Reports indicate students get more out of other methods when Brain Gym is added.

—LARK CARROLL

Resources

The Educational Kinesiology Foundation
   P.O. Box 3396
   Ventura, CA 93006-3396
   Tel: 1-800-356-2109
   Web site: www.braingym.com
   Lists Brain Gym instructors, provides copies of the newsletters *Brain Gym Journal* and *Edu-K Update,* and offers schedules of courses.

Further Reading

Dennison, Gail E., and Paul E. Dennison. *Brain Gym.* Ventura, Calif.: Edu-Kinesthetics, Inc., 1986.

———. *Brain Gym: Teacher's Edition.* Rev. ed. Ventura, Calif.: Edu-Kinesthetics, Inc., 1994.

———. *Edu-K for Kids.* Ventura, Calif.: Edu-Kinesthetics, Inc., 1987.

———. *Personalized Whole Brain Integration*. Ventura, Calif.: Edu-Kinesthetics, Inc., 1985.

Dennison, Gail E., Paul E. Dennison, and Jerry V. Teplitz. *Brain Gym for Business*. Ventura, Calif.: Edu-Kinesthetics, Inc., 1995.

Hannaford, Carla. *Smart Moves: Why Learning Is Not All in Your Head*. Arlington, Va.: Great Ocean Publishers, 1995.

Contact Improvisation

 Contact improvisation is a form of dance that explores the relationship of mind and body during interactive touch and improvised movement. Although it is generally performed in group classes and jam sessions and involves ensemble exercises, training in this practice focuses on the skills and the attitudes required to create a duet without cues from a choreographed scenario or speech. In fact, music often is not used in contact improvisation. The process starts by tuning the partners' capacity to "listen" and respond to touch and leads to dancing that ranges freely from gentle gestures to acrobatic movements. In a typical dance, the partners lean, roll, and fall on and with each other; each may also lift or invert the other. At any level of expertise, the dancing builds a momentum that encourages trust, risk-taking, and physical dialogue from participants. Contact improvisation is best known as a component of professional dance, but awareness of its psychological and physical benefits has made it increasingly popular as an "art sport" for amateurs. During the past few years, it has also been approached as a mode of mind-body healing and as an adjunct to the martial arts of Asia.

History

Although contact improvisation is now included in the repertoire of many dancers, it originated in the 1960s amid a wave of experiments that challenged the traditions governing the conception and presentation of dance. Stylized movement, mythic narrative, and stage spectacle were jettisoned in an effort, led first by the Merce Cunningham ensemble and later the Judson Church Group, to find ways to connect dance to the realities of contemporary life. Judson Church productions featured movement taken from work, sports, and the martial arts and often investigated ordinary activity, such as sweeping a floor. What was eventually called contact improvisation first appeared in 1972 in "Magnesium," a piece presented by Steve Paxton, a choreographer and dancer who had been a member of both Cunningham and Judson Church. The dancers of "Magnesium" did not attempt to "perform" anything; they instead reacted to one another, improvising their movements and going with the flow of the experience. Later in 1972, Paxton presented a performance evolved from "Magnesium," which retained the use of a group of improvising dancers but focused on the interaction of mixed- and same-sex partners. This performance became the prototype for his subsequent work in contact improvisation.

Assisted by teachers such as Nancy Stark Smith and Daniel Lepkoff, Paxton offered workshops and performances in contact improvisation. By the late 1970s Paxton's group had its own publication, the *Contact Newsletter*, later renamed the *Contact Quarterly*, and was becoming a major force in the development of postmodern dance. Dance companies that based their work on contact improvisation were mushrooming in the United States, and by the early 1980s dancers in cultural centers throughout the world, especially Amsterdam, Berlin, and London, were adapting its principles.

Contact improvisation entered the world of body-mind therapy through an outpouring of popular support. It had been attracting a huge amateur following during the 1970s and 1980s and gradually made its way into the curricula of many colleges and universities. In this context of self-discovery and liberal arts study, contact improvisation began to be viewed as a technique accessible to those interested in enhancing their understanding of body-mind communication. For some, contact improvisation became a complement to the practice of t'ai chi, aikido, or yoga. For others, it offered a means of helping children, senior citizens, and people with disabilities. Today three organizations, Touchdown, DanceAbility, and Mobility Junction, are at the forefront of the work being done to incorporate contact improvisation into therapy programs for people with special needs.

Basic Principles

Despite the diversity of its sources and improvised structures, contact improvisation has a remarkably consistent look and feel, whether done by professional or amateur dancers. This is because, like a conversation, it has a few ground rules that participants understand and follow as they meet and exchange responses. Trust is a top priority. The dancers need to release tension and uncertainty and meet one another in an open, relaxed way, otherwise they will not be able to establish the connection that is essential to the process of reciprocal improvisation. Trust and physical listening are key factors in determining the actions of the dancers. They drop concern for the look of the body in order to concentrate on the flow of energy between themselves and their partners. The outcome is a collaborative process described as "a cross between jitterbugging, wrestling, and making love." Dancers focus on the physical sensations of touching, leaning, supporting, and falling with one another. Awkwardness matters only if it is a symptom of one dancer's lack of focus and withdrawal from the spontaneous release into the here and now of physical experience. The emphasis on being present in the moment links contact improvisation to the martial arts, yoga, and meditation. All these disciplines encourage the individual to let go of blocks that prevent him from apprehending the energy that constantly courses between mind and body.

Practice

Students work with one another, learning to establish connection through light physical touch and to move together in a shared kinesphere. A kinesphere may be pictured as a bubble of space in which the body moves. It is usually envisioned as the 360 degrees of space encircling an individual, but in contact improvisation the kinesphere is the joint creation of dancers who become adept at falling and rolling together, sliding off each other, spiraling around, and leaning into each other. They learn to find "tables," or body surfaces, on one partner that can support the balanced weight of the other.

The structure of a class in contact improvisation depends on the teacher's particular interests and on the needs and abilities of individual students. Beginning-level classes concentrate on the basic skills for performing duet and group improvisation. Exercises in touch increase the skin's ability to register information about the speed and angle of movement. Other exercises help the body to release and become receptive. Students learn to roll and slide on the floor and on each other with ease, to use the body's surfaces for support, to flow with the momentum of movement, to reverse and invert the body's orientation, and to circle and spiral in space.

More complex duet and group improvisation is the focus of classes at the intermediate and advanced levels. Mastery of an exercise known as "flying" is often the last skill to be taught. The dancers vault in the air, are caught by their partners, and perch momentarily over the head of their partner. Gender equality is valued at this as at all levels of training: men lift women and vice versa.

A portion of each class is generally reserved for free-form dancing by students. The action is likely to begin in a round robin. Some members of the group improvise as the others form a circle around them. As the dancing proceeds, the organization of the round robin becomes increasingly fluid. People join and leave the dancing at will, improvise with various partners, or dance alone.

Benefits and Risks

Though injuries are rare in contact improvisation, it is a strenuous activity and many participants take the precaution of wearing kneepads. It is also advisable to review one's personal boundaries before taking up this therapy. Those with a history of trauma or abuse may find it disturbing.

Advocates regard contact improvisation as a unique blend of sport, art, and meditation and credit it with numerous health benefits. It can release tension, promote an overall sense of well-being and ease, boost vitality, and aid concentration. Further, as a nonsexual form of intimacy, it affords a safe way to sort through volatile issues of gender, trust, bonding, control, and spontaneity in human relationships. Some proponents add that contact improvisation is most effective and complete when experienced as a metaphor for the movement and change that pervades all aspects of late twentieth-century life.

—PAUL LANGLAND

Resources

Contact Collaborations
c/o Forti Studio
537 Broadway
New York, NY 10012
Provides information about contact improvisation training and performance; maintains a video archive of contact improvisation.

Contact Quarterly
P.O. Box 603
Northampton, MA 01061
Tel: (413) 586-1181
A journal with articles on contact improvisation and an international directory of contact improvisers.

Movement Research
296 Elizabeth St.
New York, NY 10012
Provides information about contact improvisation classes.

Further Reading

Novack, Cynthia J. *Sharing the Dance: Contact Improvisation and American Culture.* Madison: University of Wisconsin Press, 1990.

Continuum

Continuum, a movement program developed by Emilie Conrad-Da'oud in 1967, encourages participants to resonate with the motions and rhythms of our primordial origins, which are subtle, undulating movements pulsing in the fluids of our bodies. One of the benefits of this practice is to facilitate the release of mental and physical illness from the body and promote health through engagement on a biological level.

History

Continuum springs from the work of one woman, Emilie Conrad-Da'oud, who was born in New York City in 1934. A classically trained dancer, she spent five years as a choreographer in Haiti in the late 1950s. Upon her return to the United States in 1960, Conrad-Da'oud remained fascinated with the throbbing drum rhythms of Haitian music and dance. She wondered if the richness of Haitian dance might draw from roots deeper than culture, and whether its power might stem from a biological source.

Guided by all that she had absorbed from the richness of the sacred dances of Haiti, Conrad-Da'oud spent seven years deconstructing their movements and exploring their origins. Inspired by Damballah, the snake deity from the vodou religion of Haiti, she gained insight into the powerful origins of these movements. As a serpent with its belly to the earth, Damballah brought the undulating movements of the water to land, and it was these motions that Conrad-Da'oud recognized in Haitian sacred dances as a link between humankind's water-based origins and our current, land-based lives.

From 1974 to 1979 Conrad-Da'oud's work was researched by Dr. Valerie Hunt, professor of kinesiology at UCLA. Hunt's findings questioned conventional notions of movement education at the time. She found that through a practice such as continuum, we can access our own cellular world, or effect changes in our bodies on a cellular level, and encourage our bodies' capacity to innovate when faced with injury or illness.

Many movement education programs deal with the body as an object, whereas continuum presents it as a process. Continuum explores the body on a fluid and cellular level, believing the body is not bounded by form; there is a constant exchange in our fluids and cells with those of the environment, and we are in continual participation with the planetary process.

These ideas have influenced the fields of dance, physical therapy, and deep tissue therapy, as well as disciplines such as chiropractic, physical fitness, and somatics. People from many different disciplines in the alternative health community explore continuum and apply to their own practices the idea of the human being as a fluid, innovative, boundless being, with movement inherent to our very selves.

Theory

The continuum program represents Conrad-Da'oud's distillation of Damballah's wave-like motions with our own human biology. A human's first environment, in the uterus, is liquid. According to Conrad-Da'oud, our fluid origin is inseparable from our surrounding environment. In other words, the fluids of the biosphere resonate with the fluid of our bodies, and we are in concert with our world. For these reasons, continuum holds that human beings are primarily aquatic and become terrestrial.

Conrad-Da'oud also sees human beings as "biomorphic," which means that we include all life-forms. We are all part of a larger process, along with other animals, plants, and Earth itself. Conrad-Da'oud emphasizes that the human body emerges from the matings of earlier life, from protozoa to mammals, the vestiges of which lie within us, along with the vastness of biological intelligence.

Continuum encourages participants to explore themselves as biomorphic beings and to establish a mental and physical rapport with the various life-forms within them. Participants allow their primordial movements—which curve, arc, and spiral—to emerge. Through rapport with our biological heritage, Conrad-Da'oud has found that our complex fluidity can provide an environment for creativity and innovation to occur. In relation to "healing," the suggestion is made that innovation can create neural pathways that can bypass trauma, allowing life to move on in new and surprising ways.

Practice and Benefits

Conrad-Da'oud's work involves a great deal of attention to the movement of breath. All movement begins with inhaling and exhaling. By invoking a softening of the breath, participants of continuum disrupt habitual patterns and encourage an increased mobility of breath to access greater flexibility and adaptability. This new dexterity of breath invigorates nerve fibers and connective tissues that have become entrenched in the old patterns. Ultimately, these breathing exercises increase our capacity to receive cellular nourishment and bring about a healing environment to areas that have become barren and atrophied.

Physical and emotional trauma and genetic deformities sometimes leave the body with limited functionality. Among the paralyzed, for example, the traditional neural pathways have been injured. By breathing in a manner that creates a wavelike motion, we can cause micromovements to spread into dormant areas, often returning function to areas that traditional medicine cannot affect.

Continuum, more than anything else, provides a context for questioning and comprehending not just physical movement but all aspects of our functioning. Our whole thinking-feeling-moving-electrochemical-electromagnetic organism participating within its biological and cultural environment can be lived as one unbroken movement. Participants come to understand that our responsibilities, the significance and meanings we give our world, can be seen as one process of flowing movement.

—COMPILED IN CONSULTATION WITH EMILIE
CONRAD-DA'OUD

Resources

Continuum Studio
    1629 18th St., Suite 7
    Santa Monica, CA 90404
    Tel: (310) 453-4402
    Fax: (310) 453-8775
    Offers workshops in continuum.

Eurythmy

Eurythmy is a movement art that translates verbal and musical sounds into movement of the human body. According to eurythmy, there are three basic ways in which life expresses itself: movement, form, and language. By integrating these elemental expressions of life and creating a harmonious expression of them, eurythmy is believed to reach the spiritual nature behind all living things, giving this nature a clear voice and a visible reality.

History

Eurythmy was conceived in 1912 by Rudolf Steiner, the Austrian-born founder of the spiritual movement known as Anthroposophy. *Eurythmy* is a Greek term meaning "harmonious rhythm" and was chosen because Steiner saw rhythm as the very basis and center of life. Around the time that he began to consider the notion of eurythmy, Steiner founded the Anthroposophical Society, a movement intended to help further his teachings, particularly his belief in the existence of a spiritual realm that can be perceived by people with highly developed mental faculties.

A philosopher and visionary, Steiner asserted that all human beings—with proper training and preparation—have the potential to participate in the spiritual world. To this end, he devised a system of education called the Waldorf School movement, which uses such disciplines as eurythmy to teach individuals from the earliest age about their inner spirituality and their relationship to the world around them. Eurythmy also can be performed on stages before audiences or employed as a therapy for treating various types of illness. There are currently more than thirty eurythmy training centers located throughout the world.

Basic Principles

In eurythmy the human voice and language are often used as the basis for movement. Human sound can be thought of as carrying all of life within it. The name of a thing, a person, or an experience can be seen as more than just a separate description. The sounds chosen to represent something can be seen as a reenactment of the unique spiritual and physical qualities of the thing in question, as holding the essential qualities of the thing itself. When eurythmy is performed, the gestures are not symbols; they are expressions of the essence of the thing itself.

The human voice is a remarkable instrument, capable of transforming our inner experiences into another medium—sound. When the sounds of language and song are intoned, they set into motion unique yet invisible waves or gestures through the air. In eurythmy these gestures are artistically expressed to reveal the outer forms belonging to each consonant or vowel, each musical tone or interval.

Philosophy

For Steiner, eurythmy was not a physical illustration or interpretation of language and music, but instead a true expression of sound through the body. Claiming to see a shifting field of energy around each human being, Steiner identified a system of body movements that correspond to the shapes of the energy field as it responds to each spoken word and musical sound. To the uninformed, eurythmy may seem to be a mix of mime, dance, and sign language performed to music, singing, or spoken word. Steiner, however, declared that eurythmic movements are equivalent to sound, not artistic representations of it. To him, eurythmy is one means of assisting humankind in returning to an earlier state in which people were more aware of their inner being and the invisible processes of the world. In *An Introduction to Eurythmy,* Steiner stated: "The seeds of movement are manifest in the human larynx and its neighboring organs when someone speaks . . . or when he produces musical sounds. If one had some artificial device by which one could see at such a moment how the air mass is stirred to rhythmic vibration by the incipient movements of the larynx and its neighboring organs, he would realize . . . how the entire man is revealed through it."

Practice

In studying eurythmy, a person learns about the different qualities found in the sounds of language and tones of music. Classes begin with movement exercises that help students better understand and feel more comfortable with space, with people around them, and with their own movements. Subsequently, one is taught specific movements or gestures that correspond to each letter of the alphabet. Initially, movements are acted out in silence, and later they are performed in collaboration with live music or spoken words. In a speech eurythmy class, students examine the elements of language Steiner felt appeared in poetry, drama, and fiction. In a tone eurythmy class, they study the gestures Steiner believed were inherent in music. Performance of eurythmy on a stage can incorporate colorful costumes and dramatic lighting, which heighten the mood created by the actors and musicians.

Benefits

Students who have studied eurythmy at Waldorf schools reportedly benefit from improved coordination, agility, flexibility, and a greater sense of physical well-being; for these reasons, eurythmy is also commonly used as therapy. Group practice creates a strong sense of teamwork, as individuals jointly overcome their reluctance to use physical expression in public. Furthermore, since eurythmy is taught as a means to explore the psyche, this very personal, revealing experience can have the effect of bonding those who undergo the process with others. Steiner insisted that the most important benefit is mental: decreased dependence on the world of the senses and increased perception of the spiritual world.

—Beth Dunn-Fox

Resources

Anthroposophic Press
  P.O. Box 960
  Herndon, VA 20172
  Tel: (703) 661-1594; 1-800-856-8664
  Fax: (703) 661-1501; 1-800-277-9747
  Publishes many Rudolf Steiner texts, including several on eurythmy. A catalog is available on request.

Eurythmy Association of North America
  c/o Maria Ver Eecke
  Editor, *Eurythmy Newsletter*
  Tel: (845) 356-1380
  Web site: www.eurythmy@bestweb.net
  Publishes quarterly newsletter with information on courses for professional eurythmists and interested nonprofessionals.

Eurythmy Spring Valley
  260 Hungry Hollow Road
  Chestnut Ridge, NY 10977
  Tel: (914) 352-5020
  Fax: (914) 352-5071
  e-mail: info@eurythmy.org

Provides a professional training program accredited by the Association of Eurythmy in Dornach, Switzerland. Weekly courses and summer workshops are also offered for those interested in experiencing eurythmy for refreshment and self-development.

Waldorf Schools in North America
  Web site: www.io.com/user/karisch/waldir.html
  Waldorf schools, many of which offer eurythmy classes for children, teens, and adults, are located throughout the United States and Canada.

Further Reading

Steiner, Rudolf. *Curative Eurythmy.* Hudson, N.Y.: Anthroposophic Press, 1984.
———. *Eurythmy as Visible Speech.* Hudson, N.Y.: Anthroposophic Press, 1984.
———. *An Introduction to Eurythmy: Talks Given Before Sixteen Eurythmy Performances.* Hudson, N.Y.: Anthroposophic Press, 1983.
———. *A Lecture on Eurythmy.* London: Rudolf Steiner Press, 1977.

Gurdjieff Movements

 The Gurdjieff movements were developed by the Armenian teacher George Ivanovitch Gurdjieff as a way for his pupils to experience in movement the reality of his teaching. Practice of the Gurdjieff movements has meaning only when undertaken in the context of an entire program of activities and study of the system of Gurdjieff's ideas. The movements aim to bring together the mind, body, and feelings through the performance of different exercises, rhythmic sequences, series of postures, and dances.

History

George Ivanovitch Gurdjieff was born in 1872 in Alexandropol, now known as Gumri, in what is now Armenia. He was raised and educated in Russian Armenia at a time and place in which there was a confluence of new technologies and scientific ideas of the West with the traditions, thought, and religions of the East.

In his autobiographical account, *Meetings with Remarkable Men* (published posthumously in 1963), he writes of his father, a well-known *ashokh*, or bard, who was part of an oral tradition stretching back to the distant past. The legends that he heard from his father left a mark on his whole life. His tutors, men of science and religion, trained him for both the priesthood and medicine, and he pursued his studies with burning interest. In *Meetings with Remarkable Men*, Gurdjieff describes several close escapes from death as well as encounters with "magic" and other manifestations of realities beyond the explanations of science and logic. As he came of age in the midst of these unfathomable mysteries and inexplicable events, Gurdjieff felt dissatisfied with the answers of contemporary knowledge and began his search for other sources of wisdom. He and fellow seekers of truth—young people with questions similar to his own, including engineers, doctors, archaeologists, and musicians—journeyed for several years through central Asia and northern Africa to find the answers to their questions about the meaning of life. Eventually they found a school in a remote, nearly inaccessible monastery, whose exact location remains a mystery. It was here that Gurdjieff first witnessed sacred dances.

Gurdjieff came to Moscow in the early 1900s with a teaching that attracted groups of artists and intellectuals, including P. D. Ouspensky (1878–1947), one of his best-known disciples. As the Russian Revolution drew near, Gurdjieff and a small group of followers moved to Tiflis (now Tbilisi, Georgia) and established the Institute for the Harmonious Development of Man. It was here that he first taught sacred gymnastics, now known as the movements. He was joined at this time by the composer Thomas de Hartmann and his wife, and by the Russian painter Alexandre de Salzmann and his wife, Jeanne, a teacher of Dalcroze eurythmics, a study of the relationship between music and movement. When World War I made it impossible for Gurdjieff to continue his work there, he and his pupils continued their journey to Essentuki, Russia, in 1917, to Istanbul, Turkey, in 1920, and finally to France. In 1922 he reestablished the Institute for the Harmonious Development of Man at the Chateau du Prieuré at Fontainebleau, near Paris. During the 1920s and 1930s Gurdjieff further developed many of the central methods and practices of his teaching, including the movements. His work began to attract people throughout Europe, and in 1924 he visited America for the first time.

During the years between 1924 and 1935, Gurdjieff spent less time at the institute, focusing most of his energy and attention on writing. After 1935, assisted by Jeanne de Salzmann, he expanded the work of the institute in France and visited the United States three more times, expanding his work there. He died in Paris on October 29, 1949.

For forty years after Gurdjieff's death, his primary pupil, Jeanne de Salzmann, guided the ongoing efforts of Gurdjieff Foundation groups throughout the world. She oversaw the publication of his writings, and between 1950 and 1984 she produced a series of documentary films of the movements as an archive of Gurdjieff's teaching. Today movement classes are part of a program of activities conducted at the Gurdjieff Foundations in Paris, London, New York, Caracas, and other major cities. The Gurdjieff work remains an oral tradition, passed from teacher to pupil in a living chain of transmission.

At the heart of Gurdjieff's teaching is the perspective that human beings are a vital link in a universal process. Unfortunately, they are "asleep" as to their unique cosmic place and as to the full potential of their individual essential natures. Each person is like someone who lives in the smallest room of her house, never suspecting there are other rooms filled with treasure.

According to Gurdjieff's teaching, what is needed in order to discover each person's own hidden treasure is a new kind of attention that comes from the physical and emotional sides of one's nature as well as from the mind. Gurdjieff was a merciless critic of the usual kind of education, which he said only "stuffs" the mind with unrelated information and opinions. He constantly told his pupils that they should verify for themselves everything he taught and accept nothing until they had personally experienced its truth.

Practice

With the aim of an education for the whole human being, Gurdjieff introduced the study of ideas, group meetings, practical physical work, and the movements. Participation in the movements is one of the primary means through which students are able to experience the power that mechanical habits such as posture, tension, and facial expression have over their inner states. The practice of experiencing one's actual way of being, or self-study, according to Gurdjieff, is the beginning of self-knowledge and inner freedom. Practice of the movements offers the opportunity for such study and the foretaste of such a liberating knowledge.

The task of the dancers is to learn to participate with the whole of themselves. What is seen is the movement itself, as if the series of postures were the outer image of an inner and subtler energy. Understood in this way, one realizes that the aim of the movements is not to create a psychic state of some kind, but to develop a specific attention leading to an immediate and practical experience of the inner structure of the human being and of the cosmological order to which humanity belongs.

Movements classes are composed of students working together in a group, with more experienced pupils directing and guiding the course of each class. There are exercises of different qualities, including movements of forceful dynamism and quiet prayer, men's and women's dances, and exercises that demonstrate the cyclic movements of mathematical laws. Each dance or exercise is composed of sequences of fixed postures executed in specific rhythms and tempos in which a demand is made to stretch the attention beyond its usual limits. Practicing these exercises, one finds it possible to truly inhabit the body; from there, one may then open to the transformative power that an improved quality of attention can bring.

The music used to accompany the sacred dances comes from various sources. Gurdjieff had a keen sensitivity to and memory for the music he had heard since his early childhood and during his travels in Asia. Between 1919 and 1924, he began to write music for the sacred dances in close collaboration with the composer Thomas de Hartmann. Later, de Hartmann and others expanded this literature, and pianists ac-

During his youth, Gurdjieff traveled to regions of Central Asia in search of answers to the questions that tormented him. In remote monasteries, he first witnessed certain sacred dances that made a lasting impression on him. This is dramatized in Peter Brook's film *Meetings with Remarkable Men*, when the young Gurdjieff asks, "What is the meaning of these movements?" An older pupil answers, "They tell us of two qualities of energy moving without interruption through the body. As long as the dancer can keep in balance these two energies, he has a force that nothing else can give."

companying today's movements classes play these earlier compositions as well as improvise music based on similar scales and harmonies. The task of the pianist, like the pupils working in the class, is to seek to understand the meaning of each exercise as it is being practiced.

Benefits

The study of the Gurdjieff movements, when undertaken in conjunction with the study of his system of ideas, offers the means for inner discovery and development. Through this practice, the mind and the feelings are able to combine with the movements of the body to express the potential of the whole human being.

—THE GURDJIEFF FOUNDATION OF NEW YORK

Further Reading

Gurdjieff, G. I. *Beelzebub's Tales to His Grandson.* Aurora, Ore.: Two Rivers Press, 1993. (A facsimile of the original 1950 edition published by Harcourt Brace and reissued by E. P. Dutton in 1964.)

———. *Beelzebub's Tales to His Grandson.* New York and London: Viking Arkana, 1992. (A revised translation of the original.)

———. *Meetings with Remarkable Men.** New York: E. P. Dutton, 1963; New York and London: Arkana, 1985.

———. *Life Is Real Only Then, When "I Am."* New York: E. P. Dutton, 1978; New York and London: Viking Arkana, 1991.

———. *Views from the Real World: Early Talks in Moscow, Essentuki, Tiflis, Berlin, London, Paris, New York, and Chicago as Recollected by His Pupils.* New York: E. P. Dutton, 1973; London: Viking Arkana, 1984.

Ouspensky, P. D. *In Search of the Miraculous: Fragments of an Unknown Teaching.* New York: Harcourt Brace and World, 1949.

———. *The Psychology of Man's Possible Evolution.* New York: Knopf, 1954.

*The film *Meetings with Remarkable Men,* created by Jeanne de Salzmann and Peter Brook, is available on videocassette through Corinth Video.

Pilates Method of Body Conditioning®

The Pilates Method of Body Conditioning® consists of a series of exercises designed to develop a complete and balanced individual by strengthening and stretching the body while fully engaging the mind. Founded more than seventy years ago by Joseph Pilates, this method has become quite popular among dancers and professional athletes. While the exercises may appear to be only physical, there is a conscious aspect that is essential. Students use concentration and mental focus to control body alignment and breathing and to perform exercises with grace and control. The exercises are intended to create a graceful efficiency in one's everyday movements. Many practitioners also report a direct "mental rejuvenation" as a result of performing these exercises.

History

Joseph H. Pilates was born in Germany in 1880, a frail and sickly child who suffered from rickets and asthma. Determined to be strong and healthy, Pilates worked extremely hard at bodybuilding, and by the time he was fourteen years old, he had become so physically fit that he was able to pose for anatomical charts. He then went on to become a boxer, diver, skier, and gymnast.

In 1912 Pilates moved to England, where he continued his boxing training and taught self-defense classes. During World War I he was interned with other German nationals on the Isle of Man. While there he began devising his personal exercise methods and started designing special equipment. He also helped rehabilitate injured internees and encouraged others to practice his technique in order to stay healthy.

Pilates left England for America in 1923, and on the way he met and married a woman whose own ideas about exercise fused with and encouraged his. Together they founded the first Pilates studio in New York City.

For many years the Pilates Method was extremely popular among dancers and professional performers in New York City, while it remained virtually unknown elsewhere. Dancers embrace the method for its ability to fine-tune the body, giving the dancer great strength and energy while maintaining long, lean muscles with tremendous flexibility. In more recent years this system's popularity has grown to encompass people of all ages and all stages of fitness. Today physical therapists, chiropractors, and other medical professionals are recommending and adopting Pilates as a means of rehabilitation and preventive medicine, and certified studios now can be found throughout the world.

Philosophy

Joseph Pilates believed that fitness required more than just physical education. He believed in the development of the whole person—body, mind, and spirit—and referred to his unique system of exercise as the "art of contrology." In his book *Return to Life,* he states, "Contrology develops the body uniformly, corrects wrong postures, restores physical vitality, invigorates the mind, and elevates the spirit." With improved physical functioning, one's endurance improves, allowing more time and energy for what he called "playing," spending quality time with family and friends, enjoying a movie or a

play, or reading a book. Pilates believed that having increased energy for such activities would undoubtedly have a positive effect on one's mind and spirit.

Basic Principles

Control, centering, precision, and flowing movement are the key principles of the Pilates Method. Throughout a session, one concentrates on all of these aspects. To be effective, the movements must be performed correctly according to precise standards. For this reason, concentration is considered as important as the physical movements. The mind focuses on controlling all aspects of the movement: maintaining body alignment; doing exercises exactly as indicated by the instructor; using graceful, flowing movements; and keeping the breath flowing. An essential element of the Pilates Method is the concept of the body's "center," referred to as the "powerhouse of the anatomy." This circular "belt" around the body encompasses the lower back and abdominals; an immediate benefit one feels as a result of practicing Pilates is strength in the abdominal muscles and relief of chronic lower back discomfort.

Practice

Today the Pilates studios and classes look strange yet elegant with equipment, mats, and various apparati, all built to Joseph Pilates's specifications. Although there are several machines used, the main piece of equipment is known as the universal reformer. It looks similar to the frame of a single bed with a sliding carriage attached to four springs. After adjusting the number of springs to regulate the resistance, the student pushes or pulls against a metal bar or straps. The exercises are done sitting, lying down, kneeling, and standing. Emphasis is not on maximum resistance but on the student's ability to work with and control the springs. The springs help with a stretching and contracting action in the muscles.

Individuals may begin practicing Pilates at any level of fitness. The exercises are learned slowly, and strength is built gradually. Students are encouraged to progress at their own rate. Once fundamental exercises have been mastered, new and more challenging ones are introduced, each in a particular order, thus building up a repertoire of exercises. There are hundreds of various exercises and, depending on the individual's progress, as many of these will be taught as deemed necessary by the instructor.

At the initial session, the client's physical history is discussed. A certified instructor then takes the student through the initial series of exercises from beginning to end. An experienced instructor will be able to assess a person's particular strengths and weaknesses quickly and gauge what exercises are to be included in, or omitted from, the personal routine. From the beginning, basic principles are taught, including how to engage lower abdominal muscles, how to roll through the spinal column evenly and smoothly, and how to maintain correct body posture and alignment.

While there is a specific sequence to the system, lessons are customized to suit the individual, with special problems taken into account. Each person does a complete series of exercises on specialized equipment and on a flat cushioned mat; in Pilates, the apparatus work and mat work are of equal importance. Within each exercise, repetitions are kept to a minimum, focusing on quality rather than quantity. This allows for a high level of concentration and precise, careful movements and ensures that muscles are never worked to exhaustion. The instructor often sets the rhythm, keeping the workout dynamic and energetic, yet always gentle and never hurried. One rarely hears music or chatting because students are encouraged to concentrate fully on the exercises and on their breathing. Many studios offer small group classes with rarely more than four students per instructor. Once a student has learned to perform the basic exercises correctly and confidently, he can choose to supplement studio time with work done at home on a cushioned mat. Students can generally expect results after approximately ten consistent lessons, although some react more quickly.

The Pilates Method always considers the body as a whole rather than separate body parts. Every exercise will engage the entire body while paying particular attention to one main muscle group. At the end of each session, the whole body is stretched and strengthened equally. Although a person's heart rate may increase, the Pilates Method is complementary to rather than a replacement for aerobic exercise.

Benefits

Depending on the individual, benefits of using Pilates exercises may include improved posture, leaner muscles, improved overall strength (especially in the abdominal region), greater flexibility, general ease of movement, relief of chronic aches, more energy and endurance, and a higher level of concentration and focus in all aspects of one's life. An added benefit is that students invariably leave a Pilates studio feeling invigorated.

—LEAH CHABACK, CERTIFIED INSTRUCTOR AND TEACHER TRAINER

Resources

The Movement Center
　39 Broadway
　Kingston, NY 12401
　Tel: (914) 331-0986
　A certified, fully equipped Pilates studio that offers private, semiprivate, and group lessons.

The Pilates Studio
  2121 Broadway
  New York, NY 10023
  Tel: 1-800-4-PILATES (474-5283)
  e-mail: mrpilates@aol.com
  Web site: www.pilates-studio.com
  A certified, fully equipped Pilates studio.

Further Reading

Friedman, Philip, and Gail Eisen. *The Pilates Method of Physical and Mental Conditioning.* New York: Warner Books, 1981.

Pilates, Joseph, and William John Miller. *Return to Life Through Contrology.* Boston: Christopher Publishing House, 1960.

ROM Dance

 ROM dance is an exercise and relaxation program created for people with chronic pain and other physical limitations. ROM is the acronym used in physical therapy to describe the range of motion as flexibility of joints. These exercises, recommended by doctors and therapists, are combined with the basic principles of t'ai chi ch'üan, an ancient Chinese exercise practiced for health and longevity. T'ai chi ch'üan trains the participant to be calm while alert, to be both strong and flexible, and to relax in the midst of activity. These elements are applied to ROM dancing, teaching the participant to move gently and slowly in order to maintain the ability to move in spite of pain. It also allows the participant to develop sensitivity to subtle changes in the body that may eventually reduce pain and limitations. Through regular practice, this slow, fluid exercise is purported to enhance mental focus, body awareness, and imagination.

History

ROM dance was created in 1981 by Diane Harlowe, M.S., an occupational therapist and researcher, and Tricia Yu, M.A., a t'ai chi instructor and health educator, at St. Mary's Hospital in Madison, Wisconsin. Patients had complained that their exercises were boring and monotonous. Harlowe and Yu designed this unique routine of stretches and movements to encourage their patients to keep moving every day.

The program had the following objectives: assisting and inspiring the participants in following any medical recommendations for involvement in daily exercise/rest routines; increasing frequency, enjoyment, and perceived benefit of involvement in daily exercise and rest; enhancing the ability to cope with stress and pain through use of relaxation techniques; improving body awareness; and promoting a general sense of well-being.

Originally designed as an eight-week community health education program, it is now taught by physical and occupational therapists, nurses, dance and recreation therapists, and t'ai chi ch'üan instructors in hospitals, senior centers, nursing homes, outpatient clinics, private homes, and rehabilitation clinics.

Basic Principles

The seven major ROM dance principles are adapted from the ancient body-mind principles of t'ai chi ch'üan. Attention to the present awakens all the senses of the ROM dance practitioner as she is guided to look, listen, smell, and feel all the physical sensations coming to and from the body-mind. Diaphragmatic breathing and postural alignment help relax and nourish the body and mind. As a result, the respiratory and musculoskeletal systems function more fully and easily than before. Moving more slowly than normal enhances awareness of movement sensation and builds strength as well as sensitivity in the body and the mind. Avoiding unnecessary tension or force creates relaxed movement, which encourages healthy functioning of the circulatory and nervous systems. Exercising the imagination by reciting poetic images from nature while doing the ROM dance seems to evoke soothing, nurturing, healing feelings of warmth and a sense of personal involvement and - well-being.

Practice

ROM dance, which takes about seven minutes to complete, can be performed either sitting and standing. It incorporates movement in all ranges for the large joints, and includes a special exercise routine for the small joints of the hands.

The program includes instruction in both exercise and relaxation. It is designed to be practiced as a daily routine to help maintain flexibility. The relaxation and pain management training provides participants with strategies for relaxing both during periods of rest and when dealing with stress or pain in the middle of daily activities.

Benefits and Risks

The program can help people with a variety of disabilities maintain a range of motion and cope with stress and pain. It can also be used as the warm-up and cool-down phases of more extensive exercise programs.

ROM dance is based on movements usually recommended for rheumatoid arthritis. It has also successfully contributed to the treatment of fibromyalgia, psychiatric and neurological conditions, Parkinson's disease, stress, chronic or severe pain, lupus, and cancer, among other conditions.

Those interested in learning and practicing ROM dance should be advised that it is not a substitute for medically recommended

exercise therapy unless approved or modified by a physician or therapist. Also, the following risks should be noted: people with severe neck problems or hip replacements should check with their doctors before attempting the movements; dancers should avoid straining or forcing any movements and should personally modify them when necessary; and those using this dance program should always apply proper body mechanics when standing and sitting.

Because the movements of ROM dance are gentle and take only a few minutes a day to perform, nearly everyone—including individuals in wheelchairs—can do them. The program may improve flexibility and mobility while promoting a general sense of relaxation in a safe, slow, and gentle manner.

—PATRICIA YU, M.A.

Resources

The ROM Dance Network
P.O. Box 3332
Madison, WI 53704-0332
Tel: (608) 242-9133
Fax: (608) 242-9140
Links practitioners and professionals, disseminates information and instructional materials, and organizes seminars and training workshops. Provides the ROM Dance Multimedia Instructional Kit, available to both professionals and individuals for personal home practice. It includes videos for both standing and wheelchair exercise, guided relaxation and music audiotapes, and a text for instructors.

Skinner Releasing Technique

 The Skinner releasing technique (SRT) is a movement discipline used to alleviate physical pain and tension. Based on the philosophy that all human beings have the potential to move with natural grace, SRT taps into intrinsic, primal coordination and the experience of movement at a deep kinesthetic level by using movement along with poetry, music, and imagery. It encourages people to understand how their bodies move and to visualize how their bodies can function without discomfort.

History

Joan Skinner danced in the companies of Martha Graham and Merce Cunningham during the late forties and early fifties. Between ballet class in the morning and modern dance class in the afternoon, she began to explore dance technique on her own in her apartment in Greenwich Village, New York. Skinner used an old banister as a barre and set up mirrors so that she could see herself at the three-fourths angle from the front and back simultaneously. She kept a notebook in which she posed questions about the techniques she was learning in her dance classes. Teachers at that time used the commands "pull up—grip—hold on," and she wondered how one could breathe as nature intended while gripping and holding. Then, after suffering a back injury that would not heal, she was advised to consult an instructor who specialized in the Alexander technique—one of only three such instructors in the country at that time. The Alexander technique made sense to Joan because it did not compress the body with gripping but opened and extended it in a multidirectional way. It facilitated natural breathing, and it

took the pressure off her injury so that it could heal.

After leaving New York, Joan spent three years working alone to develop what is now known as SRT. She began by applying the Alexander principles to ballet barre movements. In searching for that multidirectional balance, the barre exercises broke down to where she spent time balancing on one leg without gripping and holding the balance. In the beginning this meant losing her balance, then getting back on the leg. The work then became kinesthetic—that is, she began perceiving movement at a subtle level of the muscular sensation.

When she joined the University of Illinois in 1966 to teach a traditional modern dance class, she introduced her new knowledge and techniques to her students, using images and metaphors for kinesthetic experiences. They responded powerfully to the imagery and would drop the structure of the class to stay with an image. Joan realized that something important was happening to them, so she allowed the class to become less structured, a concept that formed the foundation of SRT.

Practice

A typical class includes three parts: tactile studies; floor work with guided imagery; and movement studies for the group, guided by the instructor. Music and sounds are interwoven throughout the session. The SRT pedagogy progresses from introductory work through ongoing levels to advanced.

Tactile studies in SRT help students experience kinesthetically the releasing of fixed tension patterns in the shoulders, back, or legs. Almost everyone has acquired patterns of tension, sometimes hidden, in the body during the process of growing up under numerous stresses. Trained dancers often find these tension patterns in their bodies underneath their training. The tensions are blocks—distortions of the alignment of the natural body. Releasing these blocks allows for realignment of the body, making it possible to move with greater flexibility, range, speed, and strength.

A unique aspect of SRT is its integration of technique with creative process through the use of imagery. If an instructor wants to focus a class on the concept of "autonomy of the limbs," he might begin with a tactile study focusing on the hip joint. The instructor guides student partners to gain a physical experience of increased freedom of movement at the hip by instructing one partner to rotate and extend their partner's leg while their partner is passive, relinquishing control of the leg. Eventually the active partner is instructed to let go of the leg, allowing the passive partner to continue the movements alone. Later in the class, the same concept is developed through the use of a metaphor, a poetic image given by the teacher that stimulates an improvised exploration. To begin this creative process, students lie on the floor while the teacher, using a procedure similar to relaxation technique, verbally guides students into a state just under conscious control. This state is free of anxiety and allows the sharpening of sensory perception. In this state, one can be physically transformed by a mental image. Propelled by the image, students begin to move up from the floor, to improvise from the image of freeing the legs, and eventually to dance as the concept of "autonomy of the limbs" plays through the body-mind.

Basic Principles

The objectives of the technique are similar to traditional dance techniques: optimal alignment, flexibility, strength, coordination, balance, speed, clarity of articulation, and control of nuance. But the means are distinctly different in that the nature or essence of a movement finds its own form, fostering creativity.

SRT deals with the universals within all dance forms. The individual discovers how she can move with the essences of basic body movements, such as turning or spinning, rather than a specific stylized form of the movement. Gradually, practitioners are encouraged to improvise in more complex and challenging ways with the movement, while simultaneously focusing on a principle; for example, no one segment of the body compresses against any other segment. Thus the practitioners develop maximum technical freedom without being constricted within a specific dance style and ideally can adapt to any form.

Some professional dancers use SRT as a practice to enhance their study of a specific dance technique. Some practice SRT as their only dance technique. Many declare that their technical progress speeds up and their growth as artists deepens with these SRT experiences. Nonprofessional dancers who study SRT are frequently artists in other media: musicians, painters, and poets, as well as doctors, psychologists, physicists, and pregnant women. SRT's organic, holistic approach to body-mind integration becomes part of a way of life. The technique gives the individual an understanding of the uniqueness of her own body and the way in which a movement flows through it.

Benefits

As it is the primary objective of the discipline to maximize the movement potential of all its practitioners, it can be useful to people of all ages. The use of guided imagery allows individuals to explore important issues and encourages people to get in touch with their creative and expressive selves. Individuals report reduced levels of stress, relief of chronic pain, improved alignment, and increased flexibility and strength, as well as increased energy and vitality.

—*Joan Skinner*

Resources

The New York Public Library for the
Performing Arts
    Dance Collection
    c/o Lincoln Center Plaza
    New York, NY 10023-7498
    Tel: (212) 870-1657
    Provides information about SRT.

Skinner Releasing
    Emily Herb, Administrator
    University of Washington Dance Program
    Box 351150
    Seattle, WA 98195-1150
    Tel: (206) 233-8803
    Fax: (206) 726-0616
    e-mail: ejherb@aa.net
    Manages workshops and seminars on the
    practice of SRT. Offers listings of certified
    teachers of SRT worldwide.

Further Reading

Books
Knaster, Mirka. *Discovering the Body's Wisdom.*
New York: Bantam Books, 1996.

Journals
Davidson, Robert. "Transformations: Concerning
Music and Dance in Releasing."*Quarterly
Dance Journal,* Winter 1985.

Skinner, Joan, Bridget Davis, Sally Metcalf, and
Kris Wheeler. "Notes on the Skinner Releasing Technique." *Quarterly Dance Journal,* Fall
1979.

Skura, Stephanie. "Releasing Dance Interview
with Joan Skinner." *Quarterly Dance Journal,*
Fall 1990.

Spatial Dynamics^{SM}

 Spatial Dynamics^{SM} is a discipline that concerns itself with
the human being's movement
and interaction with space
through spatially oriented movement activities. By focusing on how the body moves
through space, an individual develops
awareness of the potential of the body. It is a
core premise of Spatial Dynamics that this
awareness influences psychological, emotional, intellectual, and spiritual development.

History

In the mid-1970s a young clinical psychology student named Jaimen McMillan was
struck by the disconcerting similarity in the
postures and movement patterns of patients
suffering from similar complaints. In the
case of autistic children, where it could be
determined that they had never been exposed to others with the same disorder, their
movement repertoires were so similar as to
appear almost rehearsed. It was clear that a
particular condition affected the movement
patterns of the patients. McMillan wondered
if one could possibly work in the opposite
direction. If, indeed, the disorder had a negative effect on a patient's movement patterns, could practicing more wholesome
movement patterns have a positive effect on
the person's disorder? McMillan's initial attempts in this direction yielded encouraging
results.

It became clear to him that in order to use
spatial movement therapeutically in an appropriate and scientific way, one's own
movements had to be worthy of imitation,
one had to develop new concepts of space
and new ways of perceiving movement, one
had to know which effects a given movement elicited, and one had to work from a
holistic movement picture of the balanced

individual. Attracted by the artistry and up-rightness of the discipline of fencing, McMillan began his movement research through extensive training with the saber and attained "fleeting moments of mastery." In comparing his experiences with those of others who had achieved success in their fields, he considered a common factor largely overlooked in the study of sport, physical education, therapy, and movement in general: the concept of enlivened space.

His inclination to experience and understand enlivened space led him to begin rigorous training in various disciplines, including two ancient martial arts and yoga, which incorporated Eastern philosophies that allowed him to develop mental power and experience the effects of concentrated space. He also studied water, sound, sculpture, projective geometry, and eurythmy, which helped him learn about fluidity of movement and the processes of change through movement.

McMillan was also influenced by the work of such revolutionary twentieth-century thinkers as Albert Einstein and anthropologist Edward T. Hall; in particular, their concepts of time and space. From Rudolf Steiner came the concepts of the evolution of space and the connections between the human soul and the dimensions of space. These concepts contributed to the development of Spatial Dynamics.

For the next ten years McMillan worked, traveled, and studied in Europe. He went on to receive diplomas in physiotherapy, massage, movement therapy, and Bothmer gymnastics, and continued to collect and develop suitable movement activities that aid the processes of growth, health, and integration. This body of exercises has come to be known as Spatial Dynamics.

Philosophy

In Spatial Dynamics space is perceived as a vibrant medium and movement as a dynamic force that is at our disposal to span distances psychologically as well as physically. The concept of space is further differentiated to designate an ever-widening range of possibilities for self-knowledge and interaction with others. Working first from the "body-space" in Spatial Dynamics exercises, practitioners can explore moving through the "personal," or surrounding space; to the "interpersonal," or meeting and exchange space; to the "public," or social space; and finally, to the "suprapersonal," or macrocosmic space.

Out of the totality of spatial work, many exercises and games that aid in balance, orientation, and spatial differentiation have been developed and combined. Many of the exercises are taught in slow motion so that one can learn to follow, distinguish, and control the quality of the movement. At no time, even when performed more rapidly, are they done automatically. Great emphasis is placed on the individual's need for awareness and freedom. The exercises incorporate a developmental sequence that spans the years of movement development, corresponding to the unique spatial need of any given age and stage of development. For young children, they have the quality of playful imagination and joyfulness, whereas for adults they bring calm and enable one not merely to change but to choose one's own habits.

Perhaps the most distinctive characteristic of Spatial Dynamics is the conscious interplay between the opposing forces of gravity and levity. The earth represents a force that pulls everything toward one point, which is called gravity. For practitioners, the sun represents a force that draws and lifts toward the periphery, toward infinity. This force is called levity. A third force, rhythm, is born out of the interaction between these two.

The concept of enlivened space has educational, artistic, and athletic applications. A movement artist can learn to create consciously by bringing the three above-mentioned forces (gravity, levity, rhythm) into play through deliberate differentiation. An observer perceives an athlete or dancer

The Bothmer gymnastics exercises are spatial gems developed to augment the Waldorf School curriculum for grades three through twelve. (The Waldorf School was a special institution set up by Rudolf Steiner in 1919.)

Spatial Dynamics makes use of the Bothmer exercises and in addition has expanded the range of its spatially oriented movement activities to touch the whole spectrum of life, from a unique approach to childbirth preparation all the way to working with the elderly, including preparation for death and dying.

who orchestrates these forces successfully as graceful. An actor may employ these techniques to transcend his own personality and represent the forces called for in whatever role is being played. A child who has a learning block may move to the next step in the learning process if the correct movement experiences that are missing in his development are given.

Practice

One of the goals of Spatial Dynamics is to enable people to experience, and effectively enliven and employ, their spheres of activity in daily life. As a discipline it can be practiced alone, even subtly during the course of the day, pursued one-on-one with a teacher, or carried out in larger groups. Another important aspect is its unique approach to posture as a spatial process rather than as a set position or "pose." The social aspect of the exercises is visible in group work, in which the extensions of each individual's movements create weavings of geometrical patterns with others.

Benefits

Spatial Dynamics graduates have made an impact on the field of psychosomatic illness, most notably with eating-related disorders such as anorexia and bulimia; with space-related phobias such as claustrophobia and agoraphobia; and with problems involving nervousness, lack of awareness, and lack of "presence." Movement therapists, physical therapists, chiropractors, and orthopedic doctors have implemented Spatial Dynamics principles successfully in the area of physical medicine.

—*JAIMEN MCMILLAN*

Resources

Spatial Dynamics Institute
    423 Route 71
    Hillsdale, NY 12529
    Tel/fax: (518) 325-7096
    Provides in-service training programs in the discipline of Spatial Dynamics. Annual public conferences are also held at varying locations around the country.

Further Reading

Hall, Edward T. *The Hidden Dimension*. New York: Anchor Books, 1969.

McMillan, Jaimen. *Posture: Giving Yourself Space*. Hudson, N.Y.: Lindisfarne Press, 1998.

Schwenk, Theodor. *Sensitive Chaos*. Ann Arbor, Mich.: Rudolf Steiner Press, 1972.

Steiner, Rudolf. *Man: Hieroglyph of the Universe*. Translated by G. and M. Adams. Ann Arbor, Mich.: Rudolf Steiner Press, 1972.

Whicher, Olive. *Sunspace*. Ann Arbor, Mich.: Rudolf Steiner Press, 1989.

T'ai Chi Ch'üan

 T'ai chi ch'üan is an ancient Chinese exercise art, a system of activating the body for the simultaneous development of physical, emotional, and mental well-being. Composed of a slow, continuous series of circular movements, it is said to develop balance, stamina, and grace. One of the oldest exercise arts—dating back to about 2205 B.C.E.—it was not fully established as a body-mind technique for increasing the span of a healthy life until 1100 C.E. From the Chinese viewpoint, a healthy life includes emotional stability and a high degree of mental efficiency as well as physical stamina.

History

For centuries many civilizations have devised systems to improve health and reduce occurrences of disease and illness. Believed to be one of the earliest systems of this nature, the "great dances" were devised by Emperor Yü of China in 2205 B.C.E. He maintained that these exercises, if done daily, would stimulate the body's natural circulatory process, combat disease, and keep the mind alert by tending to the activity of the stipulated patterns and rhythms. It was also believed that performing these organized and structured movements awakened "positive and agreeable feelings" in the practitioner, thereby calming the emotions as well.

As centuries passed, the exercises became more intricate than those of the previous century until, as history has it, the twelfth century, when Chang San-Feng profoundly extended the range of self-understanding physically and spiritually. He created the uniquely structured form of t'ai chi ch'üan as a set of movements that build on one another, movements that are interconnected and require the full concentration of the practitioner.

Philosophy

T'ai chi ch'üan is never to be practiced automatically, as for example the way one can recite the alphabet while one's thoughts wander elsewhere. It is a complex composition of multiple themes. The varied patterns pass from one part of the body to another so that no part is overworked and the mind stays interested. The mind directs the action and participates in it.

T'ai chi ch'üan is a long exercise, continuous for twenty-five minutes. This basic length of time is essential. According to experts, it is just long enough to overcome resistance and laziness; to develop physical strength, patience, and persistence; and to give every part of the body varied exercise, but not long enough to fatigue the body or the mind.

The way of moving in t'ai chi ch'üan looks soft, continuous, light, and fluid, giving the appearance of effortlessness. Yet in order to do it the body must be firm, stable, and strong. The mind must be alert and active. The movements of t'ai chi ch'üan are circular, made in curves, arcs, and spirals. According to t'ai chi masters, moving in circles conserves energy, creates security, and lessens nervousness.

During the process of action, muscles are never tensed to their maximum ability. The amount of effort-tension used depends entirely upon the demands of the position or movement itself. For instance, it requires more energy to stand on one leg than on two. The muscles naturally behave differently in each case. Force is never added to a movement; one tries to use exactly as much force as necessary to perform the movement. As Chinese t'ai chi masters say, "Use 1 pound to lift 1 pound." The approach of t'ai chi ch'üan is to balance force with necessity, which awakens the practitioner to the proper use of strength and helps him find a harmonious relationship with the natural force of gravity.

Balance is an essential aspect in the practice of t'ai chi ch'üan. Through the control

The symbol for t'ai chi ch'üan is a circle divided by a flowing line that represents the movement of a wave. Filling the circumference of the circle are two curved shapes of equal size: one white, representing yin, and one black, representing yang. There is a small dot of the opposite color in each shape, showing the sympathetic character of each to the other. The dynamic flow within the symbol represents movement and the continuity of the life force.

of every nuance, muscles and joints are strengthened. Proper posture and lightness of movement are inevitable results of good body balance. Balance on the physical level also contributes to mental and emotional stability.

T'ai chi ch'üan is connected and flowing. Each unit, each moment of movement, is joined to the next without a visible break. Calmness and lightness are evoked by such fluidity. There is no cessation of movement throughout the entire twenty-five-minute exercise. Stamina and endurance grow as one develops the ability to sustain an even continuity. It is a slow exercise. The breathing is meant to stay natural, the heartbeat steady. The tempo of the movement is related to a healthy heart rate. Slowness develops patience, poise, and power. But that is not to say that t'ai chi is without changes in dynamics. Changes of delicate force and strength, stillness and activity are in constant alternation throughout the form. The variation in dynamic flow produces flexibility, pliability, and resilience.

The Chinese masters recognized and worked with the mind's desire for diversity. The form was designed to engage what the Chinese believe to be the two vital energies of life, yin and yang. Yin represents all things receptive and quiet. Yang represents all things assertive and active. The many ways in which yin and yang are contrasted within the form add to the development of good coordination and heightened perception as well as memory. With the mind satisfied and the body exercised, a sense of total relaxation and well-being results.

Practice

T'ai chi ch'üan is generally taught in small classes, but some teachers also offer private lessons. It is usually taught indoors in studios with wooden floors. In temperate climates it is often taught and practiced out of doors, where students can breathe freely and fully and perhaps more easily feel themselves in harmony with their natural surroundings. Loose, comfortable clothing is worn. Students may be barefoot, in socks, or in soft Chinese slippers, depending on the surface of the floor. Music is never used when teaching the discipline, as it distracts students from the awareness of the dynamic rhythms within the form.

T'ai chi ch'üan can be practiced in every phase of life: as a child, adult, and senior citizen. While beginners are generally separated from advanced practitioners in classes, it is always possible for experienced practitioners to learn something new by starting at the beginning once again, or for beginners to learn by feeling the flow of movement of an experienced practitioner.

Benefits

Many people believe the practice of this discipline can be a calming preparation for any task. Many people report that by doing even some of the form, their mind focuses away from their anxious self, and emotional and psychological problems seem to evaporate. Other people report that t'ai chi has helped them become more mentally and physically proficient and limber than before. With quickened physical reflexes comes an easier acceptance of new ideas and a quickened capacity to discard old habits. Emotionally, self-consciousness is diminished and self-assurance awakened. Many practitioners assert that practicing the form has helped them develop patience, awareness, and endurance.

—SOPHIA DELZA

Resources

T'ai Chi Ch'üan/Shaolin Ch'üan Association
3720 Illinois Ave.
St. Charles, IL 60174
Tel: (630) 443-0070
Web site: www.taichi-shaolin.com
Conducts demonstrations, seminars, lectures, and a certification program for members. Publishes annual booklet on the practice of martial arts.

T'ai Chi Foundation, Inc.
5 E. 17th St.
New York, NY 10003
Tel: (212) 645-7010
Founded in 1979, this educational organization strives to make the practice of t'ai chi ch'üan more accessible to Western society through promoting international conferences. In addition, it operates a resource center that provides information about this discipline.

Further Reading

Delza, Sophia. *T'ai Chi Ch'üan: Body and Mind in Harmony.* Rev. ed. New York: State University of New York Press, 1985.

Emerson, Margaret. *Breathing Underwater: The Inner Life of T'ai Chi Ch'üan.* Berkeley, Calif.: North Atlantic Books, 1993.

Hooten, Claire. *T'ai Chi for Beginners: 10 Minutes to Health and Fitness.* New York: Berkley Publishing Group, 1996.

Part 11:

Martial Arts

Martial arts are forms of combat that advocate the integration of mind and body as the basis for the study and practice of physical forms of self-defense. Although many different styles of martial arts have evolved over time, many of those practiced today are similar in their belief that the highly charged, dynamic quality of a physical confrontation is a powerful metaphor for life. Today martial arts are practiced the world over by people who enjoy the vigorous physical conditioning they demand, as well as the inner path of psychological and spiritual transformation and growth they offer. A list of martial arts and countries where they developed appears on page 246.

Three Theories

It has been suggested that hunting skills comprised the early forms of combat for primitive man. As these techniques were used, their degree of sophistication generally increased. However, the origins of the martial arts remain speculative and open to controversy among writers, historians, and researchers. Three general theories seek to explain how martial arts developed throughout time.

One theory holds that ancient fighting techniques of the Greeks and Romans spread into Asia following the routes of commerce and trade. Indeed, some elements of combat can be found in literary writings and sculptures of Greece and Rome. Despite this, the complexity of specific Asian martial arts techniques appears to be lacking in literary descriptions or sculptured poses uncovered thus far in archaeological investigations.

A second theory maintains that martial arts can be traced to either China or India. A common myth credits Bodhidharma, a prince of India and founder of Buddhism in China, with teaching specific exercises to monks at the Shaolin Temple that later evolved into formal

AIKIDO

CAPOEIRA

JU JUTSU

JUDO

KARATE

KENDO

KUNG FU WU SU

TAEKWONDO

combative techniques. Under close scrutiny, this theory contradicts historical fact and has lost favor with experts and historians.

The third theory argues that similar techniques of several martial arts that differed coincidentally evolved in parallel form in widely separate regions of the world. Unique characteristics of these similar techniques later evolved as a function of certain conditions, such as social structure and physical demographics. As examples, slaves from Africa who were brought to Brazil initially developed capoeira techniques in chains and restraints, which limited the development of hand strikes while emphasizing kicking movements from a handstand position. In China, individuals who were taller developed systems that emphasized kicking (northern region) while individuals of shorter stature resorted to systems that stressed close-range hand movements (southern region). In the Philippines, Chinese merchants from the Fukien province taught kuntao to the royal families of the people of Mindanao as a token of their friendship and good faith. The "hard" style that evolved here reflected the more external, combative focus of the Filipino martial arts in general.

Central to the problem of documentation is the fact that martial arts were often shrouded in secrecy. Experienced teachers did not reveal their knowledge readily. Secret teachings were not passed on to students until after many years of training and dedication to the art and teaching alike. If no suitable successor to the tradition could be found, the art often died with the master. Information was also often transmitted orally (as opposed to any documentation in written form), leading to further gaps in any traceable history.

Today the martial arts of Asia have emerged as a significant component of American culture. It is difficult to find an individual who does not have some sense of familiarity with or recognition of these ancient disciplines when reference is made to them. Following World War II, a number of servicemen who had been exposed to these esoteric practices endeavored to pass on their teachings to other Americans. Fueled by developments in media presentations, the growth of interest in martial arts—seldom even mentioned forty years ago—has been quite phenomenal. Depiction of martial arts in films, television, and popular magazines is now commonplace.

Basic Principles

The physical foundations of the martial arts as a whole have roots in self-defense movements that make use of punches, hand strikes, blocks, and kicks; jumping, grappling, and rolling techniques; and chokes, joint manipulations, locks, and throws. Aside from empty-hand techniques, many systems of martial arts make use of weapons, which might include a staff, stick, blade, or projectile instrument. Martial arts disciplines that stress these combative components are often labeled "external."

Other martial arts disciplines emphasize an esoteric component in their teachings that has been described as internal in nature. These practices and exercises include specific types of breathing techniques, performance of unique rituals, use of special hand-body configurations, chanting or recitation of specific combinations of letters or words, cultivation and manipulation of internal energy, and sitting, standing, and movement meditation exercises. These more esoteric practices are taught for improving physical performance, enhancement of health, and psychological and spiritual development. Practice of traditional, regimented, prearranged forms often serves to unify both external and internal aspects of martial arts.

Each of the different systems of martial arts has defining characteristics that identify the nature of the art. For example, t'ai chi ch'üan is a Chinese art that consists of smooth, flowing, gentle movements with no hesitation observed between various postures and rounded, curling gestures that involve kicks, strikes, and evasive actions. Originating in Africa, capoeira is now practiced widely in Brazil and is characterized by a dancelike, acrobatic movement style accompanied by music and song and takes the form of a game being played as a performance. Another example is aikido, a contemporary Japanese art of self-defense based on principles of nonresistance to and harmony with one's opponent that makes use of circular movements to gain control of an attacker's momentum, thus neutralizing aggressive actions.

Learning Martial Arts

While each discipline of martial arts is unique, some general principles underlie the pursuit and study of all the disciplines. Instructions are often given in a group setting, with classes being taught anywhere from three to seven days a week for one, two, or even more hours per session. An instructor or set of instructors will lead the class and often insist on the display of proper behavior, attitudes, moral conduct, and discipline throughout the class. Training can be demanding physically and mentally and requires dedication and perseverance to progress through a defined ranking system.

Benefits and Risks

Millions of people worldwide study martial arts disciplines. They report many positive effects, including an increase in mental clarity and means of achieving self-discipline, maximum physical fitness, general well-being through proper breathing techniques, an outlet for aggression, increased personal power through internal energy development exercises, and increased self-confidence from the knowledge of valuable self-defense techniques.

People with severe physical limitations may have difficulty participating in the more vigorous "external" forms of martial arts. Choosing which martial art to study should entail some knowledge of the physical techniques involved; the mental, emotional, and spiritual goals stressed; and exposure to the teaching style of a particular instructor. The degree to which the philosophical aspects of a practice are emphasized will depend on the individual teacher, but the physical self-defense aspect of these disciplines remains the defining feature that distinguishes them from other body-mind disciplines.

—*MICHAEL MALISZEWSKI, PH.D.*

COUNTRY	MARTIAL ART
India	kalarippayattu, thang-ta
China	t'ai chi ch'üan, wing chun, pa kua, Hung-gar
Korea	taekwondo, hapkido, tang soo do, hwarang-do
Japan	kendo, aikido, ju jutsu, judo, karate
Okinawa Islands	Goju-ryu, Shito-ryu, Uechi-ryu, Shorinji-ryu
Indonesia	pencak silat, kuntao
Philippines	arnis, escrima
Thailand	muay Thai, krabi-krabong
Africa and Brazil	capoeira, ju jutsu
U.S.A.	jeet kune do, talahib-marga

Further Reading

Books

Draeger, Donn F., and Robert W. Smith. *Comprehensive Asian Fighting Arts.* Tokyo: Kodansha International, 1969.

Maliszewski, M. *Spiritual Dimensions of the Martial Arts.* Tokyo: Charles E. Tuttle, 1996.

Journals

The Black Book: The Quarterly Martial Arts Supplies Guide and Master's Desk Reference. Erica Talorico, editor. Bellmawr, N.J.: Marketing Tools, Inc. (204 Harding Ave., Bellmawr, NJ 08031).

Journal of Asian Martial Arts. Michael DeMarco, editor. Erie, Pa.: Via Media Publishing Company. (821 W. 24th St., Erie, PA 16502)

Aikido

Aikido is a Japanese martial art. The word *aikido* means the path to the coordination of body, mind, and spirit. It is a defensive system of continuous, circular movements meant to counter the attack of an armed or unarmed opponent. Continued practice in aikido allows one to effectively anticipate and successfully defend oneself with minimum effort against an attack.

History

The founder of aikido, Morehei Ueshiba (1883–1969), also known as O Sensei, or "great teacher," was influenced by religion and martial arts. In Tokyo in 1902, O Sensei studied kendo (Japanese sword technique) and ju jutsu, the traditional art of hand-to-hand and small weapons combat. Ueshiba would continue these studies all his life, earning several certificates in various schools. He also studied sojutsu (spear fighting), sumo wrestling, and kokodan judo.

Ueshiba studied extensively with Onisaburo Deguchi, founder of Omoto-Kyo, a religion based on the traditional Shinto religion. After his father's death, Ueshiba moved to Deguchi's organic farming community near Kyoto. There he studied spiritual works that later influenced his philosophy of martial arts. In 1920 Ueshiba opened his first martial arts school, Ueshiba Academy. By 1922 his teachings evolved into a discipline he called aiki-bujutsu, known generally as Ueshiba-ryu Aiki-bujutsu. Later the art became known as aikido, the way of harmony, reflecting O Sensei's concern with the peaceful resolution of conflict.

In the thirties and forties, the practice of aikido spread throughout Japan and was recognized by the state as a martial art. During World War II, Ueshiba retreated to the country to build a shrine to aikido. After the war, aikido's focus on conflict resolution allowed for its practice during the American occupation. In 1961 the first practice hall opened outside of Japan in Honolulu, Hawaii. Ueshiba died in 1969.

Basic Principles

The central concept of aikido is the peaceful resolution of conflict. To this end, O Sensei envisioned it as training for the spirit and mind, as well as the body. All techniques in aikido are defense techniques and guide the aggressor's attack to its conclusion, resulting in the aggressor's downfall. These techniques are meant to show the aggressor the error of his judgment and end the attack. The defender, called *nagi*, protects himself and his attacker, known as *uke*, with these techniques. Rank is given according to knowledge of technique and ability to perform basic movements. Ranking tests are given, but they are not competitive.

On a physical level, the focus and direction of *ki*, or vital life energy, is very important in practice; *ki* is developed through breathing exercises. The pelvis, center of *ki*, is the origin of all movement in aikido. From the pelvis, *ki* is channeled through the arms and legs and eventually to the hands. This process is called extension, another important principle of aikido. The embodiment of these concepts produces the flowing, circular movement that is the trademark of aikido.

Practice

All aikido practice takes place in a dojo, a room with mats on the floor and a shrine to O Sensei at one end. For practice all students wear a *gi*, a heavy white cotton kimono jacket, pants, and belt. Students in the lower ranks, known as the five *kyus*, wear white belts. Advanced students in the higher ranks, or *dans*, wear black belts. Senior students in the dojo are often given permission to wear black wide-legged pants called *hakama*. All advanced students wear *hakama*.

Etiquette is important in aikido. Class begins and ends with a set sequence of quiet bowing to the shrine, to the teacher, and at the end of class, to fellow students. Students are expected to bow to the shrine on entering and leaving the mat. Bowing is a gesture of respect rather than worship.

After opening the class, the instructor, also called *sensei*, leads the class in a warmup. Then the instructor demonstrates a technique with a senior student. In the course of most classes, a few techniques will be practiced. Often each student will take a partner and work on the technique. Both students in each pair practice being the attacker who takes the fall, and in turn play the defender. By changing roles, students learn to cooperate with each other. They are expected to adapt their practice to their partners. Injuring your partner is considered bad form in most dojos, since injury takes a student out of class. Aikido classes often are silent, which fosters students' concentration on the technique; concentration is important since all aikido techniques can injure the attacker.

The attacker's falls in aikido are called *ukemi*; these movements, like other aikido defensive techniques, are circular and flowing. *Ukemi* maneuvers are just as important as defense movements, called *nagi*. For example, the forward roll in aikido begins from standing and flows from the leading arm, across the back, down to the leg, and back to standing. This roll should always be flowing, without any jarring movement.

Benefits

Because of its psychological and physical benefits, aikido is an ideal martial art for life. Practice builds strength, coordination, and flexibility. As students advance, the tempo of practice accelerates, bringing aerobic benefits. On an intellectual level, many students find mental focus and clarity through their practice. Many of O Sensei's students have opened dojos all over the world. Today, O Sensei's son, Kisshomaru Ueshiba, heads aikido schools worldwide.

—Clio Pavlantos, M.A., CMA, Second Kyu USAF, in collaboration with Marvin Bookman, Third Dan USAF

Resources

United States Aikido Federation, Eastern Region
142 W. 18th St.
New York, NY 10011
Web site: www.usaikifed.org
Eastern United States division of the international organization founded by O Sensei and now headed by his son, Doshu Kisshomaru Ueshiba. The USAF provides lists of affiliated dojos in America and abroad. Publishes the *Federation News*, a newsletter promoting aikido.

Capoeira

 Capoeira is an ancient martial art that has its roots in African culture but developed fully and attained an immense popularity in Brazil. Like other martial arts, capoeira strives to integrate mental as well as physical strength in order to perform combat maneuvers with dexterity, skill, and grace. Yet capoeira differs from other martial arts in that rhythmic music, including singing, clapping, and the playing of instruments, is integral to the unique spirit and practice of the discipline.

History

Although there are many theories about the origin of capoeira, most scholars agree it can be traced back to certain hand-to-hand combat forms and dances of central Africa. Two African dances are most often credited with being the origin of capoeira: *sanga* and *n'golo*. Both dances exhibit characteristics that are central to the practice of capoeira today. *Sanga* was an ancient war dance, also known as a sword dance, in which warfare and dance movements were inextricably linked. The dance element is significant because the ability to leap, twist, roll, and dodge the arrows and blows of opponents is one of the most important skills of capoeira. *N'golo* was an acrobatic dance used as competition between the young males of the Mucope people in Angola.

Capoeira traveled with the Atlantic slave trade to Brazil. Among themselves, slaves trained in capoeira as a form of physical resistance, stressing the fighting aspects of the discipline. When the slave owners were present, the dance aspects of capoeira were emphasized. Slave owners outlawed capoeira and made the practice punishable by death. Well into the twentieth century, capoeira was an outlaw art performed secretly by slaves or by thieves and criminals. Roving bands of capoeiristas (those that practice capoeira) were employed as thugs and enforcers by businessmen and would attack taverns and police, further advancing the negative image of the discipline.

Through the efforts of two modern masters, Manoel dos Reis Machado (known as Mestre Bimba) and Vincente Ferreira Pastinha (known as Mestre Pastinha), capoeira eventually became an acceptable part of Brazilian life. Mestra Bimba is known as the great innovator. He invented the style called capoeira regional, which emphasizes the offensive, fighting aspects of the martial art. Known as the great traditionalist, Mestre Pastinha was a proponent of the style called capoeira angola, which aims to maintain the ritualistic, defensive, aesthetic, and philosophical aspects of the discipline.

Today many styles of capoeira are practiced throughout Europe, the United States, and South America. It is taught in private academies and in many universities. The Capoeira Foundation in New York City promotes the study, research, and performance of the art.

Basic Principles

Capoeira is based on the African cultural values from which it arose. The religious traditions and rituals of central Africa form the basic philosophical underpinnings of the practice of the art.

In the August 1988 issue of *Karate/Kung-Fu Illustrated*, scholar Alejandro Frigerio identified six characteristics of modern capoeira angola:

1. Complementation is the importance of playing with, not against, the opponent. It is similar to a "cutting session" in jazz, in which the musicians try to outplay each other with the ultimate goal of creating beautiful music. Through complementation the most creative interaction possible is achieved.
2. *Malicia* is the art of being evasive or deceptive. One aspect of *malicia* is to look vulnerable until the opponent attacks, then gracefully defend and/or counterattack. In other words one should play closed (or controlled), while appearing open (undisciplined or vulnerable).
3. It is not enough merely to defeat the opponent; one must prove superior skill by displaying it with style or beautiful movement. This style and grace are as important as the victory.
4. Both slow and fast movements are important to capoeira angola. Most movements are slow and deliberate—they teach control and precision, which then enable practitioners to perform the movements very quickly and effectively and to improvise new moves.
5. Capoeira angola is a sophisticated discipline with subtle rules and rites. If a player displays ignorance of these

There is little use of offensive hand techniques in capoeira. Some scholars have attributed this to the belief that slaves had to fight with their hands immobilized by chains and therefore developed advanced foot and leg techniques. Other commentators contend that it is more likely that the absence is based on an old central African proverb: "Hands are to build, feet are to destroy."

unwritten rules, he or she is considered an inferior player, uneducated in the proper, traditional way. Secret personal and religious rituals called *mandingas* protect a player from harm.

6. Finally, unlike other martial arts, the *jogo*, or play of capoeira, is performed for others. The viewers should be entertained by the skill, deception, and humor of the play. The practitioners of this discipline should always be aware of the effect their display has on those attending and develop their play accordingly.

Practice

The play of capoeira takes place in what is known as a *roda*, which is a circle formed by the players and onlookers. Included in the circle is the *bateria*, which is an ensemble of musicians and singers.

Music is one of the most important elements of the art of capoeira. Different songs and rhythms inspire the players to more intense levels of performance and calm them down if the dance becomes too heated. The order of songs is part of the ritual aspect of capoeira. The *berimbau*, a musical bow with one string, is considered "the soul of capoeira." Attached to the bow is a hollowed-out gourd that acts as a resonator box. Tones are produced when the bowstring is struck by a

thin flexible stick *(baqueta)*. A small rattle *(caxixi)* is also held in the hand that holds the *baqueta*. Each instrument has a prescribed position in the circle.

The ritualized practice of capoeira begins when two players enter the circle and kneel at the foot of the *berimbau*. One player sings a *ladainha*, a ritual song of commencement. If his opponent doesn't respond with a song of his own, the first begins another song, an *acorrido*, a song for going out to play. The song is then passed on to one of the musicians as the *jogo-de-capoeira* (play of capoeira) begins.

Capoeira is characterized by dynamic movements such as cartwheels, handstands, circling kicks, and acrobatics. Performers use agility, guile, and superior technique to maneuver the other into a defenseless position, rendering him open to a blow, kick, or sweep. Only one's hands, head, and feet are allowed to touch the floor. Disqualification occurs when a player is knocked down.

Improvisation is greatly admired. It allows the capoeirista to create openings and keep the action of the performance innovative and fluid. Also prized are evasive techniques and implied strikes, especially when one fighter has been maneuvered into an indefensible position.

Benefits

Capoeira aims to teach its practitioners how to face harsh experiences while remaining flexible and receptive, how to respond to violence with evasion and grace, and how to use the trials and tribulations of life to develop physical strength, spiritual strength, and wisdom in thought and action. It is an ancestral wisdom that aims to create balanced and productive bodies, minds, and lives.

Resources

The Capoeira Foundation
104 Franklin St.
New York, NY 10013
Tel: (212) 274-9737
e-mail: dancebrazl@aol.com
Provides information on capoeira, including information on instructors.

Further Reading

Almeida, Bira. *Capoeira: A Brazilian Art Form.* 2nd ed. Richmond, Calif.: North Atlantic Books, 1986.

Dimock, Anne. "Capoeira Angola." *Black People and Their Culture: Selected Writing from the African Diaspora.* Edited by Linn Shapiro. Washington, D.C.: Smithsonian Institution, 1976.

Kubick, Gerhard. "Capoeira Angola." *Angolan Traits in Black Music, Games, and Dances of Brazil: A Study of African Cultural Extensions Overseas.* Lisbon: Junta de Investigacoes Cientifica do Ultramar, Centro de Estudos de Antropologia Cultural, 1976.

Lewis, John Lowell. *Ring of Liberation: Deceptive Discourse in Brazilian Capoeira.* Chicago: University of Chicago Press, 1992.

Ju Jutsu

 Ju jutsu is a type of fighting that involves grappling, throwing, and limb twisting. Although variously spelled as jiu jitsu, ju jitsu, or even ju jutso, the name refers to the yielding principle of the art, which refers to the ability to submit to an opponent's direction of attack while attempting to control it. The Japanese character *ju* has several meanings: soft, pliable, submissive, adaptable, yielding, and harmonious. The character *jutsu* means skill or technique. Yet the common translation of ju jutsu as the "gentle art"

is somewhat misleading. Many ju jutsu techniques can be very forceful and damaging to an opponent. Sometimes great strength is needed to ensure the defeat of an opponent, though expert technique can make it appear to be effortless. Perhaps the fact that ju jutsu is an art that adapts to the opponent and the situation—using leverage, balance, and the minimum amount of effort necessary to gain an advantage over the aggressor—that has earned it the name of the "gentle art." In ju jutsu the mind is used to evaluate the opponent's weaknesses and anticipate their next move, while the body controls the opponent's balance and positioning.

History

Considered the forerunner of the popular martial arts judo and aikido, ju jutsu dates back a thousand years, being known as tai-jutsu, yawara, and hakuda during the course of its development into what is recognized today as ju jutsu. Grappling and throwing arts have long existed in Japan, and there are a number of legends about the emergence of ju jutsu.

According to one popular story, ju jutsu originated with a Japanese physician named Akiyama, who traveled to China to study medicine. While there, he learned hakuda, which consisted of kicking, striking, seizing, and grappling. Upon his return to Japan, Akiyama began to teach hakuda. According to the legend, he had few techniques, so his students grew bored and left him. Angered, Akiyama went to meditate at the Tenjin Shrine. During a snowstorm, he saw a pine tree broken beneath the weight of snow. Nearby was a slim willow tree bending under the snow, its branches so pliable that the snow slipped from them, leaving the tree unbroken. Akiyama later meditated at the shrine and is said to have come upon 303 different martial art techniques that applied the principle he had seen demonstrated by the willow. He opened a new school in which flexibility and suppleness were all-important, naming it Yoshin-Ryu, or Willow Tree School.

The 1500s are considered a turning point for ju jutsu. During this time of the art's greatest popularity, there were more than 700 schools sharing few standard techniques. No method existed that could be considered a complete and independent system of unarmed fighting.

Many sources regard the Takenouchi Ryu, founded in 1532 by Takenouchi Hisamaro, as the core ju jutsu ryu (school) from which all empty-handed (meaning without weapons) ju jutsu sprang. Ju jutsu had traditionally been taught in conjunction with, and as a complement to, archery, swordsmanship, and other forms of armed fighting. Takenouchi Ryu, also known as Kogusoku, parted with weapon-oriented training, establishing a pure method of unarmed ju jutsu.

It is doubtful that the empty-handed ju jutsu practiced today bears much resemblance to the ancient art from feudal Japan. Although Takenouchi established a formal system of unarmed combat, ju jutsu still continued to flourish mainly as a part of samurai training.

In the mid–seventeenth century, changes in ju jutsu began to emerge. Increasingly, ju jutsu systems started to develop independently from weapons training. Later, in the nineteenth century, schools opened to teach people other than samurai who were interested in studying the martial arts. The new schools of ju jutsu lacked the real combat training of the older schools, and many methods became theoretical as the need for practical application disappeared. This kind of ju jutsu came to be the most well known and eventually spread to the West. A few old schools still exist, practicing their dangerous art according to tradition. Over the years ju jutsu, like karate, judo, and many other arts, developed as a form of sporting and good-natured competition. Because of this, lethal techniques were further removed from the training programs.

Since the 1970s, when the martial arts benefited from tremendous growth due to the cinema phenomenon brought about by the films of Bruce Lee, many offshoots from the traditional styles have sprung up, and with the help of no-holds-barred contests, ju jutsu and the grappling arts are enjoying renewed popularity.

Training and Techniques

Ju jutsu does not require any particular clothing to be effective, unlike the high kicking arts that require loose clothes for proper execution. The student is expected to wear traditional clothing not for effectiveness, but out of respect for the history of ju jutsu.

Many of the training procedures date back to the early days of ju jutsu, when this discipline was still part of the samurai's training. For example, ju jutsu is practiced mostly with the partners facing each other. This custom originates from the battlefields of the old samurai. Sometimes a samurai would stand facing the enemy before his soldiers and scream out a challenge, his name, his ryu (school), or even a favorite technique. A samurai from the enemy camp would come forward and accept the challenge. Such a duel could determine the outcome of the whole battle.

While ju jutsu is often identified as pure grappling that incorporates arm locks, joint manipulation, throws, and breakfalls, the art also includes devastating kicks and punches. Training in ju jutsu progresses from the learning of basic techniques to the practice of choreographed or prearranged series of fight moves, to freestyle or improvisational practice.

The many techniques of ju jutsu include *atemi waza* (striking techniques), *tachi waza* and *nage waza* (standing and throwing techniques), and *ne waza* and *katame waza* (lying and grappling techniques). Just as in other martial arts, ju jutsu training includes prearranged fight patterns or choreography called *jigo waza* (defense techniques). *Jigo* waza is a methodical way to learn how to apply the basic techniques. *Randori,* or free sparring, is a means of learning one's strengths and weaknesses because it tests the student's fluency with spontaneous moves and responses. In *randori,* students avoid causing injury but may use any techniques at their disposal.

As the name implies, ju jutsu is not a contest of muscular strength. Excellent balance, leverage, and speed are needed to get the most out of the technique. Throws, holds, and locks are carried out in a manner that if not handled with care could be devastating to the opponent. Calling for an awareness of anatomy, ju jutsu focuses on the vital points on the body and the effective use of force on the joints and limbs. Nevertheless, competitors are taught to stop short of harming each other. Modern ju jutsu is designed to render an opponent helpless without causing injury.

Philosophy and Benefits

Because ju jutsu originated in Japan, there are similarities in etiquette and terminology with martial arts such as karate and judo. The training takes place in a dojo, or training hall. As in karate, the philosophy of ju jutsu is based on Zen Buddhism. According to this philosophy, the dojo is considered more than a place to practice. The vigorous training that occurs there helps practitioners to understand themselves.

Through competition and practice, students develop confidence and learn about commitment, determination, discipline, and conquering fear. The lessons learned in the dojo help the student to deal with conflicts and stresses that occur outside the dojo. In this way, ju jutsu training is a source of self-enlightenment.

The mental aspect of ju jutsu complements the physical aspect. The philosophy of ju jutsu stresses the power of *ki* (also known as *chi*), or inner spirit and energy. According to this thinking, each time attackers commit themselves to a movement, they are also committing their *ki.* Skilled students of ju jutsu can control this energy by applying the principle of yielding, which means using opponents' attacks and movements against themselves: if the opponent pulls, the defender pushes; if the opponent pushes, the defender pulls.

It is believed that by controlling the opponent's *ki* one can also control his mind and therefore his whole being. Because this art is potentially destructive and must be used responsibly, ju jutsu, like other martial arts, places strong emphasis on character and self-control. Students must be patient and tolerant, with the ability to resist confrontations if deemed unnecessary. By studying ju jutsu, students learn about controlling their opponents and, more important, about self-control, commitment, discipline, and rising to challenges.

—STEFAN NIKANDER

Resources

American Judo and Jujitsu Federation
c/o Central Office Administrator
P.O. Box 993312
Redding, CA 96099-3312
e-mail: ajjfdanzan@aol.com
Web site: www.ajjf.org
Founded in 1958, this is a nonprofit corporation that promotes the DanZan Ryu system of ju jutsu.

American Jujitsu Institute
c/o 1779 Koi Koi St.
Wahiawa, HI 96786
Tel: (808) 621-6274
Fax: (808) 622-2179 (call first to set up fax)
e-mail: pra0005@pixi.com
Web site: www.pixi.com/~pra0005/aji.html
Founded in 1939, AJI is the oldest martial arts organization in the United States. It sponsors tournaments and offers instruction, testing and certification, and seminars and clinics.

World Martial Arts Association
P.O. Box 1568
Santa Barbara, CA 93102
Tel: (805) 569-1389
Fax: (805) 569-0267
Promotes and teaches martial arts such as ju
jutsu, judo, aikido, and karate.

Further Reading

Ferrie, Eddie. *Ju Jitsu: Classical and Modern.*
Wiltshire, U.K.: Crowood Press, 1990.

Nakae, Kiyose, and Charles Yeager. *Jiu Jitsu Complete.* Secaucus, N.J.: Carol Publishing Group,
1995.

Palumbo, Dennis G. *The Essence of Hakkoryo Jujutsu.* Boulder, Co.: Paladin Press, 1995.

Uphoff, Joseph A., Jr. *Jujitsu: The Art of Precision.*
Colorado Springs, Co.: Arjuna Library Press,
1993.

Judo

 Judo is a modern Japanese martial art that has its roots in the ancient martial art of ju jutsu. It integrates mental as well as physical strength in order to perform a series of combat maneuvers and movements with dexterity, skill, and grace. Like other martial arts, this discipline places a strong emphasis on spiritual balance, serenity, and mental and physical fitness as an approach to life. It is characterized by techniques that are used to upset the balance of an opponent, eventually neutralizing her. Today judo is often thought of as an aggressive, competitive sport, but in its original form it was nonviolent and basically defensive.

History

The story of judo begins with Terada Kanemon, an eighteenth-century warrior who, from the many techniques of ju jutsu, developed a specific art of combat using only bare hands. He called this martial art *judo*, which means "way of gentleness." The modern art of judo, however, is attributed primarily to the work of Kano Jigoro. Born in 1860, he grew up as a member of a wealthy family in Kobe, Japan. He was very dedicated to the study of ju jutsu. Even though the discipline had a long and respected tradition as a martial art, at that time ju jutsu was used by bandits and thieves and had a negative reputation.

Kano explored ways to bring together the techniques he had learned studying with different master teachers. He wanted to create a "sporting discipline" that would educate and train young people in a time of peace. He revived the name *judo* to describe his new "martial sport."

In 1882 he opened his own school (dojo) in Tokyo. His method became very popular, and by 1889 he had 600 students. That same year he gave a demonstration in Marseilles, France; the popularity of the discipline spread, and the first dojo outside of Japan was established in Paris under the directorship of Jean-Joseph Renaud and Guy de Montgrillard.

Between 1902 and 1912 Kano was sent on official missions by the Japanese government to teach the principles and techniques of judo throughout China and Europe. Soon there were dojos throughout Japan, China, and Europe. In 1922 Kano established another school in Japan called the Kodokan, which became the official international center for all the dojos.

Although Kano did not believe that public competition was an appropriate aim of the study of judo, some students enjoyed competing with each other. Public competitions were held among European, Chinese, and Japanese dojos until the outbreak of World War II. After the war, international judo competitions resumed. Weight categories, such as those used in boxing, were established. This step gradually led to an ideological split between those who began to see judo more and more as a competitive sport and those who remained dedicated to Kano's view of judo as a personal art of training the mind and body. Today judo is one of the most widespread sports in the world, but very few dojos teach the spirit of gentleness that was at the heart of Kano's technique.

Basic Principles

Kano Jigoro believed that his art of unarmed self-defense was a means to teach a philosophy or art of daily living. A serene, disciplined mind, working in conjunction with controlled body actions, was used to bring down an opponent and, applied in a larger sense, to live life in peace and well-being. Control of body and mind results from a supple body, perfect balance, constant alertness, emotional detachment, and proper breathing techniques.

The techniques of judo are practiced with a partner and require quick shifts of body and mind. The fundamental movements derived from judo are designed to neutralize an opponent, but the overall aim of the technique, according to Kano Jigoro, is to understand and demonstrate the living laws of movement. The movements involve the body, arms, and legs. They are taught carefully and repeated many times in the course of training.

Today the principal movements of judo also include *kumi-kata*, the action of gripping an opponent; *nage-waza*, a series of throws; *katame-no-kata*, techniques of control; *osaekomi-waza*, the action of immobilizing an opponent on the ground; *shime-waz*, strangulation techniques; and finally, *kansetsu-waz*, techniques of bending and locking the joints.

Once the fundamental movements are learned, the partners practice training in a freestyle combat called *randori*. In this quick, dancelike practice, *uke*, the one who submits, is thrown to the mat and immobilized by *tori*, the one who throws. Suppleness of body, perfect balance, serenity, and alertness are all tested and developed in this practice.

Practice

Judo is taught on large, rectangular tatami mats. Traditionally the mats were made of straw, but today they are often made of pressed foam. Students are barefoot and wear a special uniform called a *judogi*. It is made of thick white or unbleached cotton. It consists of large, baggy trousers called *zubon*, a loose-fitting jacket with wide sleeves that come halfway down the forearm called a *sode*, and a belt called an *obi*.

Judo training is organized in stages. When a student passes a particular stage, he is allowed to wear the colored belt associated with that stage. A white belt represents a beginner, a black belt the most advanced practitioner.

Even though today judo is more often a test of strength between two opponents, the underlying principles of the spirit of the founder and of all martial arts are still at the core of this body-mind discipline.

Benefits

Judo is one of the more popular martial arts disciplines, and people throughout the world who practice it have reported a variety of benefits. These include a significant improvement in physical fitness, sharpened mental clarity and emotional balance, increased self-discipline, and self-confidence gained from a knowledge of valuable self-defense techniques.

—*Nancy Allison, CMA*

Resources

American Judo and Jujitsu Federation
c/o Central Office Administrator
P.O. Box 993312
Redding, CA 96099-3312

e-mail: ajjfdanzan@aol.com
Web site: www.ajjf.org
Founded in 1958, this organization promotes the teaching of ju jutsu and judo in the United States.

International Judo Federation
   21st Floor, Doosan Bldg.
   101-1 Ulchiro 1ka, Choongku
   Seoul, Korea
   Tel: (82-1-2) 759-6936
   Fax: (82-1-2) 754-1075
   e-mail: yspark@ijf.org
   Web site: www.ijf.org
   The world-governing body of judo. Provides information about competitive judo, including international and Olympic events.

World Martial Arts Association
   P.O. Box 1568
   Santa Barbara, CA 93102
   Tel: (805) 569-1389
   Fax: (805) 569-0267
   Founded in 1979, this group promotes and teaches several martial arts, including ju jutsu, judo, aikido, and karate.

Further Reading

Caffary, Brian. *The Judo Handbook: From Beginner to Black Belt.* New York: Galley Books, 1989.

Frederic, Louis. *A Dictionary of the Martial Arts.* Translated and edited by Paul Crompton. Boston: Charles E. Tuttle Company, 1995.

Tegner, Bruce. *Judo: Beginner to Black Belt.* Ventura, Calif.: Thor Publishing, 1991.

Karate

 Karate originated as a method of hand-to-hand combat, but today is also practiced as a sport and a form of self-discipline. The name *karate* derives from the Japanese characters *kara*, meaning "empty," and *te*, meaning "hand," and is therefore often translated as "empty hand." Karate students, known as *karateka*, learn highly effective weaponless ("empty hand") techniques of attack and defense using their arms and legs. The philosophy of karate is based on Zen Buddhism, which places great value on inner calm, clear thinking, self-knowledge, and a heightened awareness of one's relationship to others and the world. Therefore, karate not only is a form of physical training and self-defense but also is used to develop spiritual and mental well-being.

History

Karate developed in Asia over the course of several centuries. Its roots lie in the different forms of unarmed combat that arose among peasants who sought to protect themselves from neighboring invaders. Buddhist monks of the Shaolin Temple in the Hunan province of China also refined a method of fighting to protect themselves against troops and robbers. At Shaolin, the Zen Buddhist monk Bodhidharma equipped his disciples with the strength and discipline to approach enlightenment by instructing them to practice fighting moves. The teachings of Zen Buddhism became the basis for the mental and spiritual training that is essential to the martial arts.

The island of Okinawa, located almost midway between Japan and China, became a place that allowed traders, soldiers, travelers, and local inhabitants to exchange goods, ideas, and fighting techniques. It was here in the seventeenth century that several martial arts styles arose, collectively known as Okinawa-*te* ("Okinawan hand"). In the early twentieth century, the various styles of Okinawa-*te* were unified under the name of karate by Gichin Funakoshi (1868-1957), considered the founder of modern karate, who promoted his sport by traveling through Japan staging tournaments and demonstrations. The karate practiced at this time was used as a form of violent combat. Because of this, *karate-do* was established as an alternative to the lethal version of karate. The suffix *do* means "way" and conveys the sense that the new approach was intended for spiritual and physical development, not war. In *karate-do,* blows are never completed, but instead stop just short of impact; in *karate-do* competitions, *karateka* are evaluated on their form and the quality of their execution of prescribed moves.

By 1930 every major university in Japan had a karate club. With the outbreak of World War II, karate was taught to the Imperial Japanese army. When Japan surrendered in 1945, General Douglas MacArthur placed a ban on all martial arts training. In 1948, one year after U.S. occupation forces lifted the ban on karate instruction, Funakoshi started to rebuild the sport. He gave a demonstration at an American air base, and the impressed commanders gave permission for instruction to take place on their military bases. Funakoshi himself toured the air bases giving demonstrations. It was this effort that saved karate and introduced it to the West. Karate was officially introduced to the United States in 1953. Two years later the Japanese Karate Association was formed, and by 1957 karate had reached Europe. Millions of people currently practice karate, and the sport is known throughout the world.

Styles

Karate is not a single unified system—in fact, hundreds of styles of karate exist. Many of these styles originated in the years after karate's first introduction in Japan. Some were advanced by Okinawan masters following in Funakoshi's footsteps, while others were outgrowths from Funakoshi's karate school. However, all of the other styles are outgrowths of five major branches: *shotokan, wado ryu, goju ryu, shito ryu,* and

kyokushinkai. Each style has its own strengths, techniques, and applications. By comparing different styles, individuals seeking to study karate may find the school most suited to their ability and temperament.

Philosophy

Karate is practiced in a dojo, or training hall. The dojo is not just a place to practice fighting techniques. It is also where karateka learn to become emotionally sound and mentally disciplined. Perfecting the technique requires a long and demanding training schedule. Through triumphs and failures, *karateka* must remain committed to the study of karate and be willing to work hard.

In karate, as in all the martial arts, etiquette is an important part of training and practice. *Karateka* bow before entering the training area of the dojo as a sign of respect for their training community. Before they practice fighting, the students bow to each other. At the beginning and end of every training session, they line up and bow to the *sensei,* or master. When *karateka* bow, they are not only showing respect but also learning to display an inner calm and power that emanates an aura of inner strength and invulnerability. Practitioners of karate believe that confidence, character, dignity, and self-awareness are as important as physical technique.

The student's uniform is called a karate *gi.* A belt called an *obi* is worn by all *karateka* and marks the level they have reached in their training. The belts vary in color, with each color corresponding to a specific level of progress. When belts were first introduced, students started with a light color and dyed them darker shades each time they passed the examination and advanced to the next level. If the *karateka* studied long enough and made significant progress, the belt eventually became black.

Training

Karate employs the whole body and is used to gain and maintain physical fitness. While karate techniques stress relaxation, muscular effort is needed to accelerate the arms and legs. Physical training exercises are performed to improve stamina, power, and flexibility.

Moves include kicking, striking, and blocking with the arms and legs. The practitioner attempts to focus as much force as possible at the point and moment of impact. Blows are made to the opponent with the forearm, elbow, knee, heel, and ball of the foot. All of these parts of the body are toughened by practice blows against padded surfaces or pine boards. *Tameshiwara,* or "power breaking," is one of the most spectacular and well known of karate training techniques. This involves breaking pine boards up to several inches thick with the bare hand or foot. But like all the techniques of karate, *tameshiwara* is as much a personal measure of concentration and self-confidence as it is a test of physical strength.

Proficiency comes through drills and repetition of techniques. Extensive repetition requires patience, stamina, and discipline. The philosophy of karate is based on Zen Buddhism, which promotes these qualities and aims to bring the mind and body into harmony. A person training to perfect the basic teachings of karate develops resilience, respect, and the knowledge of self-sacrifice.

Semisparring introduces the beginner to an actual fighting situation. Under controlled conditions, students face each other, one as the attacker, the other as the defender. Moves are prearranged and may look somewhat stiff in their execution. In contrast, real fighting is fast and unpredictable. The free-form movement that occurs in real fighting is difficult to teach, so the movements are broken down into their simple components. As students progress, new techniques are learned and added to the repertoire of movements that they have mastered. In the beginning, defensive blocking and counterattacking are performed as separate movements, but as students advance, the lapse in time between the two should gradually disappear until the block and counter flow fluidly.

The karate *kata,* or form, is a series of carefully arranged offensive and defensive moves performed against imaginary opponents. Only one person performs the *kata* at a time, thus no contact is involved; in tournaments, panels of judges evaluate the execution of the *kata.* To an outsider, the *kata* appears to be a confusing sequence of movements and may resemble a dance more than a fight. Nevertheless, it is a fundamental element of karate. Besides teaching the student the basic fighting movements, the *kata* helps the student to bring her body under the control of her mind and will. At an advanced level, the *kata* training includes very quick strikes and reactions. Those who have mastered *kata* seem to be able to anticipate their opponents' movements.

In the hands of a well-trained individual, karate can be the most lethal of martial arts. To some, it is an exciting form of competition, while others enjoy it as a form of physical fitness training. But to Gichin Funakoshi, and to thousands of serious teachers and students of karate throughout the world, it is a powerful vehicle of discipline and self-knowledge.

—STEFAN NIKANDER

Resources

American Amateur Karate Federation
    1930 Wilshire Blvd., Suite 1208
    Los Angeles, CA 90057
    Tel: (213) 483-8261
    Fax: (213) 483-4060
    A national governing body for karate. The federation promotes karate with the intention of improving the physical and mental health of the public through the practice of karate.

U.S.A. Karate Federation
   1300 Kenmore Blvd.
   Akron, OH 44314
   Tel: (216) 753-3114
   Fax: (216) 753-6967
   A national governing body for karate. The federation certifies instructors, conducts classes, and organizes competitions.

Further Reading

Aiello, Jerry L. *Warrior Within: A Guide to Applying Your Warrior Spirit.* Berkley, Mich.: Aiello Group, 1992.

Aigla, Jorge H. *Karate-Do and Zen: An Inquiry.* Santa Fe, N.M.: Do Press, 1994.

Funakoshi, Gichin. *Karate-Do: My Way of Life.* New York: Harper and Row, 1975.

Hassell, Randall G. *The Karate Spirit.* St. Louis, Mo.: Focus Publications, 1995.

Johnson, Nathan. *Zen Shaolin Karate: The Complete Practice, Philosophy, and History.* Boston: Charles E. Tuttle, 1993.

Nakamura, Tadashi. *Karate: Technique and Spirit.* Boston: Charles E. Tuttle, 1986.

Nicol, C. W. *Moving Zen: Karate as a Way to Gentleness.* New York: William Morrow, 1982.

Kendo

 Kendo is the Japanese martial art of swordsmanship. The name literally means "the way of the sword." It is considered the oldest of the Japanese martial arts and is based on rigorous physical and mental training and self-discipline. Essential to the practice of kendo is the knowledge and anticipation of the opponent's thoughts in order not only to defend oneself from the attack of others, but also to better understand oneself and others in daily life.

History

Kendo has a long and respected tradition in Japan, with techniques as old as swordsmanship itself. They were first used by the *bushi,* or warrior class, which developed in the northern provinces of Japan in their battles with the Ainu tribes. Throughout Japanese history the techniques have been called *ken-jutsu, heiho, toho, gekken, hyoho, to-jutsu, tachi-uchi,* and *hyodo,* and were passed on from father to son and from teacher to student through oral tradition.

The samurai, an elite class of *bushi,* started training in these techniques in the tenth century. It is estimated that from the start of this training until 1876, more than six hundred different schools of swordsmanship flourished throughout Japan. In 1876 the first Meiji emperor forbade the samurai to carry swords due to the many fights and political intrigues between the samurai and the noble class.

The exact origin of modern kendo is credited to a variety of sources. According to Louis Frederic in his *Dictionary of the Martial Arts,* Sakakibara Kenkichi, an expert of the Jikishin kage school of swordsmanship, improved a technique using the *shinai,* or bamboo sword. He gave demonstrations of his new technique throughout Japan in 1873. Sakakibara's desire was to revive the art of Japanese swordsmanship without its violent applications. The name *kendo* was given to the new peaceful discipline by the Abe-ryu, or school headed by the Abe family. Modern kendo, or Japan kendo style, developed through a collaboration by the six leading ken-jutsu schools at the end of the feudal era in 1876.

In 1909 the first academy of kendo was founded in Tokyo. Both men and women were taught, and the new martial art gained a large following throughout Japan. Its study was primarily confined to Japan until 1955, when it was introduced on an organized scale to France and the United States. In

1970 the first international tournament was held in Japan.

Since that time kendo has gained a high reputation internationally and is practiced throughout the world. It is practiced in thirty-seven countries today, and there are thirty-four member countries in the International Kendo Federation, which sponsors an international competition every three years.

Basic Principles

The goal of kendo is to overcome the opponent by overcoming the self. This involves tremendous self-discipline and intense mental concentration, often in the face of great physical pain. Unlike tai chi ch'üan or aikido, which admonishes the practitioner to "go with" the opponent, the philosophy of kendo teaches the student to approach each conflict as a battle to the death: only the strongest will remain alive when the fight is over.

To dominate the opponent, the *kendoka*, someone who practices kendo, must unite her *ki* with the *ki* of the universe. According to Japanese belief, *ki* is the vital life energy flowing through all things and all people. Kendo philosophy states that the power of *ki* can be channeled and directed through concentration. This ability to channel the *ki* is first realized through the kendo stance, in which the *kendoka* absorbs the *ki* from the earth by pulling it up through the soles of the feet into the legs, torso, and eventually the top of the head. The spine must remain straight in order to avoid impeding the flow of *ki*. The effect of a bent spine on the flow of *ki* can be compared to the effect of pinching or bending a garden hose to stop the flow of water.

Even more fundamental than the stance is the flow of breath, which is slow and deep. It is pulled through the nose into the *tanden*, or *hara*, located about three inches below the navel, midway between the navel and the spine. The *tanden* is considered the physical and psychological center of the human being. It is here that individual *ki* and universal *ki* unite to form a powerful fighting energy. At the moment a blow is struck, the attacker releases a powerful sound called *ki-ai*, which is the concentration and focus of *ki* toward the *kendoka's* goal.

The focus of the eyes is another way in which the *kendoka* seeks to dominate her opponent. The *kendoka* must "see through" her opponent, penetrating to the mind with her eyes. This allows the *kendoka* to predict her opponent's next move. At the same time the *kendoka* must "see as far away as possible." By seeing "far away" the opponent becomes like a person seen against a mountain—a small insignificant dot that cannot stop the *kendoka* from achieving her goal.

Mental energy is paramount to the training in kendo. Only through mental concentration can total control and power be achieved. Yet the *kendoka's* mind must be like that of a baby, soft and focused. In this way the *kendoka* can stay totally concentrated in the moment and be prepared for any attack.

Practice

A typical kendo class is a rigorous, ritualized workout that usually lasts for two hours. The dojo (training hall) is a large, open room with a wooden floor. At one end of the room is the *joza*, or altar. Each class begins and ends with a bow to the *joza* as a sign of respect, specifically to the *sensei*, or master teacher, but metaphorically to all ancestors and all knowledge that have gone before.

Students wear the armor and traditional dress of samurai warriors: navy blue *hakama*, or wide skirtlike pants, and *gi*, or jacket. In the feudal era, only samurai were entitled to wear the *hakama*, a symbolically pleated garment. Each of the five front pleats represents a virtue from the *bushido*, or samurai code of honor. The first pleat stands for humility, the second for justice, the third for courtesy, the fourth for knowledge, and the fifth for trust. The two back pleats represent

Precision, speed, and coordination are the qualities admired in a kendo attack. Bruce Robertson-Smith, a first-degree black-belt student, explains that scoring a point in kendo is not as clear-cut as scoring a point in soccer or basketball. Three judges, standing in a triangular formation around the contest area, must all agree that the *kendoka* has earned the point.

Earning a point involves many things. First of all, the *kendoka* must strike the exact target that he calls out at the instant of the attack. Kendo recognizes nine target spots on the body: the right, left, and middle of the forehead; right and left forearms; the right, left, and center of the torso; and the center of the throat. Only the point or upper third of the *shinai* can effectively be used to strike a target area. The movement of the attack must be aesthetically pleasing, much like the criteria for earning points in competitive gymnastics. Finally, the energy expressed through the *ki-ai* must be full and strong. These criteria, known as *kikentai-no-ichi,* literally translated, mean "life force-sword-body-one."

yin and yang, the two opposite cosmic energy principles that unite symbolically in one straight line down the back of the *hakama.*

A *taiko* drum on the *joza* is beaten to signify the beginning of class. After the initial bow, students generally form a circle to perform basic warm-up exercises. Then *suriashi* (footwork exercises) are practiced while walking the length of the dojo. The exercises progress from slow to fast and from simple to complex, beginning with the basic kendo sliding step, by which the foot never leaves the ground, to complex patterns involving multiple changes of direction and thrusts of the *shinai.*

The class proceeds to *waza,* or techniques. *Waza* include instructions in how to hold the *shinai* and how to attack. Beginning with a single target, the training advances to multiple targets, all of which must be quickly and precisely hit during the length of one long exhalation.

In more advanced classes the teacher will eventually signal that it is time to put on the steel-grilled head masks called *men.* At that point students line up, in order of their ranked ability, with the highest-ranking students nearest the *joza.* They sit in *za-zen,* a traditional kneeling posture in which the mind, breath, and body are brought to a state of calm readiness. Gloves and mask rest in front; the *shinai* is placed to the left of the body. The *sensei* puts on a protective head scarf and mask, and then upon verbal cue all the students do the same.

Now in full armor, the *keiko,* or practice, begins with a bow to the *joza,* the *sensei,* and the opponent. Beginning with specific thrusts and advancing to series of thrusts, the *keiko* eventually progresses to full contact, where *kendokas* practice a series of fights, each lasting about three minutes. The *keiko* continues until the *taiko* drum is beaten once again.

The students return to their line of rank and repeat in exact reverse order the ritual movements that began the *keiko*: bowing, removing the *men* and head scarf, and finally kneeling again in *za-zen* for a brief period of meditation. Classes often conclude with the *sensei* giving a "teaching" on the spirit of kendo.

Benefits

Because of its psychological and physical benefits, kendo is one of the most popular martial arts in Japan. Practice builds strength, coordination, and flexibility. On an intellectual level, many students are able to sharpen their mental focus and clarity through practice. Through the rigorous training and self-discipline of kendo, students learn first to master themselves, and through that how to master all opponents and adverse situations. The physical, mental, and emotional knowledge gained can be applied to all endeavors in life. Many of the political and industrial leaders of modern Japan study kendo.

—*NANCY ALLISON, CMA; WITH DANIEL T. EBIHARA, AND BRUCE ROBERTSON-SMITH*

Resources

Canadian Kendo Association
  205 Riviera Drive
  Markham, Ontario L3R 5J8
  Canada
  Tel: (416) 445-1481
  Fax: (416) 445-0519
  Provides information on kendo in Canada.

Eastern Kendo Federation
  c/o Mozart H. Ishizuka
  445 Fifth Ave., Suite 21E
  New York, NY 10016
  Tel: (212) 679-1230
  Fax: (212) 679-1236
  Offers information about dojos in the New York area.

Great Lakes Kendo Federation
  c/o Dr. Tsuyoshi Inishita
  2423 Fenwick Road
  University Heights, OH 44118
  Tel: (216) 321-1187
  Disseminates information about kendo in the Midwest.

Pacific Northwest Kendo Federation
  616 S.W. 135th St.
  Seattle, WA 98146
  Tel: (206) 246-2239
  Provides information on kendo in the Northwest.

South East Kendo Federation
  2830 Carolyn Drive
  Smyrna, GA 30080
  Tel: (404) 434-7166
  Furnishes regional information on kendo practitioners.

Southwest Kendo Federation
  c/o Charles Riddle
  12101 Randy Lane
  Burleson, TX 76208
  Offers resources to those practicing kendo in the American Southwest.

Further Reading

Kiyota, Minoru. *Kendo: Its Philosophy, History, and Means to Personal Growth.* New York: Columbia University Press, 1995.

Sasamori, Junzo. *This Is Kendo: The Art of Japanese Fencing.* Rutland, Vt.: Charles E. Tuttle, 1964.

Kung Fu Wu Su

 Kung fu wu su refers to a multitude of Chinese martial arts and gymnastic movements, and encompasses nearly four hundred disparate styles. It includes combative styles such as hung gar and more defensive styles such as t'ai chi ch'üan, and even includes acrobatic exercises. Advanced practice of kung fu requires almost lifelong study combined with knowledge of Chinese culture, customs, and history.

History

Some forms of kung fu wu su date back approximately five thousand years. The form that is the basis of most forms practiced today is said to have been perfected by Buddhist monks, who practiced it to protect themselves from bandits and brigands in ancient China. The system itself is so potent that China's first great monarch, Huang Ti, known as the Yellow Emperor, had it systematically taught to his troops to improve their fighting ability. Kung fu, as we know it today, flourished in both northern and southern China, but throughout the years evolved in different ways. Generally speaking, southern styles emphasize hand techniques, while northern styles emphasize leg techniques.

The term *kung fu wu su* has a direct translation from its Chinese characters, and a philosophical meaning derived from that translation. *Kung* means "discipline technique;" *fu* means "person;" *wu* means "martial art;" and *su* means "technique" or "skill." But the word as a whole encompasses much more. The philosophical idea of kung fu is to develop three distinct but necessary characteristics: *dar* (character), *tse* (mental ability), and *tee* (physical ability). The aim is to live a positive and harmonious life.

The concept of self-defense is as old as humanity, but the first definitive martial arts systems evolved in China. It is assumed that the Chinese had already cataloged and codified a basic system of self-defense as early as 4,500 years ago, a system they called kung fu or wu su. In time Taoist monks began to experiment with various divergent styles, beginning with five animal styles: crane, tiger, snake, dragon, and monkey. The second great transformation in the system came from India, when a traveling Buddhist monk, Bodhidarma, introduced advanced breathing techniques and meditative exercises, which were incorporated into kung fu about 550 years ago. This reinforced what came to be known as the Shaolin style, named after the temple where it was taught. Bodhidarma was enshrined by his Chinese name, *dor-mor*, for adding to and strengthening an already established system.

China's history has been tumultuous, and conflict and warfare eventually disrupted the tranquillity of the Shaolin Temple. The Shaolin Temple era ended with the Ming dynasty (1368–1644 C.E.), when the reigning emperors began to regard the two Shaolin temples, one in southern China and one in northern China, as a threat to their authority. They effectively embarked on a campaign that led to the destruction of both temples. Shaolin monks scattered throughout Asia, teaching kung fu wherever they went.

Styles

The differing styles of kung fu evolved through need or observation. For example, besides the animal styles, which are based on observation of animal movements, there are also styles based on natural phenomena, such as moving shadow. Other styles are based on distinct physical features like white eyebrow, a state or condition such as drunken monk, or even a physical substance like green jade.

Twenty-five groupings in kung fu identify the various styles. These groupings include everything from an astrological classification, like *chee sin*, or seven stars style, to insects, like *tong lon*, or praying mantis style. All these groupings can be classified into four general categories:

1. The first classification is based on appearance. Some may emphasize the "hard" way with strong, devastating blows and movements. Others may emphasize the "soft" way, in which the opponent's strength may be used against him, but which is just as effective in subduing an adversary. For example, *gin kong* is considered a hard style because of its aggressive nature, and t'ai chi soft because of its emphasis on defensive movements. Some disciplines, such as northern Shaolin style, may be a combination of both.
2. The second classification is based on geography. *Pa kua*, a style that emphasizes distinct stepping movements, comes from north-central China. *Jow gar* and *hung dar*, styles that emphasize strong hand techniques, come from southern China.
3. The next classification is based on the character of the style. T'ai chi, with its emphasis on inner force and evasive

How does kung fu differ from other martial arts systems? There is no easy explanation. Traditionally, kung fu is considered circular in its motions, while other disciplines are more linear. This does not take into account other ways of fighting such as judo, ju jutsu, aikido, and kempo.

One of the defining differences in kung fu is that the students utilize footwear. They do not train barefoot, as in Korean or Japanese styles. Also, traditional Shaolin kung fu does not have a belt system. Since training was within the family or village group, a ranking system was not necessary. Some large schools in northern China did use a button system of ranking, which is used in certain kung fu schools today.

maneuvers, is considered an internal discipline. An example of a discipline that is external in nature is *hung gar*, because of its preference for force and rapid attack movements. A combination of both can be found in the northern Shaolin style.

4. The final classification is based on the purpose of the style. It may be the grabbing, grappling style of *chin-na fa*, or a weapon style like the steel sword, or *kong chien*. The terminology used to define each style often reflects its content.

Most styles of kung fu employ punching and kicking techniques, but others use grappling and throwing techniques, and/or ground fighting. Most utilize a variety of weapons: staff weapons such as the long, or sleeve, staff; small-bladed weapons such as the straight sword or machete, long-bladed weapons such as the spear or trident, and throwing weapons such as stars or spikes. Nearly all the styles incorporate meditation, breathing techniques, and body conditioning. The end result is a vigorous combination of external and internal methods designed to promote knowledge of self-defense and enhance general health. The overall philosophy is derived from Taoist and Buddhist teachings, theoretical concepts designed to keep both the body and mind agile and resilient.

Kung fu embodies more than just physical aspects. Ancient masters in China considered it a way of life, not just a sport or pastime. In its true essence, it is an ethical discipline that permeates every aspect of life. Since kung fu is more than a martial arts technique, any disciplined person can practice it. If one does a task well and acts in a correct and moral manner, he is said to have kung fu. The purpose of kung fu practice is to create not a fighting machine, but a complete individual—one who aspires to continual growth as a total person and who contributes to the well-being of the community.

When choosing a style to practice, consider your own needs and desires as an individual. There are kung fu schools or temples that will emphasize one style or manner of practice. Others may offer a combination of styles. Eventually, you will gravitate toward the method that is best suited to your nature.

Practice

The study of kung fu wu su in all its diverse forms can take a lifetime. A basic course in martial arts practice can take up to five years to complete. High-level studies will take longer. The length of the training depends on how much the individual student wants from the study and how much time and effort he gives to the training. The basic applications range from body conditioning to calisthenics to basic self-defense techniques. The training is all-inclusive. It can also be extensive in other areas if the student is given a grounding in philosophy, concentration, kung fu medicines, breathing, meditation, and diet. Not many temples or schools will offer such a varied and extensive program of study.

Benefits

People study kung fu for many reasons. Some seek a measure of self-protection. Others are drawn by its refined, elegant movements. Some are enthralled by the sheer power generated by its defensive and offensive techniques. Some are enticed by the arcane self-healing practices rooted in the system, such as the enhancement of *chi*, or life force, the positive energy within all of us. Some individuals seek to develop this *chi* to its highest level, to channel this energy to protect and heal themselves and others from illness. Kung fu is a system that seeks a dynamic flow between mind and body. In the beginning, it may test one's commitment to learning and mastering the different movements and their applications.

—*OSWALD RIVERA*

Resources

Chinese Kung-Fu Wu-Su Association
28 W. 27th St., 8th Floor
New York, NY 10001
Tel: (212) 725-0535
Provides information on different martial arts disciplines.

T'ai Chi Ch'üan/Shaolin Chüan Association
3720 Illinois Ave.
St. Charles, IL 60174
Tel: (630) 443-0070
Web site: www.taichi-shaolin.com
Founded in 1987, this organization promotes and offers instruction in t'ai chi ch'üan and Shaolin chuan kung fu. Conducts demonstrations, seminars, lectures, and certification programs for members, and publishes a bimonthly newsletter.

World Martial Arts Association
P.O. Box 1568
Santa Barbara, CA 93102
Tel: (805) 569-1389
Fax: (805) 569-0267

Promotes many kung fu wu su disciplines and instructs practitioners in the technical aspects of these disciplines.

Further Reading

Mitchell, David. *Shaolin Temple Kung-Fu.* London: Stanley Paul, 1990.

Parulski, George R. *The Secrets of Kung-Fu: A Complete Guide to the Fundamentals of Shaolin Kung-Fu and the Principles of Inner Power.* Chicago: Contemporary Books, 1984.

Wong, Kiew Kit. *The Art of Shaolin Kung-Fu: The Secrets of Kung-Fu for Self-Defense, Health, and Enlightenment.* Rockport, Mass.: Element, 1996.

Taekwondo

 Taekwondo is one of the most popular martial arts in the world. Its offensive and defensive movements are uniform for all of those that practice the discipline, which makes it easy to set standards of accomplishment and skill. Many people also find it an effective system of self-defense. People of all ages and walks of life have taken up this contemporary Korean martial art to improve their stamina, physical fitness, and mental acuity, and to learn to defend against attack. The practice of taekwondo has a rich heritage, and its practitioners adhere to strict ethical and moral guidelines.

History

The contemporary art and modern sport of taekwondo can be traced to *tae kyon*, a discipline characterized by its emphasis on kicking techniques. Some experts believe that tae kyon was an offshoot of *su bak,* the martial art said to have been practiced more than one thousand years ago by Hwarang warriors in Korea. The Hwarang (which means "flowering youth") were a national group of outstanding youths handpicked for training in swordsmanship and archery. The chosen youths were guided by a code of ethics known as the Code of Hwarang, prescribed by the eminent Buddhist monk Wongwang. The code dictated that followers would loyally serve the king, be obedient to their parents, be honorable to friends, never retreat in battle, and kill justly.

In peacetime there was little use for the practice of tae kyon. At the time of the Silla dynasty (688–935 B.C.E.), Korea became a highly centralized Buddhist state. The fine arts flourished, and the practice of martial arts was suppressed because of their offensive, warlike capabilities.

The contemporary art of taekwondo was founded by General Choi Hong Hi in 1946. Choi came from a military family; he studied tae kyon as a child and karate while forced to serve in the Japanese army. Originally, taekwondo was nothing more than transplanted Japanese karate with a bit of tae kyon. In fact, the term *taekwondo* (*tae* meaning "foot," *kwon* meaning "fist," *do* meaning "art" or "the way") was adopted by the Korean Taekwondo Federation as the Korean translation of karate (*kara* meaning "empty," *te* meaning "hand"). Today, however, the World Taekwondo Federation is the undisputed governing body, sanctioning all taekwondo competitions and certifying all belt-rank promotions at the black-belt level and above. In addition, the body and movement structure of the contemporary, karate-like taekwondo has been modified into a modern sport form within the past ten years. Notable changes include a higher fighting stance, faster footwork, a new set of prearranged patterns, and an emphasis on sport competition and its rules rather than on self-defense applications.

Basic Principles

While the physical movements of taekwondo are simple, dedicated practice is necessary for them to become natural and spontaneous. As a result, the practitioner develops discipline and perseverance, as progress is sometimes slow. The mental discipline, self-confidence, and self-control gained through prolonged practice bring practitioners the utmost determination and stability of both mind and body.

As a sport, taekwondo's uniform technique sets a standard for all practitioners. As a martial art, the basic techniques of taekwondo serve as a powerful system of self-defense skills. In competition, taekwondo techniques are evaluated on the practitioner's ability to perform them individually in the air, in series as self-defense techniques with an opponent, and in application through sparring.

Practice

Taekwondo is taught in a *dojang* (training hall), usually a simple room with a wooden floor. In the more traditional taekwondo dojang, one will find a *makiwara* (striking post), used to develop focus and power in striking. In the modern, sport-oriented dojang, however, this is replaced with a heavy punching bag, and various types of padding, such as chest, head, and foot protectors, and padded punching gloves are used.

At the beginning of each class, students line up in rows. The *sabumnim* (master) will then yell out a few commands, and students will bow to him, to the senior student, and to the flags of Korea and the country where the training hall is located. Then the students will stand for a few minutes in meditation, clearing their minds and relaxing in preparation for serious practice. Once these preparations have concluded, physical training begins.

Classes generally last one hour or ninety minutes. The first fifteen minutes are spent stretching the legs and hips. Students spend the next fifteen minutes practicing sets of basic blocking, striking, and kicking techniques in the air. This is followed by a fifteen-minute practice of predetermined offensive and defensive movements known as *hyung* or *poomse.* The next fifteen minutes are generally spent on the practice of basic self-defense techniques, including defenses against the straight punch, wrist grabs, and holds of various types. The next ten minutes are used for the practice of sparring, which allows students to use their skills against an opponent in a controlled environment. This is where many students feel they benefit the most from training in that they are able to see firsthand how their skills have improved. The final five minutes of class are spent in meditation to calm the mind, shed the fighting mentality, and ease back into daily activities.

The conclusion of class finds students reciting the Code of Hwarang, and bowing to their master, the senior student, and the flags once again. Practitioners then take a few minutes to sweep the dojang floor and clean any mirrors that may be present. The bowing and cleaning are humbling mechanisms. They instill in the student a sense of respect for one's elders and seniors, the training hall, and one's surroundings. It is hoped that this will carry over into the practitioner's daily life.

Benefits

As taekwondo practitioners refine their physical abilities, they improve in many seemingly unrelated areas. A relaxed state of mind, improved patience, sharpened concentration, and numerous other benefits accompany new self-defense skills. Above all, taekwondo students embrace the philosophical and ethical beliefs that define the discipline, beliefs that function to guide the students in their daily lives.

Since its Olympic debut in 1988, taekwondo's popularity has spread at a remarkable rate across the world. Proficiency in basic techniques takes only a few years. While the earning of a black belt takes roughly three or four years, it is typically thought to be just the beginning of a lifelong journey toward self-actualization.

—MARK WILEY

Resources

International Taekwondo Association
P.O. Box 281
Grand Blanc, MI 48439
Tel: (810) 232-6482
Promotes the practice of taekwondo in the United States.

Korean Ki Do Federation HQ
Seoul, Kang Nam Gu, Non Hyun Dong
122-2 Nam Yang Bldg. 300
Korea
Tel: (02) 540-2156-7
Provides information for international organizations and associations.

United States Taekwondo Association
220 E. 86th St.
New York, NY 10028
Tel: (212) 772-8918
Disseminates information about taekwondo in the United States.

United Taekwondo International
4707 48 St., 2nd floor
Camrose, Alberta T4V 1L2
Canada
Tel: (403) 672-3500
Offers information about the practice of taekwondo in Canada.

Further Reading

Books
Cho, S. Henry. *Taekwondo: Secrets of Korean Karate.* Rutland, Vt.: Charles E. Tuttle Co., 1992.

Corcoran, Jon, and Emil Farkas. *The Original Martial Arts Encyclopedia.* Los Angeles: Pro Action Publishing, 1993.

Draeger, Donn F., and Robert W. Smith. *Comprehensive Asian Fighting Arts.* Tokyo: Kodansha International, 1980.

Haines, Bruce. *Karate's History and Traditions.* Rev. ed.. Rutland, Vt.: Charles E. Tuttle Co., 1995.

Park, Y. H., and Jeff Leibowitz. *Fighting Back: Taekwondo for Women.* East Meadow, N.Y.: Y.H. Park Publications, 1993.

Shaw, Scott. *Hapkido: Korean Art of Self-Defense.* Rutland, Vt.: Charles E. Tuttle Co., 1996.

Journals

Young, Robert W. "The History and Development of Tae Kyon." *Journal of Asian Martial Arts* 2, 2 (1993): 44–69.

PART 12:

Yoga

Yoga is an ancient Hindu method of body-mind integration used to achieve spiritual enlightenment. Literally translated from Sanskrit, the language of the Hindu spiritual texts, *yoga* means "union." This union refers to the joining of the individual human spirit with the motivating spirit of the universe.

Over thousands of years many methods of reaching this desired spiritual union evolved. These methods include such activities as the study of metaphysics and philosophy, meditation, the development and cleansing of the physical body, and living a life of service and devotion. As practiced in the United States today, most yoga classes focus on hatha yoga, the method of developing spiritual enlightenment through physical mastery of the body. Hatha yoga practice includes stretching, flexing, and balancing the body in many different positions, internal cleansing techniques, and breathing exercises. In many yoga classes, such as those offered in health clubs or recreation centers, the physical aspects of hatha yoga are often more emphasized than the spiritual. With or without the spiritual goal, the many forms of yoga now practiced offer a means of gaining and maintaining physical, emotional, and mental health and well-being.

The History of Yoga

Archaeologists and yoga scholars believe that images found on ceramics during excavations in India's Indus River basin are of yoga asanas, or postures, and show that the practices of yoga flourished in India as far back as 3000 B.C.E. Sometime between the fifth and second centuries B.C.E., the Indian philosopher Patanjali gathered many of the basic techniques and concepts of raja, or kingly yoga, into a book called *The Yoga Sutras*. The most common forms of yoga practiced in the West today are derived from the concepts and practices that Patanjali recorded.

INTEGRAL YOGA

IYENGAR YOGA

KRIPALU YOGA

Yoga was incorporated into the Buddhist religious tradition by Buddhism's founder, Prince Siddhartha Gautama. The young Indian prince was well versed in the theories and practices of yoga when he left his home in search of the cause of human suffering. The solutions he found form the philosophical basis of Buddhism. Followers of Gautama, also called the Buddha, or "enlightened one," lived peacefully in India until around the third century B.C.E., when the political climate became less tolerant of non-Hindus. It was at this time that the monks and disciples of Buddhism began to migrate in large numbers across the Asian continent.

Over time the Buddhist monks became a vital part of the cultural fabric of their adopted countries, and the yoga-based practices they brought with them were integrated into the native religions of China, Japan, and other Asian countries. In each country distinctive variations of the original Indian yogic practices developed. In his three-volume work, *The Complete Yoga Book,* James Hewitt states that ancient yogic techniques traveled in similar ways as far east as Siberia, mixing with Inuit shamanic practices, and as far west as the Middle East, where they were incorporated into Islamic Sufi practices. Both Hewitt and the scholar Mircea Eliade believe that Indian yogic practices also influenced the mystic sects of Christianity.

The philosophy and practices of yoga have slowly infiltrated Western culture throughout the twentieth century. With the British colonial expansion into India, knowledge of the physical, psychological, and metaphysical practices of yoga increased. The World Parliament of Religions, held in Chicago in 1893, brought many yoga teachers to America for the first time. In 1911 the American writer William James described in his classic study of the psychology of religious experience, *On Vital Reserves,* the considerable benefits one European friend received through the practice of yoga. By the 1930s Indian practitioners of yoga, such as Paramhansa Yogananda, were lecturing in England and in the United States. By 1946 Paramhansa's book *Autobiography of a Yogi,* describing the concepts and meditative practices of yoga, was available throughout the English-speaking world.

In the 1950s and 1960s yoga practices become more popular throughout the United States, with many books published on the subject and many schools established. In 1970 Swami Rama, founder of the Himalayan Institute in Pennsylvania, was the subject of research at the Menninger Foundation in Topeka, Kansas. According to *Yoga Journal International,* he shocked researchers with "his abilities to stop his heartbeat for extended periods of time and to remain fully lucid while his brain registered the delta waves normally associated with sleep." It was this research that first drew the attention of much of the mainstream Western scientific community to the link between human consciousness and physical functioning.

Today many Westerners practice yoga on a variety of levels—from full body-mind-spirit union to the maintenance of physical well-being. Many types of yoga classes are available in most major cities and even in smaller towns. There are a multitude of training programs in which yoga practitioners, from beginner to advanced, can develop their practice.

The Spiritual Goal of Yoga

To understand the practice of yoga, it is helpful to understand something about its spiritual goal. The spiritual goal of yoga is closely connected with the Hindu philosophical view concerning the relationship between spirit and matter. According to that view, the spirit animating the universe and the spirit animating every individual human being are one and the same. Every single thing on this planet, from the simplest blade of grass to the most complex human being, is, according to the Hindu view, a materialized form of this same spirit.

The desire motivating this spirit, as Mircea Eliade describes in his widely respected book *Yoga: Immortality and Freedom,* is simply "to be known." This spirit incarnates and reincarnates into more and more complex forms of matter according to a moral code known as the law of karma. When the spirit reaches human form, it has the ability to realize its true nature as part and parcel of the whole. This is a long and varied process involving many changes of human consciousness or awareness. *Samadhi* is the Sanskrit word that describes the blissful state of human consciousness attained when the individual human spirit experiences itself once again as part of the universal cosmic spirit.

The Nine Systems of Yoga

Reaching samadhi requires great discipline and much dedication. Over thousands of years many different systems of yoga practices evolved to suit the needs and personalities of different people. The different systems often share so many concepts and techniques that it is difficult to find one classification method on which all yoga scholars, and certainly all yoga teachers, would agree. However, the following represents the nine generally recognized paths to the goal of *samadhi.*

1. Raja yoga, also known as royal, kingly, classical, ashtanga, or eight-limbed yoga, is the path of mental mastery. Mental mastery here refers to the basic yogic belief that the disciplined focus of mental energy is the necessary basis for spiritual awareness. Raja yoga recognizes that this energy cannot be tapped unless the body is strong, healthy, relaxed, and balanced. Students work through the first seven limbs, or stages, which cover physical stretching, strengthening, toning and cleansing exercises, breathing exercises, ethical and philosophical inquiry, and meditation practices to reach *samadhi,* which is considered the eighth limb.
2. Hatha yoga, the path of bodily mastery, is the best-known and most practiced form of yoga in the West. Perhaps because of its focus on the body itself, the benefits of hatha yoga may be felt most easily without having to accept the spiritual component. For this reason many scholars believe that the practices of hatha yoga are merely a preparation for raja yoga. Hatha yoga practices include *asanas,* or postures, in which one balances, stretches, and strengthens the body; *kriyas,* or methods of cleansing the internal body; and *pranayama,* or special breathing exercises. Together these constitute a thorough method of

hygiene that cleanses and tones the internal organs and glands and the musculoskeletal, respiratory, digestive, and nervous systems.

3. Mantra yoga is the practice of influencing consciousness through repetition of certain syllables or phrases known as mantras. The word or phrase is considered to be a mystical distillation of the cosmic energy of the universe. It can be repeated aloud or silently in the mind. In Western scientific terms, spoken mantras may be understood as sound vibrations affecting one's emotions, similar to the way music often does. Transcendental Meditation, which was brought to the West by Marahishi Mahesh Yogi, is a form of mantra yoga.

4. Yantra yoga uses visual images as the focal point for concentration in order to affect consciousness in the same way that mantra yoga uses sound. Yantra images may be sculptures or paintings of deities or teachers, but more often they are mandalas—symbolic, geometric images of the relationship between the individual and the universal energy. Traditional mandalas are ornate paintings incorporating many Hindu or Buddhist deities in a sort of map of the spiritual universe, but simple abstract images are also common in the West today.

5. Kundalini or *laya* yoga is a method in which cosmic energy is depicted as a sleeping serpent coiled three and a half times around the base of the spine. In this image the mouth of the kundalini, or serpent, is grasping the *sushumna*, a narrow nerve channel through the spine. Difficult asanas, strenuous pranayama, mantras, yantras, muscular contractions or locks called *bandhas*, and concentrated meditative practices are all used to encourage the kundalini to climb up the *sushumna* through the seven chakras, or spiritual centers, that correspond to physical places along the length of the spine. As the kundalini passes through each center, it purifies the channel and awakens specific physical and psychic powers. While the traditional practices of kundalini yoga are often considered dangerous, the imagery associated with the chakra system is frequently used in other systems of yoga and has affected the development of many Western body-mind disciplines as well.

6. Jhana yoga, the path of spiritual knowledge and wisdom, emphasizes philosophical inquiry and meditation to reach spiritual enlightenment. For instance, students are encouraged to reflect on the nature of the world, reality, and the meaning of life, as well as their true selves. This is the path of intellectual pursuit and does not involve the body directly. A follower of jhana yoga would be comparable to Albert Einstein. Einstein was not a yoga practitioner, but the way he focused his intellect to inquire deeply into the nature of the universe had the disciplined and dedicated quality of a yogic meditation. Interestingly, Einstein's groundbreaking theories about the relationship of energy and matter set in motion a shift in Western physics that continues to move ever closer to the Hindu philosophical view of the universe.

7. Bhakti yoga is the path of love and devotion. It emphasizes living a life that demonstrates one's pure and selfless love of the divine. The Hindu god Krishna is often a focus for this form of yoga in India. Rites include singing songs and dancing dances of devotion. Members of the Krishna Consciousness Movement are among its devotees. While it has traditionally been one of the most popular paths for the people of India, Westerners are generally less comfortable with its practices.

8. Karma yoga, the path of selfless action and service, might be exemplified by Mahatma Gandhi or Mother Teresa. Even though Mother Teresa practiced Catholicism, the way in which her devotion to her religion led her to serve humanity is similar to the way in which a follower of karma yoga is taught to dedicate all of his actions to the good of others.

9. Tantric yoga as a general term can refer to any method of yoga using physiological techniques such as hatha or kundalini yoga, but is more specifically used to describe the path of union through harnessing sexual energies. In tantric yoga sexual union is seen as a way to spiritual illumination. Its practices include asanas, pranayama, mantras, and yantras employed in preparation of and during sex, which is performed as a ritual uniting of the male and female aspects of the one universal energy. (The Hindu spiritual texts have many names for these aspects, which are represented in Hindu art as gods and goddesses in the act of sexual embrace, but they are more familiar to Westerners through their Chinese names of yin and yang.) Because tantric yoga is an ecstatic path that embraces the earthy aspects of life, it has often been abused as a spiritual path, but the goal of tantric yoga, like the goal of all yogas, is spiritual union, and when practiced in earnest requires the same discipline and dedication.

The Yoga Experience in the West

Most yoga practiced in the West today primarily combines elements of hatha, mantra, and raja yoga. Because of the enormous overlap of the elements of various yogic systems, jhana, karma, kundalini, and/or yantra yoga may also be combined. Classes are generally taught in groups, but individual lessons are available. They are generally taught indoors, but some ashrams, or teaching centers, offer classes outdoors, where the energy of the sun and fresh air can enhance the pleasure and effectiveness of the exercises. Often the room will have an altar where flowers, incense, candles, a mandala, or photo of the founder of the school will rest. Students and teacher generally wear comfortable cotton clothing, which allows for the flow of air to the skin.

Yoga classes may be extremely vigorous and fast paced or very gentle and slow moving, depending on the tradition of the school and teacher. Many yoga classes will begin with the chanting of a mantra. The Hindu sacred syllable *om* is often used. The purpose of chanting is to utilize the power of sound vibrations to focus and influence consciousness.

Classes generally proceed to a series of asanas. Hundreds of asanas and many different techniques have been developed by different gurus, or teachers. Whether the class is vigorous or gentle, students will be urged to focus their attention on the initiation, sequencing, and quality of movement as they enter, hold, and leave each pose. Each pose has a specific purpose and name. For example, the cobra pose, named for the characteristic pose of the animal, is a backward lengthening and bending of the spine performed while lying on the stomach. It is used to develop flexibility in the spine, strength in the abdomen, and openness in the personality and spirit. Focusing on the flow of breath while in the pose calms the nervous system and mind, gently preparing the body and mind for deeper meditation.

Yoga therapy is an emerging field of physical therapy most often practiced on a one-on-one basis. It is not a complete method as are the nine ancient systems, but it uses the therapeutic properties of yoga breathing, posturing, and meditative techniques to aid the healing process. Yoga therapy functions much like a visit to a doctor or therapist, at which certain exercises are prescribed to treat particular symptoms, and verbal dialogue between the therapist and client addressing the body-mind nature of the ailment may ensue.

The asana portion of the class is generally followed by a series of pranayama, or breath-control exercises. Through pranayama, yoga students aim to create steady, flowing movement of *prana*, or life force, through the system. As the breathing becomes deeper, more controlled, and rhythmical, the mind becomes calm and focused.

With a cleansed and strengthened body and a calm and focused mind, the student is better prepared to begin meditation. The meditation portion of the class is designed to create a heightened sense of peace and awareness and to focus, empty, and control the mind. It is through the practice of meditation, after many years of long and disciplined study, yogis believe the state of *samadhi* may be reached.

Benefits

With or without the goal of *samadhi*, the benefits of yoga can be numerous. Many practitioners attribute health, vitality, and peace of mind to the practice of yoga. Western scientific studies have shown it to be effective in strengthening muscles and bones, improving circulation and respiration, reducing blood pressure and heart rate, relieving stress and physical pain, sharpening intellectual functioning and motor skills, and aiding in relief from physical and emotional addictions.

With the plethora of classes and approaches available, it is important to take the time to find a well-trained teacher in a style and class of yoga that is compatible with the goals and temperament of the student. Once found, the potential benefits of yoga seem to be limited only by the dedication of the student.

—NANCY ALLISON, CMA, WITH CONSULTATION BY LILLO (LEELA) WAY

Resources

Himalayan International Institute of Yoga, Science, and Philosophy
   78 Fifth Ave.
   New York, NY 10011
   Tel: (212) 243-5995
   Offers courses and lectures on all aspects of yoga practice and workshops for yoga teachers. The school is dedicated to helping individuals develop physically, mentally, and spiritually.

The International Association of Yoga Therapists
    109 Hillside Ave.
    Mill Valley, CA 94941
    Tel: (415) 381-0876

International Sivananda Yoga Vedanta Centres Worldwide
    Sivananda Ashram Yoga Camp
    673 8th Ave.
    Val Morin, Quebec J0T 2R0
    Canada
    Tel: (819) 322-3226; 1-800-263-YOGA
    Fax: (819) 322-5876

Yoga Journal
    2054 University Ave.
    Berkeley, CA 94704
    Tel: (510) 841-9200

Further Reading

Arua, Pandit U., et al. *Yoga Sutras of Patanjali with the Exposition of Yvasa: A Translation and Commentary.* Vol. 1. Honesdale, Pa.: Himalayan Publishers, 1986.

Eliade, Mircea. *Yoga: Immortality and Freedom.* New York: Pantheon Books, Bollingen Series LVI, 1958.

Hewitt, James. *The Complete Yoga Book.* New York: Schocken Books, 1977.

Satchidananda, Yogiraj Sriswami. *Integral Yoga Hatha.* New York: Holt, Rinehart and Winston, 1970.

Vishnudevananda, Swami. *The Complete Illustrated Book of Yoga.* New York: Harmony Books, 1980.

Integral Yoga

 Integral yoga is a modern approach to the ancient body-mind discipline of yoga. Its practice combines six ancient methods to help individuals discover inner peace and happiness: hatha yoga, which uses body postures (*asanas*), breath control (*pranayama*), and relaxation techniques; karma yoga, which teaches selflessness for the good of others; raja yoga, which stresses concentration and meditation on ethical perfection; *japa,* or mantra, yoga, which uses the repetition of sounds to help focus the mind in meditation; bhakti yoga, which stresses love and devotion to God, or the Divine Being; and jhana yoga, which encourages self-inquiry and the investigation of the meaning of life and the nature of knowledge and reality.

History

In the early part of the twentieth century, Swami Sivananda Saraswati (1887–1963) of Rishikesh, India, developed an approach to yoga that integrated several of the ancient methods of yoga. Several of his disciples spread this approach to yoga around the world. One of them, Swami Satchidananda, founded Integral Yoga International (originally the Integral Yoga Institute) in the United States in 1966.

For the past forty years Swami Satchidananda has promoted world peace through ecumenism—the recognition that, intrinsically, all religions embrace the same ultimate truth and belief in one God, which may be worshiped variously through many names and forms. He frequently conducts Light of Truth Universal Services, where clergy of all faiths worship together, each according to his or her own tradition.

Integral Yoga International now has more than forty Integral Yoga Institutes and Integral Yoga Centers throughout the United States and abroad. The headquarters of Integral Yoga International is Satchidananda Ashram–Yogaville, located in Buckingham, Virginia. The center encompasses almost 1,000 acres of woodland and fields. Here people of all faiths and backgrounds come together to study and practice the principles of integral yoga.

The focal point of Satchidananda Ashram–Yogaville is the Light of Truth Universal Shrine (LOTUS), which embodies Swami Satchidananda's teachings and his efforts to foster world peace and religious harmony. Inside the shrine each major faith is represented by an altar, on which rests a carved inscription from the scripture of that particular faith. Other known faiths and those that may one day develop, but which are still unknown to us, are also represented by illuminated arches. The theme of LOTUS is "Truth Is One, Paths Are Many," and this aphorism may also be extended to integral yoga. Integral yoga is a system that synthesizes the various yogic approaches with one goal in mind: to help the individual experience physical, mental, and spiritual harmony.

Basic Principles

The goal of integral yoga is to help people achieve what practitioners believe is the birthright of every individual—to realize the spiritual unity behind the diversity of life and to live harmoniously as members of one universal family. This goal is achieved by maintaining a well-balanced life with a body of optimum health and strength, the senses under total control; a clear, calm, well-disciplined mind; a sharp intellect; a will that is strong yet pliable; a heart full of unconditional love and compassion; an ego as pure as crystal; and a life filled with supreme peace and joy. Integral yoga strongly encourages such principles as truth, nonviolence, and universal brotherhood.

—THE REVEREND KUMARI DE SACHY, ED.D.

Resources

Satchidananda Ashram–Yogaville
   Route 1, Box 1720
   Buckingham, VA 23921
   Tel: (804) 969-3121
   Fax: (804) 969-1303
   Headquarters for Integral Yoga International. Provides teacher training courses, silent retreats, and classes and workshops in hatha yoga, meditation, yoga philosophy, vegetarian diet, and other various branches of yoga. These are offered regularly, year-round. Guests are welcome to visit the ashram.

Iyengar Yoga

 Iyengar yoga is a specific approach to the ancient body-mind discipline of yoga. It was developed in the 1940s by B. K. S. Iyengar, whose approach incorporates all of the methods of classical, or eight-limbed, yoga. Yoga begins with the study of universal and individual ethical values. This is followed by the physical practice of stretching, strengthening, toning, and cleansing the body through postures. After a time breathing exercises are introduced. This foundation leads to the various stages of meditation. Iyengar yoga is unique in its specific approach to asana, or body postures, and pranayama, or breathing practices.

History

B. K. S. Iyengar was born on December 14, 1918, in Karnataka in southern India. At the age of sixteen Iyengar moved to Mysore to live with his uncle, Shree T. Krishnamacharya, who had founded a yoga school. Iyengar's early experiences with yoga postures were tremendously painful and made him aware of his own stiffness. Through perseverance Iyengar found he was able to do more and more, achieving a remarkable skill in his own practice. Soon he was performing demonstrations and teaching at his uncle's school. In 1943 he married a woman named Ramamani, who inspired him to develop his unique approach to the practices of asana and pranayama.

After his marriage Iyengar moved to Pune, in the state of Maharastra. There he established his own yoga school, which is currently operating as Ramamani Iyengar Memorial Yoga Institute, in memory of his beloved wife, who passed away in 1973. Iyengar's renown as an accomplished yogi began to spread in India and in the West.

The first U.S. teacher-training center for the Iyengar method was formed in San Francisco in 1976 following a visit by Iyengar to Berkeley, California. The center was run by his students at that time. Presently there are schools teaching his approach worldwide. Teacher training includes classes in anatomy, physiology, kinesiology, yoga philosophy, and student-teacher relationships as well as asana and pranayama. Iyengar's students call him *guruji,* an Indian term of affection for a beloved teacher. He has written five books on yoga. He continues to teach in India, the United States, and throughout the world today.

Philosophy

Iyengar yoga relies on standing asanas more than other styles of yoga do. Students first learn to balance in the field of gravity and develop a richer contact with the earth through the feet. Iyengar believes that active development of the posture inherent to human beings—that of standing on two legs—enhances the understanding of other types of poses. Experience gained in the practice of standing poses is used in all other types of asanas—seated, twisted, inverted, and back bending.

Another unique aspect of Iyengar yoga is the use of props such as chairs, weights, benches, mats, belts, and blankets, which help stretch and strengthen the body. Teachers accommodate students with special needs through the effective use of props. In his teaching, Iyengar saw that students new to yoga tend to struggle at a muscular level, which creates a disturbance in the breath. He found that a prop used for support could alleviate muscular effort, thus helping the student achieve freedom of breath. This encourages quieting of the mind and senses, bringing the student to a state of meditation in the asana.

In Iyengar yoga, the asana practice can be quite rigorous. Yoga asanas sometimes resemble typical Western exercises or stretches. Thus, according to Iyengar, a change is required in the typical Western mind-set, a movement away from a mechanical, purely physical practice toward an integrated, mindful approach. Yoga describes the body as consisting of five layers: anatomical, physiological, psychological, intellectual, and bliss. Iyengar stresses that yoga develops all five layers, not just the physiological layer.

—*Janet MacLeod*

Kripalu Yoga

 Kripalu yoga is a modern approach to the ancient body-mind discipline of yoga. It was developed by Amrit Desai, a practitioner inspired by Kripalvananda, an Indian master of kundalini yoga. The kripalu approach combines asanas, or postures, which involve folding, stretching, bending, and balancing the body in a variety of positions; pranayama, or breath control; and meditation. Kripalu yoga is meant to give practitioners peace of mind and good health, and to develop spiritual awareness so that their inner divinity, which according to Hindu and yogic tradition is inherently present in everyone, can manifest itself.

Practice

The discipline is taught in three specific stages. The first stage is called "willful practice." Practitioners to learn to perform the postures correctly; to learn to take deep, full breaths; to coordinate their breaths with the movements; and to pay close attention to body alignment.

When students have mastered this first stage, they move on to the second, called "will and surrender." In this stage, postures are performed with the concentration focused fully on the body and the physical sensations that are being experienced. Practitioners hold the postures longer than in the first stage, providing a physical challenge that allows practitioners to face their own physical and mental resistances. Devakanya G. Parnell, director of resident yoga education at the Kripalu Center in Lenox, Massachusetts, has described it this way: "When you come to your toleration point during prolonged holding, you encounter your self-perceived limitations and learn how to consciously transcend them." This aspect of kripalu yoga is meant to help students with similar experiences in everyday life. It helps build confidence and self-reliance.

The third and final stage is reached when practitioners perform postures in a spontaneous flowing pattern, following their bodies' intuition and desires. This is known as Meditation in Motion™, the hallmark of kripalu yoga practice, in which the practitioner is able to sustain a tangible relationship with her own divine nature. At this level practitioners have truly released all of the obstructions that keep them from recognizing their essential divine nature.

Benefits

In addition to its spiritual goals, regular practice of kripalu yoga has a variety of health benefits. It can reduce stress, increase flexibility, and enhance one's sense of well-being. Practitioners consider this a method for uncovering physical, emotional, and mental tensions, allowing for insight into these problems and for relaxation.

Resources

Kripalu Center
  P.O. Box 793
  Lenox, MA 01240-0793
  Tel: (413) 448-3152
  Toll-free: 1-800-741-SELF (741-7353)
  A spiritual retreat center that offers workshops in yoga, meditation, and holistic health. Weekend, weeklong, and monthlong programs are available.

PART 13:

Meditation

Meditation, the art of turning one's attention inward in order to achieve more lucid consciousness, is a technique of character development most closely associated with Asian cultures. Since the 1960s, meditation has become more widely practiced in the West. Westerners are meditating to relieve stress, to assist in the healing of physical disorders, to increase athletic performance, to learn how to improve their concentration, and to enhance their experiences in psychotherapy. Meditation is also used in the practice of yoga and the martial arts, and as a form of inward personal discipline that many pursue as lifetime spiritual practice. As an imported product from Asian cultures, its study and practice has also led Westerners to a greater appreciation of their own contemplative traditions.

RELAXATION RESPONSE

TRANSCENDENTAL MEDITATION

The History of Meditation in the West

Practiced in the East by Asian and Indian cultures for thousands of years, meditation has been known by Western travelers to Asian countries for centuries. Meditation was also an integral part of European Renaissance culture and occult Christianity, which helped spread the practice to the West. This was particularly true among the mystical religious schools, such as the Rosicrucians.

In the New World, German mystical communities settled in the original thirteen colonies, especially in Pennsylvania, where persecuted religious groups could practice freely in an atmosphere of tolerance. Some of these groups practiced ascetic forms of meditation informed by Eastern religion and philosophy.

By the mid–nineteenth century, New England transcendentalists, such as Ralph Waldo Emerson and Henry David Thoreau, had read the few Eastern scriptures in circulation at the time and integrated ideas about meditation and yoga into their own literary and philosophical meditations. The transcendentalists used a walking form of meditation they called sauntering. They also practiced looking within one's self, or quiet contemplation, while immersed in nature. By the last quarter of the nineteenth century, international movements such as the Theosophical Society, which was first founded in the United States in 1875 and then reestablished in India in 1878, were disseminating information about Eastern contemplative practices to a public eager for the exotic as well as for alternative sources of spiritual discipline.

Formal training in Asian meditative techniques did not come to the United States until 1893, when the first wave of Asian teachers spoke to American audiences at the World Parliament of Religions, held in Chicago. In the aftermath, Swami Vivekananda of the Ramakrishna Vedanta order in India began teaching meditation to New Englanders who were attending Miss Sarah Farmer's Greenacre School of Comparative Religions in Portsmouth, New Hampshire.

Americans heard a firsthand account of Buddhist forms of meditation when Anagarika Dharmapala lectured at Harvard University and at Mrs. Ole Bull's Cambridge Conferences on Comparative Religions in 1904, and when the Zen abbot Soyen Shaku gave teachings across the United States in 1906. During the 1920s and 1930s spiritual leaders and visionaries such as Paramhansa Yogananda, George Ivanovitch Gurdjieff, and Jidhu Krishnamurti spread Asian teachings on meditation in the West. European and American writers such as Aldous Huxley and Gerald Heard popularized the meditative tradition of Hindu Vedanta in southern California during World War II. Swami Akhilananda taught Vedantic meditation in Boston during the same period.

Zen meditation became particularly popular in the 1950s among poet Gary Snyder and other members of the beatnik generation. Writers such as J. D. Salinger and psychotherapists including Karen Horney became followers of the lay Zen teacher Daisetz T. Suzuki, who by then was lecturing in New York. Zen meditation was further popularized through the writings of the psychotherapist and ex-Episcopalian priest Alan Watts during this same period. Public espousal of the Zen way by such intellectuals helped shift meditation into a position where it could be detached from questions of faith and approached as a countermeasure to materialism and stress. This view of meditation became a principal focus of the counterculture movement of the 1960s, when thousands of young people took up Asian spiritual practices in an effort to liberate their minds from the strictures of the established society.

Since that time, there have been two major developments regarding meditation as a practice and as a subject of scientific research: First, a uniquely American spiritual tradition of meditation now distinct from Asian sources has evolved. Second, the practice of meditation in various forms is making its way into the health care system and into scientific laboratories, where rigorous investigation is now being carried out by a new generation of young scientists who are also meditation practitioners.

Understanding Meditation

One way to understand the many different forms of meditation now flourishing in American culture is to consider from what tradition a particular form of practice comes. This is because there is no application of any kind of technique without some kind of philosophy to explain what is happening to consciousness as a result of the practice. For example, Transcendental Meditation represents the tradition of Vedantic Hinduism according to the teachings of the Indian guru Maharishi Mahesh Yogi. Here, in the Hindu tradition of Vedanta, the practice of meditation is understood in terms of self-realization, particularly as the experience of awakened consciousness, where one is said to realize that the subjective self and the Absolute Self of the universe (*Atman*), or pure consciousness (*chit*), are one and the same.

The different branches of Buddhist meditation strive for a completely different state of consciousness. Theravada Buddhist meditation seeks *nibanna* (nirvana), a "burning out of the flame of sense desire," while Mahayana Buddhist meditation strives to reach emptiness (*sunyata*). Both forms of Buddhism believe that there is no such thing as an underlying permanent self, which means that the experience of enlightened consciousness in meditation is quite different from that of Hindu Vedanta.

Two other significant forms of meditation, ones that have direct clinical application in medicine today, are Herbert Benson's relaxation response program at the Harvard Medical School/Mind-Body Medical Institute, and the Stress Reduction Clinic at the University of Massachusetts Medical Center, run by Jon Kabat-Zinn. Both programs, well organized and educational, have been franchised out to schools, prisons, hospitals, and other therapeutic programs.

Benson's program began with an intensive study of Transcendental Meditation and then shifted to the study of meditation practiced by monks of Tibetan Buddhism, which is a combination of Hindu Tantra, Indian Mahayana Buddhism, and Bon, the native religion of Tibet. Benson now teaches a generic form of meditation he calls the relaxation response. In Kabat-Zinn's program, patients referred to the stress-reduction clinic are trained in Vipassana (or mindfulness meditation), which comes from Southeast Asia; specifically, it is the Theravada tradition of Burmese Buddhism. At the same time, many meditators in the West practice Zen sitting, the Japanese form of Mahayana Buddhism, which originally came through China and Korea from India.

Aspects of Meditation

While there is no typical meditation session, Benson believes he has isolated the generic first steps common to all meditative and contemplative practice: a quiet environment, a relaxed position, and focus on the slow repetition of a sound or word. To this he has added readings from the inspirational texts of a practitioner's religious tradition.

A normal meditative session might last twenty minutes and be practiced once or twice a day. The subject usually sits comfortably in pleasant, quiet surroundings, preferably in a room with lowered illumination. The session might begin with a moment of deep relaxed breathing. Then, the subject might contemplate an object, such as a candle flame, while paying attention to the cycle of one's breath. The task might be to keep the mind clear of attachment to any thoughts. It might be to just witness what goes by in the field of consciousness without thought or judgment.

The difficulty in concentrating experienced by a beginning meditator should not cause alarm or frustration. Concentration merely means returning to the task without judgment. Each time the mind wanders, free of guilt or recrimination, one simply returns the mind to its original focus. Eventually, the surface of the mind becomes quieter and quieter, until sustained concentration becomes possible. Reentry into normal waking reality should be gradual and as relaxed as in the beginning. A typical session might then end with some gentle stretching.

Potential Benefits

Physiologically, it is believed that relaxed forms of meditation lead to a decrease in heart rate, a decrease in blood pressure, an increase in breathing volume but a decrease in number of breaths taken per minute (typically sixteen in-breaths and out-breaths in the normal waking state; four in the meditative condition), increased alpha waves as recorded on an electroencephalogram, and synchronization of measured brain waves between the cerebral hemispheres.

Benson believes meditation activates the parasympathetic nervous system, which quiets the nerves. Practiced twice daily for twenty minutes, meditation produces a thermostatic effect, allowing the stressed nervous system—normally in a state of fluctuation—to have a standard by which to adjust itself. Studies have shown that when the practice finally takes effect, antihypertensive medication can be cut in half, cramping in mild to moderate premenstrual syndrome can be modulated, standard light therapy for psoriasis can have an accelerated effect, and so on.

There are many forms of meditation other than quiet sitting, however. Each form has its own pattern of physiological effects, sometimes quieting the nervous system, sometimes arousing it. In walking meditation, the subject perambulates around slowly, remaining exquisitely mindful of each step. There is continuous but slow movement meditation in traditional sequences, as in Chinese qigong and t'ai chi ch'üan. Meditation is associated with rapid breathing, as in certain forms of kundalini yoga. In general, different types of philosophical teachings usually lead to radically different patterns of physiological response, which makes generalizations about meditation as a generic practice very difficult.

In most cases it is not the kind of meditation one does that counts, but rather the similarity of outcomes among different kinds of techniques that leads to moral and aesthetic improvement, an enhanced sense of well-being, and enriched relationships. These are the criteria against which successful practice, either under an advanced teacher or by oneself, should be measured.

— *Eugene Taylor, Ph.D.; and Marilyn Schlitz, Ph.D.*

Further Reading

Books

Benson, Herbert, and Miriam Z. Klipper. *The Relaxation Response.* New York: Avon Books, 1976.

Epstein, Mark. *Thoughts Without a Thinker: Psychotherapy from a Buddhist Perspective.* New York: Basic Books, 1995.

Kabat-Zinn, Jon. *Wherever You Go, There You Are: Mindfulness Meditation in Everyday Life.* New York: Hyperion, 1994.

Murphy, Michael, and Steven Donovan. *The Physical and Psychological Effects of Meditation: A Review of Contemporary Research with a Comprehensive Bibliography.* 2nd ed. Edited with an introduction by Eugene Taylor. Sausalito, Calif.: Institute of Noetic Sciences, 1996.

Prabhavananda, Swami, and Frederick Manchester, eds. *The Upanishads, Breath of the Eternal: The Principal Texts.* New York: New American Library, 1957.

Suzuki, Daisetz Teitaro. *An Introduction to Zen Buddhism.* Edited by Christmas Humphreys, with a foreword by C. G. Jung. London: Rider, 1983.

Taimni, I. K. *The Science of Yoga: The Yoga-Sutras of the Patanjali.* 4th Quest Book ed. Wheaton, Ill.: Theosophical Publishing House, 1975.

Journals

Tricycle, a magazine of Buddhism in America, which began publication in 1991.

Relaxation Response

 The relaxation response is a body-mind process character-ized by significant physical changes, such as lower blood pressure, decreased heart rate, and increased body temperature as well as a general sense of intense calm. Through an examination of the psychological and physiological aspects of meditation, Herbert Benson, M.D., found that the relaxation response could be brought about by the use of meditation, yoga, repetitive exercises, hypnosis, prayer, and other forms of stress management.

History

In the late 1960s, Benson, a Harvard cardiol-ogist, began to study the physical effects of meditation. Later he traveled to India to study Tibetan monks who meditate every day. Dr. Benson was one of the first scientists to study advanced meditators using Western scientific methods. He measured some of the physical changes, such as blood pressure and body temperature, that occurred as the monks meditated. He found that while the monks were in a meditative state their body processes slowed. He documented the fact that meditation was associated with lowered blood pressure and heart rate and an in-crease in body temperature, all of which are associated with calmness. He labeled these meditation-induced physical changes in the body the *relaxation response.*

Theory

Studies prove that when people relax the body, they can potentially prevent some of the harmful effects of psychological stress. Hundreds of scientific studies have shown that there are negative effects from psycho-logical stress; these effects are mental or intellectual, behavioral and physical. Psy-chological stress can make it harder to think effectively and behave appropriately and can also cause physical changes associated with the development of medical illness.

The relaxation response is the opposite of the stress response, or what has been termed the *fight-or-flight response.* When most animals in the wild are faced with life-threatening situations, their bodies respond with a predictable arousal pattern that pre-pares them to either fight a threat or run away from danger. In humans, this response prepares the body for vigorous muscular ac-tivity by stimulating the sympathetic ner-vous system to increase heart rate, blood pressure, and muscle tension. The fight-or-flight response was necessary for the sur-vival of humans when confronted by wild beasts. Today the same response is stimu-lated to varying degrees when we are faced with everyday stresses, most often threats to our ego, such as taking tests or being late.

Benson's studies suggested an important symmetrical relationship between the fight-or-flight response and the relaxation re-sponse. Whereas repeated or prolonged elicitation of the fight-or-flight response has been associated with medical illness related to stress and arousal, repeated or prolonged elicitation of the relaxation response has been associated with the prevention of stress-related disease.

Through his work with Tibetan monks, Benson theorized that the positive effects of meditation could be acquired without the belief in Eastern religions or altered states. The most important thing was that patients learn to generate the calming effects associ-ated with the relaxation response. The way in which an individual learned to generate the effect was unimportant. He then set out to devise a general strategy that would bring about the desired response. He found that the relaxation response would occur using many different disciplines, including yoga, repetitive exercise, hypnosis, and other forms of stress management. Benson and his colleagues concluded that only two specific steps were necessary to produce the relaxation response: the first is to focus attention on a single repetitive word, sound, prayer, phrase, image, or physical activity; the second is to passively return to a specific focus when distractions occur.

Practice

In a typical training session, the client enters the therapist's office and is instructed to sit in a comfortable chair. The therapist then begins giving the following guidance in a quiet voice:

1. Sit quietly in a comfortable position and close your eyes.
2. Deeply relax all your muscles, beginning at your feet and progressing up to your face. Keep them deeply relaxed.
3. Breathe through your nose. Become aware of your breathing. As you breathe out, say the word "one" silently to yourself. For example, breathe in . . . out, "one;" in . . . out, "one;" and so on. Continue for twenty minutes. You may open your eyes to check the time, but do not use an alarm. When you finish, sit quietly for several minutes, at first with closed eyes and later with opened eyes.
4. Do not worry about whether you are successful in achieving a deep level of relaxation. Maintain a passive attitude and permit relaxation to occur at its own pace. Expect other thoughts. When distracting thoughts occur, ignore them and continue repeating "one." With practice, the response should come with little effort. Practice the technique once or twice daily, but not within two hours after any meal, since the digestive processes seem to interfere with the subjective changes.

The potential role of meditation in overall health is often misunderstood because of its association with mystical Eastern traditions. While Eastern cultures accept the concept that regular meditational practice can result in positive psychological benefits, these cultures also believe that it can result in an altered state of consciousness or a change in the perception of reality. Because meditation is so heavily associated with altered states, the Western medical community has been slow to acknowledge that patients may be able to use the practice of meditation to produce positive healthful effects.

Benefits

The relaxation response has been associated with improvements in many medical conditions, including hypertension, cardiac arrhythmia, chronic pain, insomnia, side effects of cancer therapy, side effects of AIDS therapy, infertility, and preparation for surgery and X-ray procedures.

—*RICHARD FRIEDMAN, PH.D.; PATRICIA MYERS; AND HERBERT BENSON, M.D.*

Resources

Mind/Body Medical Institute
    Beth Israel Deaconess Medical Center
    Harvard Medical School
    110 Francis St.
    Boston, MA 02215
    Tel: (617) 632-9530
    Provides a well-respected treatment program that teaches how to elicit the relaxation response.

Further Reading

Benson, Herbert. *The Relaxation Response.* Richmond, Va.: Outlet Books, Inc., 1993.
———. *Timeless Healing.* New York: Fireside, 1996.
Benson, Herbert, and William Proctor. *Beyond the Relaxation Response.* New York: Putnam/Berkley, Inc., 1984.

Transcendental Meditation

 Transcendental Meditation (TM) is a simple technique used to help individuals access their inner creativity and wisdom while also improving their physical health. According to TM theory, which is based on the ancient Vedantic tradition, certain meditation techniques can quiet the mind, allowing the body to enter a state of deep relaxation. *Veda,* meaning "knowledge," is a science of life and consciousness that is rooted in ancient India. TM was introduced in 1957 by Maharishi Mahesh Yogi. He has since traveled the world, promoting and teaching TM. As a result, more than five million people from different countries, religions, and educational backgrounds have learned the TM technique.

History

Maharishi Mahesh Yogi was born in 1918 in India. *Maharishi,* meaning "great sage," is a title of honor. The Maharishi graduated in 1941 with a degree in physics from Allahabad University in India. Shortly thereafter, he met Swami Brahamananda Saraswati, a renowned spiritual leader in India, and asked to study with him. The Maharishi was accepted and became his disciple for more than thirteen years.

After Swami Brahamananda Saraswati died in 1953, the Maharishi spent two years in seclusion in the Himalayan Mountains, where he developed the system of Transcendental Meditation. In 1957, at the eighty-seventh birthday celebration of his teacher, the Maharishi announced his plan to spread TM around the world. To accomplish this, he founded the Spiritual Regeneration Movement in 1959. His reputation greatly increased in the early 1960s, when his teachings gained the interest of the musical group the Beatles and other celebrities from the West. Subsequently, TM became more popular in the United States. The Maharishi toured the United States in 1967 and delivered lectures at several prominent universities. By the 1970s TM had spread to more than one hundred countries.

Currently, people participate in the Maharishi's teachings to different extents. Many students follow the Maharishi's versions of various branches of Vedic science, including systems of medicine, architecture, and prediction. For them, the Maharishi's teachings influence various aspects of their lifestyles. His teachings have also inspired a political movement, organized in sixty countries as the Natural Law Party. Many other people study only the meditation technique without changing their lifestyles or political beliefs. They attend classes in which the TM technique is taught and use the skill to help achieve their own personal physical, emotional, and spiritual goals.

Basic Principles

According to the Maharishi, consciousness is not merely a function of the human nervous system; it is actually a field in nature, just like gravity or electromagnetism. This field pervades the physical universe and is the source of the creativity and intelligence in nature, as well as in an individual's life. Although this model of consciousness is derived from the Vedic tradition of ancient India, some have noted its similarities to a contemporary Western scientific theory known as the unified field of natural law, which concerns all matter and energy in the universe.

Vedic science claims that the human brain and nervous system can function as instruments capable of directly experiencing the unbounded field of consciousness. Practitioners believe that when a person is in a quiet, settled state, the mind will naturally move toward experiencing this field. TM is a technique to transcend the superficial, active level of the mind, allowing it to experience this latent and unlimited source of energy, creativity, and intelligence.

Coming from India, where meditation techniques abound, the Maharishi was frequently asked if all meditation techniques—and therefore all benefits of meditation—are the same. He asserted that there are profound differences among practices. Most meditation techniques, the Maharishi said, involve concentration or control of the mind. He advocated a departure from these methods. To the Maharishi, control of the mind actually stops the process of transcending normal consciousness. Instead, meditation should be completely natural and effortless, requiring no concentration or control of the mind. Meditation should simply allow the mind to follow its own natural tendency toward the expanded field of consciousness, a field of bliss and inner happiness.

Practice

Even though the process of TM is designed to be simple and effortless, the method is very precise. Learning to meditate in the Vedic tradition has always involved personal instruction from an expert or guru. Therefore, TM practitioners believe that those who are interested in meditating should learn from a qualified teacher.

A seven-step course in Transcendental Meditation is offered by hundreds of Maharishi Vedic universities and schools throughout the world. The course consists of two lectures on the principles of TM and four days of instruction in meditation—about two hours each day. After the course is completed, additional personal instruction is also available.

TM is practiced for fifteen to twenty minutes twice a day. A person begins meditation by sitting in a comfortable position with the eyes closed. Then, mantras—often meaningless syllables or phrases—are silently repeated. Proponents believe that meditation quiets the mind, which helps the body enter a unique state of relaxation, deeper than ordinary rest with eyes closed. As a person begins to relax his mind, he begins to experience finer levels of thought. Ultimately, a person transcends the finest level of thought and experiences the source of thought, the field of pure consciousness.

Benefits

There has been a significant effort among advocates of TM to integrate traditional teachings with Western science. Since the mid-1970s, hundreds of research studies have been conducted that confirm that TM can yield both psychological and physical benefits. It has been found to reduce stress, anxiety, and depression and increase creativity, happiness, and self-esteem. Meditation can also increase one's energy, improve memory, alleviate insomnia, and lower high blood pressure.

Some students use the technique to improve memory and accelerate their problem-solving skills. TM can improve job satisfaction and productivity in the workplace. It may also serve as an important component of programs designed to help people recover from drug or alcohol addiction. In each of these cases, the TM technique is used as a practical skill to help people in their daily lives.

—COMPILED IN CONSULTATION WITH ROBERT ROTH

Resources

Maharishi University of Management
    1000 N. 4th St.
    Fairfield, IA 52557
    Tel: (515) 472-7000
    Web site: www.miu.edu
    An accredited university offering standard academic disciplines in addition to Transcendental Meditation.

Maharishi Vedic University
    1401 Ocean Ave.
    Asbury Park, NJ 07712
    Tel: (908) 774-9446
    Offers a program of instruction in the Vedic sciences.

Transcendental Meditation Program
    Tel: 1-888-LEARN TM (532-7686)
    Web site: www.tm.org

Further Reading

Denniston, Denise. *The TM Book: How to Enjoy the Rest of Your Life.* Fairfield, Iowa: Fairfield Press, 1986.

Roth, Robert. *Transcendental Meditation.* New York: Primus, 1987.

Yogi, Maharishi Mahesh. *Science of Being and Art of Living.* London: SRM Publications, 1967.

Part 14:

Psychophysical Evaluation Frameworks

Psychophysical evaluation frameworks are organized theoretical structures and notation systems that correlate body movement with psychological attributes and patterns. These frameworks see the process of movement as a complex and multifaceted affair. Each method combines, in its own way, an objective approach to observing and recording the subtle aspects of movement with an appreciation for the subjective elements of the experience of moving. Because each method aims to create a comprehensive model of all the possible combinations of movement elements, these frameworks can be applied to many athletic and aesthetic activities, therapeutic modalities, and educational programs for diagnostic as well as prescriptive purposes.

The majority of psychophysical evaluation frameworks in use today are inspired by the work of Rudolf Laban (1879–1958), an Austro-Hungarian movement theorist. The methods included in this section are distinguished by their founders' efforts to collect first all the variations of movement they could observe before developing theoretical frameworks linking physical movements to psychological characteristics. They recorded these observations by means of various abstract-symbol systems that developed along with their theoretical concepts. From data collected, the various frameworks were then formulated, creating a comprehensive map of the possible range of movement patterns and their relationship to patterns of emotional life.

ENNEAGRAM

KESTENBERG
MOVEMENT PROFILE

LABAN MOVEMENT
ANALYSIS

MOVEMENT
PATTERN ANALYSIS

What These Frameworks Have in Common

The frameworks described in this section are linked by several basic concepts. First and foremost is the belief that physical movement is reflective of inner psychological patterns, preferences, and coping mechanisms. While some frameworks like the Enneagram model focus more on behavioral actions, the Laban-based models, including Laban movement analysis, Kestenberg movement profile, and movement pattern analysis, base their observations specifically on the qualitative changes in movements through space over a period of time.

These frameworks are also linked by the belief that each person has preferred movement repertoires that are unique and special to her. Health, growth, and understanding are often facilitated by experiencing behavioral actions, movement qualities, combinations, and patterns outside this preferred movement repertoire. In this way these frameworks are related to the ancient and contemporary holistic body-mind disciplines that see physical, emotional, and spiritual health in terms of balance and harmony.

Using the Frameworks

The modes of practice of these particular disciplines are extremely varied. In fact, a client doesn't so much "practice" them as make use of the information and new insights they provide. In some cases it is possible to visit a practitioner of one of these disciplines for a personal assessment. For example, you can go to an enneagram seminar and find out your place in that method's map of the gestalt of human consciousness. Or you can learn about your own decision-making process by having your movement pattern analyzed by a certified movement pattern analyst.

It is more likely, though, that if you were to go to a dance teacher, sports coach, or massage or movement therapist, she might be working with one of these psychophysical evaluation frameworks. The teacher, coach, or therapist is the "practitioner" of this discipline. The framework provides a model within which to assess your condition, understand the whole physical and psychological dynamic of your situation, and plan a step-by-step program to help relieve your pain, improve your performance, or assist you in reaching your goals.

—NANCY ALLISON, CMA

Further Reading

Fouts, Roger, and Stephen Tukel Mills. *Next of Kin: What Chimpanzees Have Taught Me About Who We Are*. New York: William Morrow and Company, Inc., 1997.

Moore, Carol-Lynne, and Kaoru Yamamoto. *Beyond Words: Movement Observation and Analysis*. New York: Gordon and Breach, 1994.

North, Marion. *Personality Assessment Through Movement*. London: Macdonald and Evans, 1972.

Enneagram

 Enneagram is a model of human personality that provides nine personal strategies, or ways of being in the world, called types. In Greek *ennea* means "nine" and *gram* means "graph" or "model." The system provides a framework, language, and conceptual vocabulary for understanding people and behavior. In offering personality descriptions that account for differences among people, the model greatly enhances people's ability to understand themselves and to appreciate that others approach the same situation from different perspectives. When used effectively, the enneagram system opens up new possibilities for people in management, leadership, teaching, learning, and personal growth.

History

Many ancient sacred traditions such as esoteric Christianity, Sufism, and Judaism describe variants of the enneagram model. This implies an old, common source for the current model. Other strands lead into the modern-day enneagram. For instance, the Platonic tradition from ancient Greece, in which the philosopher Plato describes nine perfect essential states of being and a tenth state called unity, is a philosophy that resonates with the enneagram as well.

In the twentieth century George Ivanovitch Gurdjieff (1872–1949), the spiritual philosopher and teacher, brought a nine-pointed star diagram to the West, purportedly from Sufi sources. Gurdjieff used the star, and the internal-flow pattern that unites the points in a specific way, in his private teaching work. According to Gurdjieff theory, by using the star he was able to describe the changing attitudes and perceptions that occur when people feel secure or stressed. Gurdjieff painted a huge enneagram on the floor of the Institute for the Harmonious Development of Man, the name of his school where students practiced movements aimed at developing personal awareness.

Oscar Ichazo, a European born in the early 1930s and a noted contemporary enneagram author who claimed to have learned the system from Sufi masters in Afghanistan, added the next step to the enneagram system. He named the central focus of each of the types after Christianity's seven capital sins—anger, pride, envy, avarice, gluttony, lust, sloth—and added two more, deceit and fear. This frame of reference has become widespread, but it does not imply that it is a system of Christian psychology.

In 1972 the first teacher of the enneagram in the United States, a Chilean psychiatrist named Claudio Naranjo, a student of Ichazo's, taught the system to a group of psychologists, psychiatrists, and students in Berkeley, California. This group painstakingly aligned the central features of the enneagram types with the *Diagnostic Survey Manual*, a canon in the psychological community used by all American and Canadian clinicians for diagnostic purposes. While the *DSM* describes pathologies (deviations from normal psychological functioning), the enneagram describes in general terms the broadly correlating characteristics of normal and high-functioning people. For example, in enneagram theory, point six represents constant fear and vigilance; enneagram practitioners believe that this corresponds with the psychological term *paranoid*. In a like manner, every point on the enneagram correlates to a contemporary psychological pathology.

Naranjo's other contribution was to explore the enneagram using panels of the types. In this method groups of people of the same personality type work together to explore the intricacies of the inner structure of their thought and behavior patterns. These early panels provided the empirical proof for the key distinguishing characteristics of the types.

The first books on enneagram theory were published in the United States in the mid-1980s. Today research on the correlation between the enneagram model and Western psychological theory is being conducted at Loyola University in Chicago, at the Center for Integral Studies in San Francisco, and less formally in many other seminaries and graduate schools.

Basic Principles

To survive in the world, we need to exhibit traits and characteristics that will enable us to make our way and form relationships. Personality is about defense mechanisms, characteristic habits of thought, emotions that underpin thoughts, interpersonal aptitudes and abilities, and a way of handling the body to manage energy. Although all of us have access to each of these areas, in many instances one area predominates and we fall into basic physical, mental, and emotional types. The enneagram recognizes these distinctions, too, and the diagram is organized in triads that are made up of these distinct energies—the emotional triad, the mental triad, and the instinctual/body triad.

In traditional psychology, personality type has been identified through pathology, or deviations in personality makeup. Many psychologists and psychiatrists believe that if a person can understand how his personality disintegrated, he can be helped to reintegrate himself. Psychotherapists are trained to find how the personality defense mechanisms have broken down, rather than to concentrate on what is working.

The enneagram system provides a new way to understand ourselves. The model offers a format for normal and high-functioning people to examine what their reactive or habitual behavior patterns conceal. Enneagram theory pinpoints nine patterns of avoidance: error, emotional needs, failure, ordinariness, connection, deviance (being different), pain, vulnerability, and conflict. Our sense of self is manufactured largely out of one of these avoidances in our emotional experience. When we face up to, process, and integrate those aspects of ourselves we have been denying, the self can emerge as a whole, and the grace of compassion for self and others becomes possible.

The system offers the choice for proactive, rather than reactive, behavior and the opportunity to cease going on "automatic" without realizing what one is doing. Knowledge of enneagram type (e-type) frees us to expand the way we think about ourselves, to find compassion for ourselves and others, to manage emotional energy with more skill, and to end habitual behavior.

Practice

The key to using the enneagram system is recognizing one's type. To do this, a group of interested people will typically see a videotape or listen to an audiotape describing the nine types. There are obvious dangers and consequences of mistyping and stereotyping. As people (especially youths) become more knowledgeable about their own personalities, they need to be honest and objective about their own defining characteristics. If after this process they are still unsure of their enneagram type, a one-on-one interview is available to help them identify their type.

Enneagram consultants do not tell people their type. Although multiple-choice tests are sometimes used to help determine type, consultants believe that knowledge of type is useful only if it is part of a process of self-recognition and self-discovery. The forty-five-minute individual interview is designed to unobtrusively elicit patterns of thought and emotion, deeply held inner motivations, and habits. The questions asked and the manner in which they are asked have been developed from thousands of interviews conducted by the Center for Enneagram Studies in Berkeley, California. Through this process the enneagram system brings many people revelatory understanding of their in-

There are currently many enneagram centers and hundreds of enneagram teachers throughout the United States and the world. In 1994 the First International Enneagram Conference was cosponsored by and held at Stanford University in Palo Alto, California. In 1996 the First National Enneagram Institute for Educators was cosponsored by and held at the Milton Academy in Milton, Massachusetts, which is becoming a laboratory for enneagram applications in education, particularly learning and teaching styles.

dividual beliefs, values, and ideas. Finding one's e-type is only the initial step; learning how to work with one's strategy, and to grow in understanding, compassion, and acceptance of oneself and others is the journey. To this end, the body-mind methods of the many sacred traditions, such as heightened self-knowledge, breathing practices, meditation, and developing a sense of groundedness, are all helpful.

Benefits and Risks

People who use the enneagram system have reported that it enriches and facilitates interactions among people and offers opportunities for more thoughtful, effective, and honest relationships. Business managers, educators, and students feel that the system helps them develop a sense of their motivations and the patterns behind their thoughts and actions.

There are dangers inherent in the system, however. Stereotyping, or not seeing the individual in the type, is a distinct danger. A shallow understanding of the system on the part of the practitioner, whether teacher or student, ignores the facets that account for individual differences. Perhaps the gravest danger in the system lies in people prematurely mistyping themselves and others.

—*JANET LEVINE*

Resources

The International Enneagram Association
    849 Independence Ave., Suite B
    Mountain View, CA 94043
    Tel: (415) 903-8300
    Fax: (415) 967-0995
    Offers a full listing of enneagram centers and teachers both in the United States and internationally.

The National Educators Institute for Enneagram Studies
    Janet Levine, Program Director
    Milton Academy
    170 Centre St.
    Milton, MA 02186
    Tel/fax: (617) 696-9410
    e-mail: Jlevinegrp@aol.com
    Web site: www.enneagram-edge.com
    Provides information about training in the enneagram system for the educational sector.

Further Reading

Books

Levine, Janet. *The Enneagram Intelligences: Understanding Personality for Effective Teaching and Learning.* Westport, Conn.: Greenwood Publishing Group, 1999.

Naranjo, Claudio. *Enneatype Structures.* Nevada City, Calif.: Gateways, 1990.

Palmer, Helen. *The Enneagram.* San Francisco: Harper San Francisco, 1988.

———. *The Enneagram in Love and Work.* San Francisco: Harper San Francisco, 1994.

Riso, Don Richard. *Personality Types: Using the Enneagram for Self-Discovery.* New York: Houghton-Mifflin, 1987.

Rohr, Richard, and Andreas Ebert. *Discovering the Enneagram.* New York: Crossroad, 1992.

Journals
The Enneagram Monthly. Troy, New York.

Kestenberg Movement Profile

 The Kestenberg movement profile (KMP) is a method of psychological assessment based on observations of patterns of movement. While observers have long recognized that bodily movement styles often reflect various aspects of personality and feelings, a framework was needed to unravel the mind-body connections in a systematic fashion. Such a framework was developed in the 1960s by Dr. Judith S. Kestenberg and the Sands Point Movement Study Group, consisting of Drs. Hershey Marcus, Jay Berlowe, Esther Robin, Arnhilte Buelte, and Martha Soodak. A new generation of students, including Susan Loman, Mark Sossin, and Penny Lewis, continues to develop the approach in the twenty-first century. KMP provides a methodology and theory for observing and interpreting body movement patterns and has been used effectively for evaluation as well as prescriptive purposes by psychologists, anthropologists, and dance/movement therapists.

History

Judith Kestenberg first observed the close integration of body and mind in Vienna in the 1930s while studying patients with neurological brain damage. Later, as a child psychiatrist in New York, she speculated about ways in which psychological disturbances might be expressed in body movement. In 1953 she began what was to be a twenty-year–long study of the movement patterns of three newborns. Unfamiliar with any system of movement notation, she recorded the babies' movements by moving her pen in accordance with their motions. Her pen traced rhythmic and semirhythmic lines across the paper, creating tracings that looked like electrocardiogram graphs. However, it was not yet clear to her how these data could be interpreted.

In 1960 the Sands Point Movement Study Group—four psychiatrists, a movement specialist, and a dance therapist—eager to learn together and cross disciplinary lines, gathered to study movement in a more systematic way. They were led to the work of the movement specialist Rudolf Laban, who had emphasized that movement patterns are closely associated with styles of thinking and feeling. For example, Laban pointed out that people who "tackle" decisions tend to prefer strong, quick, direct movements; those who slowly ponder decisions tend to prefer light, sustained, and indirect movement. He created a system of notation that allowed an observer to record, categorize, and interpret movement in relation to the mover's inner intention.

The Sands Point group studied Laban's system and adapted it to serve their interest in child development and psychological evaluations. In particular, they elaborated on Laban's observation that changes of muscle tension may reflect inner feelings and needs. They found that in children, as Laban had theorized, bound muscle tension often reflected states of anxiety or caution, and that relaxed or free-flowing movements were associated with feeling at ease.

Warren Lamb, one of Laban's students, suggested that Kestenberg's tracings of the babies' movements documented changes in muscle tension and offered a way to study changes of tension flow. Equipped with this methodology, the group discovered ten particular patterns of muscle-tension changes characteristic of children's basic everyday functioning, such as eating, crawling, or jumping. Throughout development these rhythmic patterns serve not only such bodily functions, but also other psychological needs. For instance, sucking rhythms used for nursing also serve a self-soothing function and thus are important throughout the life span. Particular rhythmic patterns typically become prominent during the early phases of development, from birth to age six, paralleling and reinforcing the process of maturation. As an example, short stop-and-go rhythms common in a two-and-a-half-year-old aid bladder control and also encourage energetic activity and competitiveness. A slow, swaying rhythm, common in three-year-olds, supports and encourages nurturing behavior and creativity.

From 1972 to 1990 additional observations were gathered at the Center for Children and Parents, a private institution in Roslyn, New York, founded by Kestenberg. These were used to refine and verify KMP and its interpretive scheme. As confidence in the profile grew, it became the basis for the evaluation of movement preferences, developmental achievement, cognitive (thinking) abilities, self-esteem, and social skills.

Basic Principles

While individuals exhibit all ten biologically based rhythmic patterns identified in the KMP, they generally favor two or three rhythmic patterns, infusing them into many of their activities. For example, some people eat with a "jumping" rhythm, gulping their food, while others "drift" along, finishing long after everyone else. Severe deficiency of one pattern may undermine the development of certain qualities, such as assertiveness or the ability to relax. By tracing a person's rhythms of tension flow, as these patterns are called in KMP, one can begin to create a profile of the subject's preferred ways of meeting personal needs.

In addition to tension-flow patterns, more than sixty-three specific movement qualities have also been studied and used to create a detailed and comprehensive movement profile for the psychological assessment of individuals. Combinations of these qualities reflect the individual's style of coping with the environment, self-image, use of psychological defenses, learning styles, cognitive thinking patterns, and ways of relating to others. Laban had theorized, and

Kestenberg's research confirmed, that in order to collect accurate, useful observations of movement patterns, it is necessary to observe more than one movement quality at a time. Observing movement from this frame of reference creates a complex palette of data from which to draw psychological implications.

The richness of the material leads the observer to the discovery of multiple interconnections between mind and body. One movement quality often underlies cognitive processes and social modes of relating. For example, an individual who favors "spreading" movements over "enclosing" motions also generally prefers to explore widely in an environment and take in many diverse perspectives. Such a person also tends to feel comfortable relating to a number of different people. One who prefers enclosing movements generally favors focused investigations and explorations and more singular perspectives, and also tends to be more comfortable relating to others on a one-to-one basis. Of course, most people have access to both patterns of movement and both modes of thinking and relating, but demonstrate distinct styles and preferences in specific contexts.

Applications

KMP can be used in natural, real-world settings as well as more controlled, therapeutic ones. Adults engaging in a conversation or children engaged in free play can be profiled. It has also been used successfully in different cultural settings.

As a preventive measure, KMP's model of childhood development suggests age-appropriate activities for children and remedial movement patterns where deficiencies are found. The profile also aids in the treatment of problems in interpersonal relations. By comparing profiles of family members, the therapist can study the areas of harmony and clash between individuals. The therapist can then analyze how certain movement patterns inhibit and mislead communication. Individuals can be made aware of the movement-level basis of their clashes and learn to build on their areas of harmony, find more compatible movement patterns, or at least understand their clashes on a more comfortable movement level.

Parents can learn to attune to their infants, use assigned movement patterns, and develop a body-level mode of communication. The process of becoming attuned with others can begin quite early. Kestenberg taught pregnant women to trace the tension flow rhythms of fetal movements. This facilitated getting to know and relating to the baby before birth, and bonding with it after birth.

KMP also serves as a guide for dance/movement therapists who utilize movement as a form of treatment. Psychologists, physical therapists, and physicians who also examine the language of the body have found KMP effective as part of the diagnostic process and in the determination of appropriate avenues of therapy.

—JANET KESTENBERG AMIGHI AND SUSAN LOMAN

Resources

Allegheny University of the Health Sciences
  1505 Reay, Mail Drop 905
  Bellet Bldg., 10th Floor
  Philadelphia, PA 19102
  Tel: (215) 246-5020
  Offers a program in KMP.

Antioch New England Graduate School
  40 Avon St.
  Keene, NH 03431
  Tel: (603) 357-3122
  Provides a training program in the Kestenberg movement profile.

The Laban-Bartenieff Institute for Movement Studies
  234 Fifth Ave., Room 203
  New York, NY 10001

Tel: (212) 477-4299
Teaches the Kestenberg movement profile to qualified individuals.

Further Reading

Books

Kestenberg, J. S. *Children and Parents: Psychoanalytic Studies in Development.* New York: Jason Aronson, 1975.

Kestenberg, J. S., and M. Sossin. *The Role of Movement Patterns in Development II.* New York: The Dance Notation Bureau Press, 1979.

Kestenberg, J. S., J. Amighi, S. Loman, P. Lewis, and M. Sossin. *The Meaning of Movement: Developmental, Multicultural, and Clinical Perspectives as Seen Through the Kestenberg Movement Profile.* New York: Gordon and Breach, 1998.

Lewis, P., and S. Loman. *The Kestenberg Movement Profile: Its Past, Present Applications and Future Directions.* Keene, N.H.: Antioch New England Graduate School, 1990.

Journals

Loman, S., and H. Merman. "The KMP: A Tool for Dance/Movement Therapy." *American Journal of Dance Therapy* 18, 1 (1996): 29–52.

Laban Movement Analysis

Laban movement analysis (LMA) is a system that provides a comprehensive language to describe, interpret, and study movement. Central to LMA is the idea that movement is an outward expression of inner intentions and that movement is a combination of the physical, emotional, and mental attributes of human behavior. LMA allows for the analysis and synthesis of the physical and psychological processes of moving. As such, its language is applicable to many fields of body-mind study.

History

Rudolf Laban, artist, scientist, and philosopher, was born in 1879 in what was then Bratislava in the Austro-Hungarian Empire. He spent much of his life in France, Switzerland, and Germany until 1936, when artistic conflicts with the National Socialist Party (the Nazi Party) forced him to relocate to England, where he remained until his death in 1958.

From 1913 to 1917 in Ascona, Switzerland, Laban began developing an abstract-symbol system that depicted movement. Originally this system provided the impermanent art of dance with a means for documentation and historical preservation. But Laban's broad range of interests, coupled with his scientific approach to the study of movement, led him to develop a system of notating all types of movement.

Between 1920 and 1936 Laban was most active in Berlin. He established two dance companies, Tanzbuhne Laban and Kammertanzbuhne Laban. His system of notation was published in 1928 as *Kinetography Laban*, and became known as *Labanotation* in the United States. Laban established dance schools throughout Germany and gained a reputation for his prolific work in developing movement choirs, orchestrating large groups of laypeople in movement displays of pageantry and community.

Laban worked in England from 1936 to 1958. His book *Modern Educational Dance*, published in 1948, became the basis for a curriculum in movement education in public schools. He also began teacher-training programs in movement with recognition from the Department of Education and Science.

Laban's legacy continues through his writings, his notation system, and his groundbreaking investigation into nonverbal expression and the creative unconscious sources of movement expression. Several of Laban's students, including Irmgard Bartenieff, Warren Lamb, Judith Kestenberg, and Anne Hutchinson Guest, have continued his work and expanded its range of application to a variety of fields. Lamb, for instance, applied the theories to the corporate sector to help professionals understand their own and others' decision-making processes. Kestenberg works with children in body/movement–conscious psychotherapy.

Philosophy

To facilitate a fundamental understanding of all human movement, the LMA system articulates and differentiates the ingredients of movement expression. These ingredients combine in infinitely varying ways to become the work actions, human behaviors, and dance styles of cultures throughout the world. Although movement is a constantly changing state, these ingredients continuously emerge as observable points of emphasis in movement patterns. LMA places these movement ingredients into four major categories: body, effort, space, and shape.

The body category focuses on how movements are executed physically. It looks at specific body parts and relationships among body parts, identifies how movements are initiated, and describes simultaneous or sequential phrasing of movement. This category also distinguishes between postural and gestural movements and examines the rhythms created as one goes from being still to moving and vice versa.

The effort category covers qualitative changes in the energy of movement. It addresses movement in terms of weight, space, time, and flow. Fluctuations of weight occur between light or strong, space is direct or indirect, time is quick or sustained, and flow is free or bound. These eight effort elements combine in a multitude of configurations that Laban described as "states" and "drives." These states and drives appear as moments of significant change and yield the endless rhythmic variation evident in human movement. For example, the language may serve to compare and contrast the percussive, strong, quick accent of a tap dancer's movement and the delicate, light, sustained, free promenade of a ballet dancer.

Space examines the way the body moves through the space around it and addresses issues of proximity, direction, pathway, location, and relationship. The LMA framework identifies a personal kinesphere as a bubble of space that travels with an individual through the general space. Proximity refers to the relative distances between people or between a person and an object. Appropriate proximity varies from culture to culture and is an important aspect of social behavior. To further delineate three-dimensional space, Laban imagined a human being standing inside various geometric forms or crystals such as a sphere, cube, octahedron (an eight-sided crystal), icosahedron (a twenty-sided crystal), or dodecahedron (a twelve-sided crystal). The vertices, edges, and facets of this crystalline architecture suggest possible pathways through space.

Finally, in shape description, Laban movement analysts observe the forms the body makes and the process of shape change as one moves between forms. LMA provides a vocabulary for identifying design elements that appear in the arrangement of body parts in relationship to one another. In addition to familiar descriptions of shape, such as curved, angular, symmetric, or asymmetric, shape is viewed as a dynamic process, the outward shape change revealing a variety of inner attitudes. The change that occurs when an individual is actively engaging or responding to the outer environment, as in building a sand castle, appears very different from a change that results from a deep sigh or other internally motivated action. This framework provides a way to describe the plasticity of the body, the forms it reveals, and the way in which its form constantly changes.

Any movement event is a complex layering of many movement elements. Variables of body, effort, shape, and space are all oc-curring simultaneously. The Laban framework provides differentiated concepts within each category. The vocabulary that results from this conceptual understanding of movement enables observers to identify the most important characteristics of a movement event and to describe how these characteristics change through time.

Practice

LMA provides a means of moving from description of movement to interpretation and creating plans for change or improvement in movement expression. In athletics, performance arts, martial arts, and fitness training, LMA is used to break down an action into its separate elements and then to determine which elements are most important in performing the action most efficiently, effectively, and/or expressively. From this assessment it is possible to move actively toward developing and refining the specific movements that contribute to virtuosity within any physical skill. In the same way LMA can also serve as a diagnostic tool in injury rehabilitation and in maximizing movement patterns for health and efficiency. Since LMA recognizes that movement can express inner intentions and psychological motivations, the system also provides concrete tools for deciphering the nonverbal language of movement expression as viewed within the fields of psychology, sociology, and anthropology. As a conceptual framework, it provides movement educators with a concrete language for the clarification of somatic goals and an assessment of progress. As a system that provides specific links between mental, physical, and emotional realms of human functioning, its range of potential application extends to any inquiry concerned with the intersection of body and mind experience.

—*Ed Groff, M.F.A., CMA*

Resources

The Dance Notation Bureau
 33 W. 21st St.
 New York, NY 10001
 Tel: (212) 807-7899
 An institute providing certificate training in
 Labanotation.

The Laban-Bartenieff Institute of Movement
Studies
 235 Fifth Ave., Room 203
 New York, NY 10001
 Tel: (212) 477-4299
 Web site: www.limsonline.org
 An institute that provides comprehensive
 training in LMA and offers a certificate
 program.

Laban Centre for Movement and Dance
 University of London Goldsmith's College
 London SE 14 6NW
 England
 Tel: 01-692-4070
 A school offering undergraduate, postgradu-
 ate, and special courses in Laban studies.

The Language of Dance Center
 17 Holland Park
 London W1135D
 England
 A school offering comprehensive training in
 Labanotation.

Motus Humanus
 Carol Lynne-Moore, Director
 P.O. Box 11036
 Denver, CO 80211
 Tel: (303) 421-2023
 An organization serving the needs of Laban-
 based movement professionals through pub-
 lications, conferences, advanced training
 seminars, and professional consultation.

Further Reading

Bartenieff, Irmgard, and Dori Lewis. *Body Move-
 ment: Coping with the Environment*. Rev. ed.
 New York: Gordon Breach Science Publishers,
 Inc., 1980.

Dunlop, Valerie P. *Modern Educational Dance*. Rev.
 ed. Boston: Plays, Inc. Publishers, 1990.
Guest, Ann Hutchinson. *Your Move: A New Ap-
 proach to the Study of Movement and Dance*. Rev.
 ed. New York: Gordon and Breach Science
 Publishers, Inc., 1990.
Laban, Rudolf. *A Life for Dance*. New York: The-
 atre Arts Books, 1975.
———. *The Mastery of Movement*. Revised by Lisa
 Ullman. Boston: Plays, Inc. Publishers, 1975.
North, Marion. *Personality Assessment Through
 Movement*. London: Macdonald and Evans,
 1972.

Movement Pattern Analysis

 Movement pattern analysis focuses on the relationship between mind and body in the
structure and coding of move-
ment. Though it can be applied to a broad
range of activities, it is generally used in
executive training programs to improve individual skills in decision making, communication, and group interaction. There is no
prescribed regimen of exercise in movement
pattern analysis. It assesses habitual structures of behavior in order to provide information that will help in the choice and
attainment of life goals.

History

Movement pattern analysis has its roots in
the system of movement analysis first developed in the early twentieth century by
Rudolf Laban, an Austro-Hungarian artist,
scientist, and philosopher. The rise of Hitler
forced Laban to flee to Great Britain where,
from 1941 to 1946, he and F. C. Lawrence, a
management consultant, conducted a study

of industrial production tasks. Their findings contradicted the mechanistic principles of time/motion study, which governed thought about efficient factory production at that time.

Laban and Lawrence approached factory work as if it were a form of dance, paying particular attention to the characteristic mental attitude needed to perform each individual movement of the tasks. They argued that this dynamic patterning, which Laban called effort phrasing, should be the basis for determining a worker's suitability to a job. Struck by the repetitive nature of factory work, they also encouraged workers to make motions that, strictly speaking, were inefficient but lent a satisfying rhythm to their tasks. Workers at factories that adopted the Laban Lawrence industrial rhythm, also called Laban personal effort assessment, increased their output, suffered less stress, and felt more complete as human beings.

At the end of World War II, Warren Lamb joined Laban's group and began to explore ways of applying effort assessment to managerial work. He observed the behavior of managers in their offices and devised a system for correlating effort phrasing with the decision-making skills required for a number of managerial activities. First marketed in the 1960s as action profiling, Lamb's method had an enormous impact on the corporate community, particularly in Great Britain. Action profiling gave companies a new, effective means for allocating responsibility and building successful management teams. In 1992 disagreements over the Laban heritage forced Lamb to leave his first organization, Action Profilers International, and rename his method *movement pattern analysis*.

Theory

Lamb's method is based on the belief that movement is a direct, faithful register of a person's inner intention, whether conscious or unconscious. The nature of the intention is evaluated through study of a particular type of movement, which Lamb named integrated movement. These movements, which seem to appear when a person is most fully revealing of his inner intentions, are distinguished by the fact that they flow throughout the entire body, moving from the core outward, or from the extremities inward.

Information for assessment of the decision-making process is derived from extended observation of integrated movements. The shape these movements take in space, rising or falling, spreading or enclosing, retreating or advancing, is noted and correlated with qualities of effort. According to Lamb, who follows Laban on this principle, effort is manifested in four qualities: flow, weight, space, and time. Each of these four attributes of movement is indicative of a specific inner attitude of the mover. For example, flow, or the ongoing quality of the movement, is indicative of an inner attitude of progression. A controlled movement reflects a sense of caution, whereas a free-flowing movement indicates an inner attitude of abandon. By attending to the relationship between effort and shape in integrated movement, it is possible to determine "where" a person is in the decision-making process. A picture of his entire decision-making process can be produced with data drawn from prolonged study. The profile is as distinctive and indelible as a fingerprint.

Practice

Movement pattern analysis is conducted like a job interview or an ordinary conversation. The client remains fully clothed and in some instances may not be aware of the precise purpose of the meeting. The movement pattern analyst asks questions concerning the client's job or life. As the conversation proceeds, the analyst assesses the client's integrated movements and records the data on coding sheets formulated by Lamb. The results are then discussed with the client and possibly with the client's employer.

When a group such as a management team is evaluated, movement pattern analysis is done in two stages. In the first stage the members of the group are approached on an individual basis and given information about their decision-making habits. In the second stage the group is studied as an entity with its own characteristic mode of behavior. This second analysis is used by the group leader and the group as a whole to determine tactics for achieving smoother, more productive teamwork.

Benefits

A profile of one's decision-making process can be an important means of self-empowerment. It allows decision making to be understood as a pattern of behavior, with strengths and weaknesses that can be examined and changed.

—WARREN LAMB

Resources

Motus Humanus
    Carol-Lynne Moore, Director
    P.O. Box 11036
    Denver, CO 80211
    Tel: (303) 421-2023
    Organizes workshops and conferences in movement pattern analysis and supervises the training of movement pattern analysts.

Further Reading

Laban, Rudolf, and F. C. Lawrence. *Effort*. London: Macdonald & Evans, 1947.

Laban, Rudolf. *The Language of Movement*. Edited by Lisa Ullman. Boston: Plays, Inc. Publishers, 1974.

Lamb, Warren. *Posture and Gesture*. London: Duckworth, 1965.

———. *Management Behavior*. London: Duckworth, 1969.

Lamb, Warren, and Elizabeth Watson. *Body Code: The Meaning in Movement*. Princeton, N.J.: Princeton Book Company, 1987.

Moore, Carol-Lynne. *Executives in Action: A Guide to Balanced Decision-Making in Management*. 4th ed. London: Pitman, 1992.

Ramsden, Pamela. *Top Team Planning: A Study of the Power of Individual Motivation in Management*. London: Associated Business Programmes, 1973.

PART 15:

Expressive and Creative Arts Therapies

Expressive and creative arts therapies are methods that use one or several of the fine arts as a means to effect changes in physical, mental, or emotional functioning. Music, painting, sculpture, dancing, mimicry, and storytelling were used by early humans to try to create order in a seemingly chaotic universe. By giving aesthetic form to their fears, hopes, and dreams, our ancestors found many ways to cope with the mysterious and sometimes terrifying forces that control the universe. Expressive and creative arts therapies are grounded in this same notion, using the evocative, organizing power of aesthetic expression to help people of all ages face challenges of healing and growing—challenges that can be as difficult in this day and age as they were for our primal ancestors.

ART THERAPY

AUTHENTIC
MOVEMENT

DANCE THERAPY

DRAMA THERAPY

HALPRIN LIFE/
ART PROCESS

JOURNAL THERAPY

MULTIMODAL
EXPRESSIVE ARTS
THERAPY

MUSIC THERAPY

POETRY THERAPY

SANDPLAY THERAPY

Learning Life Skills Through the Arts

Although the use of the fine arts for therapeutic purposes is comparatively new in Western medicine, the healing and educational power of the arts has been intuitively recognized around the world from the beginnings of human history. For ancient primal cultures and their contemporary relatives, the indigenous peoples of North and South America, Africa, Polynesia, Australia, and Asia, the arts are an intrinsic part of life. In these cultures children develop gross and fine motor skills along with a strong sense of identity as they learn to weave baskets or make pottery, clothing, or hunting equipment in the traditional patterns of their cultures.

In these cultures religious celebrations mark the seasons of the year and important events in life, such as birth, adolescence, marriage, and death. These celebrations are often communal events in which participants might prepare traditional costumes, masks, and musical instruments and take part in ritualized singing, dancing, and theatrical presentations. These activities develop physical and intellectual skills in the participants while serving on a deeper level to guide their emotional and spiritual development.

In the highly developed ancient cultures of China, India, and Egypt, the arts were an integral part of political, educational, religious, and health practices. These cultures believed that the universe was perfectly ordered by divine forces. They believed that achieving power, success, happiness, and health was a result of learning how these divine forces operate in the universe and working harmoniously with them. One way this could be accomplished was through aesthetic expression. Sound, motion, and light—the elemental materials of music, dance, and visual and performance art—were believed to follow divine cosmological laws. Artists and philosophers, who also functioned as teachers and healers in these cultures, worked to discover aesthetic theories for the arts so that artistic expressions would reflect the divine order of the universe and help people experience a sense of harmony with it. The teachers applied these laws to various artistic disciplines such as music (including chanting), calligraphy, dance, and theatrical performances.

The Changing Role of the Arts

Aesthetic modes of healing, praying, and learning continued unbroken for nearly five thousand years in the East. As Western culture evolved, the arts began to be separated from these basic human activities. Ironically, the philosophy of Plato (c. 428–348 B.C.E.), known for its promotion of aesthetic beauty, is partially responsible for this change. Plato believed humans could create a more perfect order in the universe and he put forth the idea that human behavior was created from three basic sources: desire, emotion, and knowledge. In Plato's hierarchical philosophy, reason and intellect, located in the head, were a more valuable pilot for the soul than the emotions located in the heart, or desires located in the loins or pelvis. From this point of view the physical embodiment of divine laws through art grew to be less valuable than intellectual and theoretical discussions of those laws.

As Western culture passed through the decline of Greece and the rise and fall of Rome, the arts continued to lose their primacy as a means of praying, teaching, and healing. In the Dark Ages that followed, the arts remained connected to religious activities within the Judeo-Christian tradition, but they were no longer valued as a primary method of communicating spiritual knowledge or healing. That tradition denigrated the physical body and all sensory modes of expression and glorified the human mind and intellectual thought as the one true path to spiritual salvation. The arts were treated as crafts in need of direction and control and became a mere adornment to the pursuit of spiritual excellence. Then, during the Renaissance, the arts began to fall prey to the secularized demands of commerce, where they have, by and large, remained to this day.

At the dawn of the twentieth century, however, a confluence of forces in art, politics, and health care served to partially reestablish the role of the arts as a tool for healing in the West. In the first decades of the century Sigmund Freud (1856–1939) and his colleagues, notably Carl Jung (1875–1961), began to explore the connections between physical health and the workings of the human mind and emotions. Freud's theories of the unconscious and its role in the development and behavior of human beings became the basis of an entirely new mode of treatment in Western medicine. Both psychoanalysis, as Freud termed his approach, and analytical psychology, as Jung described his, relied on the revelation of personal unconscious imagery to effect a cure. This unconscious imagery is still an important tool for many expressive and creative arts therapists.

At about the same time, Western artists such as Pablo Picasso (1881–1973), Arnold Schoenberg (1874–1951), Isadora Duncan (1877–1927), Rainer Maria Rilke (1875–1926), and Konstantin Stanislavsky (1863–1938) were becoming disillusioned with traditional art forms, which they felt were outmoded and had lost their ability to inspire. They began creating modern art forms full of vibrant, abstract images reflecting personal perceptions. By the time World War II rocked the Western world in 1939, a large body of artists in Europe and the United States was exploring the power of the arts to capture, reflect, and organize unconscious content. Many of these artists intuitively recognized the therapeutic value of their own activities, and they explored the potential of arts therapy in private teaching situations. Open-minded doctors, aware of the therapeutic successes of some of these artists, invited them into the hospitals, which were struggling to accommodate the large number of people suffering from physical and emotional trauma as a result of the war. Predominantly dancers and visual artists, but also musicians, writers, and theater artists, entered the hospital setting, and the new modalities of music, dance, art, poetry, and drama therapy were born.

After 1945 the nascent expressive arts therapies were introduced into other institutional settings such as schools, prisons, and senior citizen homes. Experiential exploration and theoretical development continued throughout the 1950s, with more and more creative artists developing unique practices and approaches to healing and changing through the arts. With the social upheaval of the 1960s and its demand for more meaningful forms of living, the creative and expressive arts were enlisted once again in growth centers across the country. At the Esalen Institute in California and the Omega Institute in New York, the arts became a means by which ever-greater numbers of people sought to expand their understanding of themselves and their role in the universe.

Today each of the expressive arts therapies (music, dance, visual art, poetry, and drama) is represented by a national organization that sets standards for the training of therapists and offers a forum for the many technical and philosophical issues confronting the field. In addition, a growing number of related creative arts practices serves individuals in their efforts to heal and grow physically, mentally, emotionally, and spiritually.

The Process of Creation as Exercise for the Brain

All the expressive arts therapies and creative arts practices share the belief that creating a work of art is in and of itself therapeutic. The process, not the end product, is the most important part of the work. For instance, creative dance sessions can extend the range of movement and develop the physical coordination of people with cerebral palsy, muscular dystrophy, or polio. Painting and sculpting can develop hand-eye coordination in the physically healthy as well as the physically challenged. Music classes that focus on the use of the voice can help people with asthma discover a new relationship to their lungs and the process of breathing.

Contemporary research into the nature of the brain suggests how the practice of creative arts brings about these seemingly miraculous improvements. Researchers have discovered that the right side of the brain controls the left side of the body and is responsible for imaginative, nonlinear thought. The left side of the brain, which controls the right side of the body, is the location of logical, rational, analytic, and verbal skills. Creative arts, which use both imaginative and analytical skills, call on both sides of the brain, developing brain cells and nerve connections that drugs and specific repetitive physical exercises simply cannot awaken.

Creating Art to Improve Social and Emotional Skills

Social and emotional skills are also explored through the process of making art. Creating a work of art requires developing an ability to turn one's attention alternately inward toward the creative impulse, and outward toward the form that is being created, and to develop a dialogue between the two. The communication skills developed in this process are similar to those needed for healthy, satisfying interpersonal relationships. In a like manner, creating a group dance, musical composition, or visual art installation can serve as a laboratory for the development of group social skills.

Whether the participant is creating alone or in a group, the form of the work being created always serves as the reference point for the developing physical or emotional skills. It is a basic tenet of all expressive arts therapies and creative arts practices that the form of a work of art reflects the inner feelings of the creator or creators. Expressive and creative arts practitioners believe we can perceive, describe, and share our conscious and unconscious feelings more effectively by giving them expression in an aesthetic form and then reflecting on that form and our process in creating it. Both the form and the process of creating it become metaphors for how we live our lives.

Reflecting on the Work

The process of reflecting on the work of art will vary depending on the orientation of the therapist, counselor, or group leader. Therapists who adhere to the Freudian model will observe and discuss the content of the work of art, interpreting it symbolically in relation to seven psychosexual stages of development of the child in relation to its parents. Therapists with a Jungian orientation will compare the content to characters and themes from world mythology, sensing in them the unfolding of an individual human consciousness in relation to the collective unconscious, a sort of world library of human experience. Followers of transpersonal psychology or humanist psychology, founded by Abraham Maslow and Carl Rogers, respectively, will probably not engage in the process of interpretation at all, trusting entirely in the ability of the individual or the group to direct their own psychospiritual healing through the process of making art.

Experiencing Expressive Arts Therapies and Creative Arts Practices

While the formalized use of expressive arts therapies began in institutional settings and remains an important part of healing and education in hospitals, prisons, shelters, and schools, it is also possible to explore these practices, individually or in a group, in private counseling or at growth centers throughout the United States today. No special talent is required, simply an enjoyment of an art form and a desire to explore and grow. Many creative arts leaders advertise workshops in magazines and newspapers. Expressive arts therapists in private practice can be located through their national organizations.

Each therapist or group leader will have her own approach to working with individuals, groups, and the specific art form. Some therapists or group leaders will focus on spontaneous creation, or improvisation, as the major activity of a session or workshop. For others the main activity may be the practice of specific movements, or playing or listening to particular pieces of music, or reading particular poems. Here the emphasis is not so much on the ability of art to capture and reflect unconscious content, but on the power of a previously created form or the experience of a particular element of artistic technique to effect a desired change in the body and mind of the practitioner. Many therapists or group leaders will combine both approaches in their creative arts sessions.

In group work the role of observer can be as important as the role of creator. Participants often observe group members in the act of creating, or view their completed works of art. Just as the ancients recognized the value of creating art, active observing has long been recognized for its cathartic and therapeutic effects on our mind and body as well. Responding verbally to a work of art can also help us learn to understand our emotions and their effects on others. By sharing our responses with the creator, we complete a loop of communication, allowing the creator to learn how others experience his creation/emotional expression.

Physical, Mental, and Emotional Benefits

Whether approached in group or individual modes, expressive art therapies and creative arts practices offer great possibilities for developing a deeper understanding and appreciation of our physical, mental, and emotional coping strategies and learning new living and communication skills. With an open heart, willing mind, and dedication to the process, the arts offer an unlimited opportunity to explore and share the unfolding of our essential humanity.

—*NANCY ALLISON, CMA*

Resources

Expressive Arts Program
   California Institute of Integral Studies
   9 Peter Yorke Way
   San Francisco, CA 94109
   Tel: (415) 674-5500
   Offers a master's degree in counseling psychology with a specialization in expressive arts therapy.

Expressive Therapies Program
   Lesley College
   29 Everett St.
   Cambridge, MA 02138
   Tel: (617) 349-8425
   Offers a comprehensive graduate program in multimodal expressive arts therapy.

International Expressive Arts Therapy Association
   P.O. Box 64126
   San Francisco, CA 94164
   Tel: (415) 522-8959
   A professional organization dedicated to multimodal expressive arts therapy.

Further Reading

Arnheim, Rudolf. *Towards a Psychology of Art.* Berkeley: University of California Press, 1966.

Berger, John. *Ways of Seeing.* Magnolia, Mass.: Peter Smith, 1977.

Dewey, John. *Art as Experience.* New York: Perigee Books, 1959.

McNiff, Shaun. *The Arts in Psychotherapy.* Springfield, Ill.: Charles C Thomas, 1981.

Art Therapy

Art therapy is a method used to help people release inner thoughts and emotions by making visual art. This process of creative expression is thought to aid a person's healing and recovery through forms of visual art such as drawing, painting, sculpture, or collage. Therapists may work with a person to decipher symbolic representations of his feelings, thoughts, or perceptions. This form of therapy may appeal to people who otherwise find it difficult to express or understand a problem or emotion. Art is used as an intuitive, physical method of manifesting hidden feelings and overcoming difficult problems.

History

Although the field of art therapy formally emerged in this century, the use of visual images to express inner emotions and master external events extends back to prehistory. Masks, ritual pottery, carefully designed costumes, and musical instruments were created as outer expressions of powerful spiritual beliefs and used in rituals, suggesting two healing aspects of art: its potential to achieve or restore psychological equilibrium, and its ability to alleviate or contain feelings of trauma, fear, anxiety, and psychological threat to the self and the community.

In the late 1800s and early 1900s, a growing number of European psychologists became interested in studying visual art made by patients with mental illnesses. In 1912 psychiatrists Emil Kraepelin and Eugen Bleuler were among the earliest to try to diagnose psychopathologies by interpreting their patients' drawings. Later Sigmund Freud reported that patients of his who were unable to describe their dreams in words would frequently say that they could draw the images. This observation encouraged the belief that artistic expression could reveal the inner world of the human psyche.

Psychologist Carl Jung's work also influenced the development of art therapy. Jung was particularly interested in the psychological meanings and uses of art expressions, including his own drawings and those of his patients. Unlike Freud, who never asked his patients to draw their dream images, Jung often encouraged his patients to draw. "To paint what we see before us," he said, "is a different art from painting what we see within." Jung believed there was an important connection between the images that people made and their inner thoughts. By studying art created around the world, Jung noted recurring and seemingly universal symbols he called archetypes. These archetypes are cultural images that represent basic elements of unconscious thought and human development. Jung's theory of archetypes became a foundation for understanding how symbolic imagery reveals meaning in artworks, and is still used by many therapists today.

In the 1940s art therapy became a profession in the United States, largely due to the work of Margaret Naumburg. She founded the Walden School in 1915, where she used students' artworks in psychological counseling. She agreed with the predominant psychological viewpoint that art expression is a way to manifest unconscious imagery. In Naumburg's view, art could provide the client a form of spontaneous expression and communication. She considered these images a form of symbolic speech.

Through the 1950s and 1960s Edith Kramer, an artist, educator, and pioneer in the field of art therapy, pointed to another important benefit of art making. She was a European artist who moved to the United States, where she began teaching art to children. While other therapists sought to decode patients' artworks, Kramer was interested in the value of the act of art making. She believed there were therapeutic benefits to the creative process itself. She stressed creativity, in addition to the communication of visual symbols, as the key to the art therapy process.

Theory

Art therapy attempts to introduce visual art making as an accessible method of communicating feelings, thoughts, and experiences. This creative process is used to aid a person's healing and recovery. An art therapist will work with her patients to help them understand their art expressions. To accomplish this, the therapist and client will review the artworks and discuss possible meanings or emotions expressed in the work. With the help of the art therapist, the patient interprets the images by trying to recognize aspects of her self in art expressions. For those clients who cannot verbally articulate the content of their images, such as children, the art therapist may look for repetition of themes over time to provide clues to possible meanings. A therapist will try to understand and clarify the meanings of images while respecting the client as a creative individual capable of contributing to her own healing process. Art therapists who practice in the United States are trained at the graduate level and receive a master's degree; a strong background in visual art and psychology is generally required to enter a graduate program.

Practice

An art therapist uses visual art media (such as drawing materials, paints, collage/mixed media, and clay sculpture) and the creative process to help a patient explore issues, interests, concerns, and conflicts through art expression. Art therapists work in a variety of ways and with many different populations. An art therapist in a hospital setting might work individually with psychiatric patients to help them use art to explore emotional conflicts or develop social skills. If a child has been traumatized by physical abuse, a therapist might use art activities to help the child explore feelings about the trauma and to reduce feelings of anxiety, fear, or depression. Art therapists often work as part of a treatment team that includes doctors, nurses, psychologists, social workers, and counselors.

Benefits

An art therapist might work with adults in a psychiatric hospital, an addictions treatment center, a shelter for battered women and their children, a school for the mentally retarded or disabled, a day care center for the elderly, a rehabilitation hospital, or a medical facility with physically ill patients. Therapists work with children, adults, families, and groups, and with a variety of patient populations. Some art therapists work as private practitioners, while others are employed by schools, hospitals, clinics, or community agencies.

Art therapy uses art making to enhance communication between therapist and client. The artworks are used as a common language through which clients and therapists can explore feelings, thoughts, and experiences. This makes art therapy a significant contribution to the field of mental health, with enhanced promise in the growth of human understanding.

—CATHY MALCHIODI, M.A., ATR, LPAT, LPCC

Resources

American Art Therapy Association, Inc.
    1202 Allanson Road
    Chicago, IL 60060
    Tel: (847) 949-6064
    Fax: (847) 566-4580
    Web site: www.louisville.edu/groups/
    aata.www

A list of approved training programs, membership information, and resources for books, tapes, and videos is available. This organization also publishes *Art Therapy: Journal of the American Art Therapy Association.*

The Arts in Psychotherapy
Elsevier Science
660 White Plains Road
Tarrytown, NY 10591-5153
e-mail: esuk.usa@elsevier.com
This journal features articles by experts in the creative arts therapies about the therapeutic use of various forms of art. It reports on national and international art therapy conferences and features book reviews.

Further Reading

Case, C., and T. Dalley. *The Handbook of Art Therapy.* London: Tavistock, 1992.

Kramer, E. *Art as Therapy with Children.* Chicago: Magnolia St. Publishers, 1994.

Malchiodi, C. A. *Breaking the Silence: Art Therapy with Children.* New York: Brunner/Mazel, 1997.

McNiff, S. *The Arts in Psychotherapy.* Springfield, Ill.: Charles C Thomas, 1981.

Ulman, E., and P. Dachinger, eds. *Art Therapy in Theory and Practice.* Chicago: Magnolia St. Publishers, 1996.

Authentic Movement

 Authentic movement is a dance-movement process practiced by individuals and groups as a way to learn from the body's own experience, insights, and imagination. It is an outwardly simple but profound process in which subjects follow their impulses for movement or stillness in an accepting rather than judgmental way. Instead of consciously choosing what movements to do, they allow their bodies to initiate movement, thereby making room for the unconscious to partici-pate. This process leads to a deepened respect for the body's wisdom and is practiced for diverse purposes such as personal enrichment, spiritual insight, artistic renewal, psychotherapy, or community ritual.

History

Mary Whitehouse, the pioneering dancer, teacher, and dance therapist, began developing authentic movement in the 1950s and 1960s. A modern dancer, Whitehouse had trained with Mary Wigman and Martha Graham. Wigman's emphasis on individual creativity and Whitehouse's interest in the psychological theories of Carl Jung provided a foundation for what is now known as authentic movement.

Whitehouse described authentic movement as that which was spontaneous and genuine to that person, rather than learned movement. It arose out of the self, and occurred when the ego relinquished control over the movement. Throughout her life Whitehouse continued to experiment with this approach to movement, and with various names for it; for example, she called it the "Tao of the body" and "movement in depth."

Janet Adler, a dance therapist well known for her work with autistic children, studied with Whitehouse in 1969. She brought her own interest in Freudian psychological theory and a deep interest in shamanism and mysticism. In the late 1970s she began to formalize a set practice and called it authentic movement. She established the Mary Starks Whitehouse Institute in western Massachusetts in 1981, two years after Whitehouse's death, as a place to study and teach this form of movement.

Basic Principles

The core element of the process shared by most practitioners is the relationship between the mover and the witness. With eyes closed or inwardly focused, the mover responds to his inner impulses while the witness watches from the sidelines without judgment. After a set time of moving, usually without musical accompaniment, a dialogue occurs between mover and witness. The purpose of the process is to honor the expression of the mover's inner experience without judgment.

Several core values are shared by most authentic movement practitioners. The first is that one's body contains wisdom and can be used as a source of insight, healing, and guidance. A second is that the mover's experience during the session—when one spends time in the body, paying attention to how the body moves—is of prime importance. The third is that authority for an individual's experience rests with the individual and not with an observer or anyone who moved with that person.

Authentic movement offers an opportunity for deep rest and recuperation of both body and soul. It cultivates the integration of one's physical, psychological, and spiritual aspects, and it invites the safe inclusion of the full range of healthy human expression—be it playful or somber, solitary or shared. Authentic movement is practiced by people varied in age, physical skill, dance or movement training, and religious belief, and for diverse purposes such as for personal enrichment, spiritual insight, artistic renewal, psychotherapy, or community ritual.

Although the name *authentic movement* is widely used to identify the process, other names are also used, such as contemplative dance, or the moving imagination. Currently, there is no central organization overseeing practitioners, although the process of building better communication between practitioners is under way.

Practice

During a session people move in a tremendous variety of ways, from extended periods of complete stillness to vigorous activity. The movement might be minute—even imperceptible—or large and highly stylized. It can be idiosyncratic, mundane, or formal; rhythmic or dancelike; familiar or foreign; homely and awkward, or graceful and elegant. No movement is inherently unacceptable unless it harms the mover or others. This very broad acceptance of movement possibilities distinguishes this practice from other forms of open improvisation. Unlike most forms of dance, there is no need to please or impress viewers or fellow movers.

To establish a safe environment both physically and interpersonally, rules about safety and confidentiality are regularly reinforced and refined. Individuals must be responsible for not hurting themselves or fellow movers (by opening their eyes when necessary, for example, or moving away from unwelcome contact), and are not to share others' experiences outside of the group. These structures and rules allow for significant privacy—both from the outer world and/or from one's fellow movers— considerable intimacy, trust, and an unusually broad freedom in movement possibilities.

Just as important is the "sharing after moving" phase that allows the participants to integrate what they have experienced. Depending on the goals of the participants, there might be analytical dialogue in a therapeutic setting, discussion of artistic ideas or images in an artistic working group or rehearsal, personal sharing in a peer group, or no discussion at all in a group practicing for spiritual purposes. This phase might take different forms for people in the same group, or different forms for one person on different days.

In choosing a facilitator, one should be conscientious and sensible. Questions about the person's background, training, and goals are appropriate. One should ask for references. It is important to feel intuitively comfortable with the teacher and to know that the goals for working together are shared.

Dance therapist Janet Adler explains the dynamics of authentic movement: "The witness, especially in the beginning, carries a larger responsibility for consciousness, as she sits to the side of the movement space. She is not 'looking at' the person moving, she is witnessing, listening—bringing a specific quality of attention or presence to—the experience of the mover.

"The mover works with eyes closed in order to expand her experience of listening to the deeper levels of her kinesthetic reality. Her task is to respond to a sensation, to an inner impulse, to energy coming from the personal unconscious, the collective unconscious, or the superconscious. . . . The mover and witness usually speak together about the material that has emerged during the movement time, thus bringing formerly unconscious processes into consciousness."

Benefits

Authentic movement is a contemporary movement practice that provides people from a wide variety of backgrounds and abilities a structure within which they can recuperate their bodies and souls. This process can lead to an enhanced awareness of one's whole self and provide insights to fundamental issues and questions relevant to one's life.

—DAPHNE LOWELL

Resources

The Authentic Movement Community Directory
   Michael Gardos Reid, Editor
   2219 Taft St. N.E.
   Minneapolis, MN 55418
   Tel: (612) 788-1822
   e-mail: 76232.1634@Compuserve.com
   Lists practitioners of authentic movement.

Further Reading

Books

Pallaro, Patrizia, ed. *Authentic Movement: Essays by Mary Whitehouse, Janet Adler, and Joan Chodorow.* Vol. 1. London: Jessica Kingsley Publishers, 1998.
———. *Authentic Movement: Moving the Body, Moving the Self. A Collection of Essays.* Vol. 2. London: Jessica Kingsley Publishers, 1999.

Journals

A Moving Journal: Ongoing Expressions of Authentic Movement. Annie Geissinger, Joan Webb, editors.

Dance Therapy

Dance therapy is founded on the principle that a vital connection exists between personality and the way in which one moves, and that changes in movement behavior can affect the emotional, intellectual, and physical health of an individual. It is used to help people attain healthy, expressive functioning, individually or in group situations. It is especially useful with people for whom verbal therapy is ineffective or overwhelming.

History

Although the roots of dance therapy are ancient, it has been recognized as an established form of therapy only since the 1940s. The rhythmic movements of dance have appealed to people throughout the ages. Dance is found in nearly every culture and civilization, serving a variety of purposes. In many cultures, dance was and still is used as a cathartic healing tool. Primitive societies used dance in rites of passage and other religious ceremonies. Dance rituals marked life transitions, helping to integrate individuals with the larger society. Many societies still use dance in similar ways. Experts agree that in early civilizations dancing, religion, music, and medicine were often connected.

In the early part of the twentieth century, radical changes in dance movement and expression resulted in what is now called "modern" dance. Up to that time Western theatrical dance had been a highly structured and regimented art form. Modern dance focuses on spontaneity, awareness of natural movement, and more freedom for personal expression. During the first half of the twentieth century, there were also new developments in psychiatry that explored nonverbal aspects of psychology and psychopathology. Eugen Bleuler in Switzerland, Jean-Martin Charcot in France, and Henry Maudsley in England were examining the unique movement behavior of people with mental illness. The field of dance therapy emerged in the 1940s and 1950s amid these innovations in dance and in psychological treatment.

The earliest dance therapists were dancers and dance teachers who were encouraged by psychiatrists to use dance as a method of communicating with withdrawn patients. Marian Chace (1896–1970) is considered an important pioneering force in the establishment of dance therapy in the United States. Chace's dance education included dance from many cultures, dance improvisation, and music theory, and cultivated in Chace an openness to many forms of dance expression. Later she established her own school in Washington, D.C., where her dance technique, which stressed improvisation and individual expression, gained a reputation for having therapeutic effects.

In 1942 Chace was invited by psychiatrists at St. Elizabeth's Hospital in Washington, D.C., to initiate a dance program for World War II veterans suffering mentally and emotionally from their wartime experiences. Chace was influenced by the ideas of American psychiatrist Harry Stack Sullivan,

among others, who stressed that personality is formed through relationships, and that relationships require communication. She believed that schizophrenics and others with mental illness who were isolated in the back wards of psychiatric hospitals could be helped through direct contact and that through movement she could open lines of communication and establish relationships with these patients. Where others had seen only bizarre, random movements, Chace saw a valuable, if distorted, form of communication. Through a technique she called "mirroring" movement, Chace established a connection with an individual by re-creating his movement behavior with her own body. Mirroring, as Chace conceptualized, is not an imitation or mimicry of a patient's movement. Rather, the therapist is trying to take on the quality of the patient's movement, to move in tune with the patient in order to better understand what he is trying to communicate and to be able to respond in kind. Through this process Chace discovered that symbols, imagery, and metaphor arose from movement that could be given verbal expression, thus providing a healing catharsis. Chace worked with individuals and groups using dance and movement as a means of communication; she took the expressive and symbolic elements of dance and merged them into a powerful form of therapy.

Other pioneers in the field of dance therapy include Franciczka Boas, Liljan Espenak, Blanch Evan, Alma Hawkins, Trudi Schoop, and Mary Whitehouse. All of these early founders of dance therapy were grounded in a modern dance tradition that stressed authentic expression of the self. Each worked independently and developed her own method that studied, interpreted, and supported movement exploration, using the dance therapy session as the "container" of emotional experience. These individuals and others helped develop a broad range of styles and clinical applications with which contemporary dance therapists continue to work today.

In 1966 a group of therapists formed the American Dance Therapy Association (ADTA) to set professional standards and establish channels of communication among dance therapists, who were working mostly independently in hospitals and clinics throughout the country. Today ADTA has more than one thousand members nationally and internationally. The association publishes the *American Journal of Dance Therapy,* holds an annual conference, and maintains a registry of dance therapists who have met educational and clinical requirements.

Basic Principles

Dance therapy relies on several theoretical tenets. First and foremost is that dance is an expressive art and as such fulfills the human being's basic need for communication. Believing that each person has a desire to communicate, the dance therapist engages those parts of the person's personality that are expressive, however subtle they may be. Dance therapists believe that the body and mind are in constant reciprocal interaction; therefore, changes that occur on the movement level can affect one's total functioning.

Movement is believed to reflect personality. Dance therapy utilizes the nonverbal dimension of personality by using the technique of mirroring, which re-creates the early experiences of the nonverbal mother-infant interaction. The relationship between the therapist and patient is central to the effectiveness of dance therapy. The dance therapist responds to the patient on a body level by mirroring, synchronizing, and interacting with the patient's movement, thus creating a strong therapeutic relationship. This helps explain why dance therapy is particularly effective with patients who are so regressed that verbal therapy is ineffective. Empathy is an important healing agent in dance therapy. By moving with the individual in similar patterns, the patient feels accepted on an emotional level.

Like dreams and the process of free association, movement can be symbolic of the underlying unconscious process. Therefore, ideas and feelings that are outside conscious awareness may emerge in movement behavior as symbols. Interpretation of these symbols can help in the process of therapeutic change.

Finally, the act of creating a movement through improvisation is inherently therapeutic, since it generates new ways of moving, which generate new experiences of being in the world with other people. Individuals often experience highly charged emotional states during a dance therapy session. Working with the individual to assess and interpret his movement verbally, the therapist creates a safe and trusting environment in which feelings are explored through dance and words together. Verbal processing helps to connect action, thought, and feeling, enabling the individual to experience greater feelings of personal integration and effectiveness.

Practice

Sessions are usually conducted in groups but can also be practiced one-on-one. Generally, the participants meet in a spacious, empty room where they feel free to move. No special dance clothing is worn. The structure of the session will vary depending on the participants involved and the orientation of the therapist. A session might begin with a warm-up led by the therapist and designed to reflect the mood of the patient or group in the moment. The therapist will be trained to pick up subtle movement cues and extend them through the mirroring technique rather than teaching dance steps or choreographed movements. Depending on the orientation of the therapist, she will continue to pick up movement and themes from the group based on improvisation or "dance in the moment." The goal of the session is not to perform or to exercise. Instead,

The professional training of a dance therapist takes place on a graduate level. Dance therapists in training study dance/movement therapy theory and practice, psychopathology, human development, and observation and research skills, and complete a supervised internship in a clinical setting. The title of dance therapist registered (DTR) indicates that the therapist has completed professional education and training as indicated by the ADTA. Academy of Dance Therapists Registered (ADTR) is a title that means qualified to teach, to provide supervision to other dance therapists, and to practice privately.

the therapist creates an environment in which any and all movement behavior is valuable. After the development of movement themes and imagery, along with free verbal associations, the session ends with some sort of structured closing.

Benefits and Risks

The goals of dance therapy include helping people achieve body-level reintegration. Individuals improve their communication skills and learn new ways to interact with others. Dance therapy also provides a safe environment in which to address emotional issues. It can help individuals with serious psychological and social difficulties, eating disorders, substance-abuse problems, Alzheimer's disease, and posttraumatic stress disorders. It can also be helpful in dealing with everyday stress as well as emotional and relationship issues. The elderly, adults, adolescents, children, and infants have all been aided by dance therapy.

—ANNE L. WENNERSTRAND

Resources

The American Dance Therapy Association
2000 Century Plaza, Suite 108
Columbia, MD 21044
Tel: (410) 997-4040
Fax: (410) 997-4048
e-mail: ADTA@aol.com
listserv: adta@list.ab.umd.edu
Founded in 1966, this membership and advocacy group sets dance therapy eligibility standards, holds annual national conferences, provides information about graduate training programs, and publishes the *American Journal of Dance Therapy*.

Further Reading

Levy, F. *Dance Movement Therapy: A Healing Art*. Reston, Va.: American Alliance for Health, Physical Education, Recreation, and Dance, 1992.

Payne, H. *Dance Movement Therapy: Theory and Practice*. London: Routledge, 1992.

Sandel, S., S. Chaiklin, and A. Lohn, eds. *Foundations of Dance/Movement Therapy: The Life and Work of Marian Chace*. Columbia, Md.: The Marian Chace Memorial Fund of the American Dance Therapy Association, 1993.

Stanton-Jones, K. *Dance Movement Therapy in Psychiatry*. London: Routledge, 1992.

Drama Therapy

 Drama therapy combines techniques from drama and theater with techniques from psychotherapy in an action-based method that helps people find solutions for social and emotional problems. This creative arts therapy helps people improve their sense of self-worth by discovering their own inner resources and by learning how to function better in groups. In its most well-known form, drama therapy uses role play to help participants learn healthier behavior patterns. Drama therapists also use techniques such as improvisation, theater games, concentration exercises, mime, masks and puppetry, scripted dramatizations, and open-ended scripts to further emotional growth and psychological integration. Drama therapy can offer individuals a vision of something outside the self and beyond a personal, subjective view of the world to expand their universe.

History

Drama has been a part of human culture since the first prehistoric cave dwellers arrived home from a hunt and acted out their daring adventures for an assembled group. Formal theater came much later, with dramas that provided moral and ethical lessons for people, as well as comedies to entertain and lighten their burdens. Religious leaders recognized the power of drama as a method of teaching their beliefs to people and added theatrical elements to their rituals. Theater practitioners have long been aware of the therapeutic value of drama.

It took a little longer for the action method of treatment combining psychology, process-drama, and theater to be formalized. Although drama therapy has been practiced in Europe, especially in England, for many years, the National Association for Drama Therapy (NADT) was not established in the United States until June 1979 at Yale University. The first annual conference was held in July 1980, which makes drama therapy the newest of the creative arts therapies. As of July 1997, there were approximately three hundred members of the NADT.

Basic Principles

NADT defines drama therapy as "the systematic and intentional use of drama/theater processes to achieve the therapeutic goals of symptom relief, emotional and physical integration, and personal growth." This creative arts therapy is used to maintain health as well as to treat such dysfunctions as emotional disorders, learning difficulties, geriatric problems, and social maladjustments. Drama therapy, as a primary or an adjunctive modality, is used in evaluation, treatment, and research with individuals, groups, and families.

Put more simply, drama therapy offers practice for living, helps clients discover their own inner resources, and promotes their ability to express their feelings. It enhances sensory awareness and helps people learn to use the imagination as a problem-solving tool. It allows a client to play a new and unfamiliar role or to play a familiar role with a new set of behaviors. For example, many people have difficulty saying no to others. A role-play scene could be set up in which the person plays a character who will not give in—who can say no. In effect, he rehearses for a real-life situation, practicing in a role what he wishes to do in reality.

Drama therapy helps people get in touch with their feelings and understand how feelings affect their bodies. For example, when angry, the body can become a tightly coiled spring. Individuals may find it difficult to express anger without violence. Exploration of such emotions and practice in dealing with life situations in a drama therapy session can help a person learn to better handle powerful emotions in real life.

A drama therapy session is a safe place to try out new behaviors or deal with existing situations in a different way without the fear of real consequences. It offers the opportunity to discuss feelings in a judgment-free environment. Perhaps one of its greatest assets is to help clients learn to identify their feelings and verbalize them. Many people think they are the only ones who have a particular problem, but they soon learn that they are not alone. Through sharing and interaction, clients realize their problems are not so different from those of others.

Practice

Drama therapists use many different techniques, from full theater performances to simple sensory-awareness exercises, depending on the people with whom they are working. A sensory-awareness exercise may involve simply passing around an unusual piece of fabric and asking, "What does it remind you of?" On the other hand, a theater performance may stimulate the whole audience to become emotionally involved with a problem and to offer alternative solutions. Some theater groups involve the audience by asking members of the audience to come up and play the role the way they think it should be done. Therapists might use clients as the actors in a play, which teaches many levels of cooperation.

Role plays are enacted to give people experience in dealing with difficult situations. Frequently, when a patient is warmed up to an issue, she becomes fully involved in the role play and has the same feelings and reactions that occur in the real-life situation. Some comments heard after a good role play are: "Now I know how my mother feels!" or "I never thought of it that way before." The experience of being in someone else's shoes can be very insightful.

In group drama therapy most therapists structure their sessions similarly, beginning with a warm-up to help the clients feel comfortable and safe. When everyone is ready, the group begins the main activity, often organized as a role play. The last part of the session involves processing the activity through sharing and discussion; this final step is just as important, if not more important, than the main activity.

In the processing or sharing part of the session, the players talk about the feelings they had in their roles during the scene. If there is an audience, they are encouraged to express their feelings and responses also. Other possibilities for the scene are discussed. How else might the scene have ended, or what else could the person have said? Everyone is encouraged to make some contribution. The processing discussion is as important as the action because it helps people realize that there is always more than one solution to a problem.

Other types of group drama therapy include theater performances dealing with specific problem issues. These are most popular in community and school settings and usually address the kinds of life choices facing students today; for instance, drug and alcohol use, sexual conduct, violence, and problems with parents, teachers, and peers. Other groups present a production that offers information and/or education on a specific subject such as AIDS, drug abuse, illiteracy, or dealing with violence. Some performers stay in role to answer questions, and others offer workshops after the performance.

Since there are many techniques and variations of drama therapy, it is suitable for all age groups and populations. Most often it is practiced in groups and can be done in a variety of settings. Drama therapists work with every population that can benefit from any of the creative arts therapies: special education classes, psychiatric patients, people recovering from substance abuse, trauma victims, dysfunctional families, the developmentally and physically disabled, prison and correctional facility inmates, anorexic and bulimic patients, AIDS patients, the homeless, the elderly, and children and adolescents. These therapists provide services to individuals, groups, and families in addition to conducting clinical research.

With some groups the therapist is brought in to deal with a certain issue or offer training to deal with specific needs of the group. A therapist may be contracted to work with a group of managers dealing with sexual harassment. All the exercises, role plays, and explorations will deal with bringing about a greater understanding of and sensitivity to that subject.

When choosing a drama therapist, verify that the person is an RDT, a registered drama therapist. This is the only valid credential for drama therapists. RDTs are registered through NADT and have met rigorous standards that include the following: expertise in dramatic, theatrical, and performance media; an understanding of psychotherapeutic process with different populations in a variety of settings; integration of the artistic and psychological aspects of drama therapy; and professional expertise in the field of mental health and/or special education.

—*Patricia Sternberg, RDT/BCT*

Resources

NADT National Office
  15245 Shady Grove Road, Suite 130
  Rockville, MD 20850
  Tel: (301) 258-9210
  The national office keeps an updated list of all RDTs, all registered drama therapists/board-certified trainers (RDT/BCTs), and other members of the National Association for Drama Therapy. The RDT registry is available and may be requested from the national office as well as further information on the organization.

Further Reading

Bailey, Sally. *Wings to Fly: Bringing Theatre Arts to Students with Special Needs.* Rockville, Md.: Woodbine House, 1993.

Emunah, Renee. *Acting for Real: Drama Therapy Process, Technique, and Performance.* New York: Brunner/Mazel, 1994.

Gersie, Alida. *Dramatic Approaches to Brief Therapy.* London: Jessica Kingsley, 1995.

Grainger, Roger. *Drama and Healing: The Roots of Drama Therapy.* London: Jessica Kingsley, 1990.

Landy, Robert. *Drama Therapy: Concepts, Theories and Practices.* 2nd ed. Springfield, Ill.: Charles C. Thomas, 1994.

Salas, Jo. *Improvising Real Life: Personal Story in Playback Theatre.* Dubuque, Iowa: Kendall/Hunt, 1993.

Schatner, Gertrude, and Richard Courtney. *Drama Therapy.* Vols 1 and 2. New York: Drama Book Specialists, 1981.

One drama therapist explains her work with substance abuse groups: "I begin by saying that drama therapy is an exploration of our strengths. I work with the imagination, helping my patients learn how to use it as a problem-solving tool." She goes on to say, "Oftentimes patients who are invited to attend a drama therapy session will say, 'I'm no actor' or 'I don't know how to act.' My answer to that is, 'It's not acting. It's human behavior and everybody does that.'" After a session with this population, she hopes to hear what she considers the ultimate compliment about the benefits of drama therapy: "I never knew you could have so much fun without being high!"

Sternberg, Patricia, and Antonina Garcia. *Sociodrama: Who's in Your Shoes?* New York: Praeger Press, 1989.

Halprin Life/Art Process

 The Halprin life/art process is an integrative approach to movement, the expressive arts, and the therapeutic arts. It is used to evoke the creative development and expression of the whole person and to foster personal, interpersonal, and social transformation. The discipline is based on the belief that dance and the expressive arts, when connected with life concerns, can have a creative and healing role for an individual, the community, and the environment.

History

Dance pioneer Anna Halprin originated the Halprin life/art process in the 1950s at the San Francisco Dancer's Workshop Company, a collaborating collective of dancers, musicians, and visual artists. Halprin tried to develop a form of modern dance that could foster the organic and authentic expression of the body, and integrate the emotions and imagination of the dancer. Beginning in the 1960s, Halprin and her company worked with leaders in humanistic psychology, exploring relationships between art and therapy. Upon being diagnosed with cancer in 1972, Halprin devoted her research and teaching to the use of dance as a healing art, working with others who were challenging cancer, and later AIDS.

Daria Halprin, Anna Halprin's daughter, was an original member of the Dancer's Workshop Company. She developed applications of the Halprin life/art process as a therapeutic and educational model to advance personal transformation. In 1978 Anna and Daria Halprin founded the Tamalpa Institute to teach the Halprin life/art process in training programs, workshops, and classes, all of which incorporate the application of the expressive arts to psychology, education, and health.

Theory and Practice

The Halprin life/art process addresses three dimensions of human experience: physical, emotional, and mental. The physical is addressed through the study and practice of basic principles of somatic awareness, movement, and dance. The emotional is addressed through the study and practice of movement, drawing, and other therapeutic processes. The mental is addressed through the study and practice of group facilitation methods, collective creativity, communication skills, creative writing, and the presentation of theory. Each of these three aspects is studied and explored from the point of view of how it interrelates with all the other aspects.

In the Halprin life/art process, expressive art activities follow the model: move/draw/dialogue. This model evokes the physical, emotional, and mental aspects of the individual, often focusing on an identified life theme. For example, working with the theme balance/off balance, a class session might start with an exploration in movement of the physical experience of being in balance and off balance. The student or client would then draw two images inspired by the movement experience, which may be consciously or unconsciously connected with a life experience. The drawings are given titles that serve as a basis for a written piece: prose, poetry, or a dialogue between the two drawings. The theme balance/off balance is encountered a second time when the student creates an expressive movement piece, which is consciously connected with the drawings and written script.

According to this discipline, an integrated and healthy life includes and honors creative expression. The Halprin life/art process is interested in how we can live artfully in our world today, and how we can bring the transformative power of art into our daily personal and community lives. Practitioners apply their work as performance artists, teachers, and therapists. As leaders in community settings, they work with people and groups facing life-threatening issues, including cancer, AIDS, eating disorders, physical and sexual abuse, homelessness, addictions, and physical disabilities. Students have applied their work to environmental and cross-cultural issues.

—DARIA HALPRIN-KHALIGHI, M.A., CET

Resources

Tamalpa Institute
  P.O. Box 794
  Kentfield, CA 94914
  Tel: (415) 457-8555

Fax: (415) 457-7190
e-mail: tamalpa@igc.apc.org
Offers training programs, workshops, and
classes in the Halprin life/art process. Upon
completion of the practitioner training program, graduates are eligible to apply for certification as an expressive arts therapist
through the National Expressive Arts Association and as a movement therapist through
the International Somatic Movement and Education Therapy Association. The institute
publishes a yearly newsletter and distributes
articles and books representing the Halprin
life/art process.

Further Reading

Halprin, Anna. *Movement Ritual.* Illustrated by
    Charlene Koonce. Kentfield, Calif.: Dancer's
    Workshop/Tamalpa Institute, 1990.
————. *Moving Toward Life: Five Decades of Trans-
    formational Dance.* Hanover, N.H.: Wesleyan
    University Press, 1995.
Halprin, Daria. *Coming Alive: The Creative Expres-
    sion Method.* Kentfield, Calif.: Tamalpa Insti-
    tute, 1990.

Journal Therapy

 Journal therapy is the act of
writing down thoughts and feelings to sort through problems
and come to deeper understand-
ings of oneself or the issues in one's life. Unlike traditional diary writing, where daily
events and happenings are recorded from an
exterior point of view, journal therapy focuses on the writer's internal experiences,
reactions, and perceptions. Through this act
of literally reading her own mind, the writer
is able to perceive her own problems more
clearly and thus feel a relief of emotional and
mental tension that has also been shown to
improve the immune system functioning of
individuals.

History

Although people have written diaries and
journals for centuries, the therapeutic potential of reflective writing did not come into
public awareness until the 1960s, when Dr.
Ira Progoff, a psychologist in New York City,
began offering workshops and classes in the
use of what he called the intensive journal
method. Progoff had been using a "psychological notebook" with his clients for several
years. His intensive journal is a three-ring
notebook with many color-coded sections
for different aspects of the writer's psychological healing. The Progoff method of journal keeping quickly became popular, and
today the method has been taught to more
than 250,000 people through a network of
journal consultants trained by Progoff and
his staff.

In the late 1970s journal writing for personal growth and emotional wellness was
introduced to a wider audience through the
publication of three books. Progoff's *At a
Journal Workshop* (1978) detailed his intensive journal process and gave instructions
on how to set up an intensive journal for
those who could not attend a journal workshop in person. A young writer and teacher
named Christina Baldwin published her first
book, *One to One: Self-Understanding Through
Journal Writing* in 1977, based on the adult
education journal classes she had been
teaching. In 1978 Tristine Rainer published
The New Diary, a comprehensive guidebook
that for many years was the most complete
and accessible source of information on how
to use a journal for self-discovery and self-
exploration.

Philosophy

In the 1980s many public school systems
began formally using journals in both English classes and other curricula as well.
These journals, often called "dialogue" or
"response" journals, offered a way for students to develop independent thinking skills

and gave teachers a method for responding directly to students with individual feedback. Although the intention for classroom journals was educational rather than therapeutic, teachers noticed that a simple assignment to reflect on an academic question or problem often revealed important information about the student's emotional life. Students often reported feeling a relief of pressure and tension when they could write down troubling events or confusing thoughts or feelings.

Probably one of the most common reports from people who write journals is that the act of putting thoughts and feelings on paper helps give useful emotional and mental clarity. However, there is scientific evidence that the relief from writing things down is more than just psychological. Studies conducted by Dr. James Pennebaker, a researcher in Texas, show that when people write about emotionally difficult events or feelings for just twenty minutes at a time over three or four days, their immune system functioning increases. Pennebaker's work indicates that the release offered by writing has a direct impact on the body's capacity to withstand stress and fight off infection and disease.

After the publication of the Pennebaker studies, the medical and therapeutic communities began taking a closer look at journal writing as a holistic, nonmedicinal method for wellness. In 1985 Kathleen Adams, a psychotherapist in Colorado and the founder/director of the Center for Journal Therapy, began teaching journal workshops designed to provide the tools that could be used for self-discovery, creative expression, and life enhancement. Her "journal toolbox" of writing techniques offers a way to match a specific life issue with a specific writing device to address it. Adams's first book, *Journal to the Self: 22 Paths to Personal Growth*, was published in 1990. Through a network of certified instructors, the Journal to the Self workshop is available throughout the United States, Canada, and several other countries.

Practice

Although many psychotherapists incorporate journal therapy into their sessions by assigning written "homework," relatively few specialize in journal therapy. Those who utilize journal writing in a session often begin by asking the client to write a short "check-in" paragraph or two on "what's going on"—how the client is feeling, what he wants to work on in the session, and what's happening in his life that impacts the therapeutic work at hand. This writing is usually shared with the therapist and an "agenda" for the session is set. The therapist then guides the client through a writing exercise designed to address the therapeutic issues or tasks that the client has brought forward in the check-in or warm-up writing or exercise. The second writing usually takes about ten minutes, and the remainder of the session is spent with the client and therapist talking about the information revealed in the longer writing. The session generally concludes with the therapist offering several suggestions for journal homework to be completed between sessions.

Journal therapy is also effective in groups, and it is common for group members to establish a sense of deep community as writings representing authentic expressions of self are shared.

At present there is one graduate educational program in poetry therapy, at Vermont College of Norwich. This program teaches techniques in journal therapy. Journal therapists first obtain an advanced degree in psychology, counseling, social work, or a related field. They may then enter a credentialing program such as that offered by the National Association for Poetry Therapy, or an independent-study program such as that offered through Adams's Center for Journal Therapy or through Progoff's Dialogue House.

Benefits

It is believed that by recording and describing the salient issues in one's life, one can better understand these issues and eventually diagnose problems that stem from them. Journal therapy has been used effectively for grief and loss; coping with life-threatening or chronic illness; recovery from addictions, eating disorders, and trauma; repairing troubled marriages and family relationships; increasing communication skills; developing a healthier sense of self-identity; getting a better perspective on life; and clarifying life goals.

—*KATHLEEN ADAMS, M.A., LPC*

Resources

The Center for Journal Therapy
P. O. Box 963
Arvada, CO 80001
Tel: (303) 421-2298
Organization dedicated to the instruction and practice of journal therapy.

The Dialogue House
80 E. 11th St.
New York, NY 10009
Tel: (212) 673-5880
Fax: (212) 673-0582
Provides several intensive workshops that utilize the journal therapy method.

The National Association for Poetry Therapy
5505 Connecticut Ave. NW #280
Washington, DC 20015
Tel: (202) 966-2536
Web site: www.poetrytherapy.org.
Multidisciplinary professional organization for students and practitioners of journal therapy.

Further Reading

Adams, Kathleen. *Journal to the Self: 22 Paths to Personal Growth.* New York: Warner Books, 1990.

———. *The Way of the Journal: A Journal Therapy Workbook for Healing.* Lutherville, Md.: Sidran Press, 1993.

———. *Mightier than the Sword: The Journal as a Path to Men's Self-Discovery.* New York: Warner Books, 1994.

Baldwin, Christina. *One to One: Self-Understanding Through Journal Writing.* New York: Evans & Co., 1977.

———. *Life's Companion: Journal Writing as Spiritual Quest.* New York: Bantam Books, 1990.

Oshinsky, James. *The Discovery Journal.* 2nd ed. Odessa, Md.: Psychological Assessment Resources, 1994.

Progoff, Ira. *At a Journal Workshop.* New York: Dialogue House, 1978.

Rainer, Tristine. *The New Diary.* Los Angeles: J. P. Tarcher, 1978.

Multimodal Expressive Arts Therapy

Multimodal expressive arts therapy integrates various forms of arts into a therapeutic relationship to foster awareness, encourage emotional growth, and enhance relationships with others. It promotes healing through the transformative power of both the arts and psychotherapy. By activating the imagination, this therapy enables self-exploration and self-understanding; by working within more than one medium, it amplifies and clarifies self-discoveries; and by expressing these discoveries through images, sound, movement, and words, it expands communication.

History

The arts have been brought together to shape and express human experience since the dawn of civilization. Paleolithic cave paintings indicate that early humans used art as a means for passing spiritual, social, and hunting skills from generation to generation. In ancient Greece, dramas incorporating music, dance, and storytelling brought crowds to amphitheaters for a collective experience of the tragic and comedic dimensions of life. Intricate hierarchies of religious and sociopolitical belief were woven into the art and architecture of medieval Europe. Today many forms of theater, dance, performance art, and multimedia installation art are used in concert to bring people together to participate in cathartic release from life's sorrows and gain a better understanding of individual and communal identity.

While multimodal expressive arts therapy draws on this entire body of the arts, it is a development of the last half century. After World War II, American veterans' hospitals integrated music, dance, and drama into an alternative method of treatment for veterans struggling to recuperate from the ordeal of battle. In Europe during the 1950s, innovative educators formulated an approach that engaged children in multiple art forms, which they believed would help foster full sensory development. Then, in the 1960s, versatile European and American performance artists began combining various forms of art to convey their messages and touch their audiences.

Changes in education, the fine arts, and medical treatment of trauma opened the way for the gradual emergence of therapy programs that take a holistic approach to both art and healing. By 1969 there was a graduate training program in expressive arts therapy at the University of Kentucky in Louisville. A decade later expressive arts therapy had become a widely recognized mode of treatment for children and adults with special needs. It had its own professional organization, the American Association of Artist-Therapists (later called the National Expressive Therapy Association), and an emergent nascent scholarly literature.

Theory

In a 1978 doctoral dissertation, *Intermodal Learning in Education and Therapy,* Paolo Knill postulated that multimodal expressive arts therapy is not simply a loose gathering of the arts under the umbrella of therapy, but rather a highly sophisticated way of bringing the imagination into the work of healing. Unlike exclusively verbal therapies, it centers on the embodiment and transformation of emotions. They are expressed in one medium, then translated into others. As one is led through a series of creative arts experiences, the imagination grows more active, and at the same time emotions are explored, clarified, and transformed, helping people to connect with themselves, with others, and with a greater sense of purpose and meaning in life.

Practice

Multimodal expressive arts therapy is generally experienced as a type of group therapy in a school, nursing home, or other institutional setting. The length and structure of sessions will vary based on the specific method of the therapist and the needs of the group or individual participant. Children may have a half-hour session, adult outpatients' sessions may last over an hour, and intensive workshops may go on for several days. The range of structure is no less broad, from sessions with a predetermined format and topic to sessions that encourage spontaneous engagement with the arts and dynamic interaction among participants.

Activity in all but the most loosely structured sessions is usually divided into three phases. A short warm-up that helps participants overcome inhibitions and tap into their imaginations is followed by a longer phase devoted to a series of art activities designed to uncover, explore, and transform the participants' feelings. In the final phase, participants reflect on the sounds, movements, images, or words they have created, as well as the process of forming them.

A session might begin by having participants stand in a circle and take turns making a movement that expresses their immediate feelings. Next, they might use oil crayons, pastels, or a felt-tipped pen first to transfer that movement onto a large piece of drawing paper, then to elaborate the graphic mark into a picture. Other transformations will probably follow. The therapist might suggest that the participants look at one another's pictures and leave a written response on a nearby piece of paper. Each participant then uses the words and phrases to compose a poem that he recites to the group. The sequential unfolding of expression, from physical gesture to recited poem, becomes the basis for a concluding discussion that might consider the interplay of emotion, bodily movement, and verbal expression or the insights gained through group interaction. Advanced art-making skills and expensive equipment are not needed to take part in multimodal expressive arts therapy.

Benefits

By engaging the imagination, multimodal expressive arts therapy promotes the creative release of emotions and stimulates the development of self-esteem and a capacity for self-healing. Since it integrates many aspects of personal growth from the sensory to the emotional to the social, multimodal expressive arts therapy is often used by individuals who are coping with physical or mental disabilities, as well as the effects of aging, loss, and isolation.

—SUSAN SPANIOL, ED.D., ATR; PHILIP SPEISER, PH.D., CET; AND MARIAGNESE CATTANEO, PH.D., ATR

Resources

European Foundation for Interdisciplinary Studies
Forchstrasse, 106
CH 8032 Zurich
Switzerland
Fax: 382-33-07
An international professional organization for expressive therapists.

Expressive Arts Program
California Institute of Integral Studies
9 Peter Yorke Way
San Francisco, CA 94109
Tel: (415) 674-5500
Offers a master's degree in counseling psychology with a specialization in expressive arts therapy.

Expressive Therapies Program
Lesley College
29 Everett St.
Cambridge, MA 02138
Tel: (617) 349-8425
Offers a comprehensive graduate program in multimodal expressive arts therapy.

International Expressive Arts Therapy Association
P.O. Box 64126
San Francisco, CA 94164
Tel: (415) 522-8959
A professional organization dedicated to multimodal expressive arts therapy.

International School for Interdisciplinary Studies
Forchstrasse, 106
CH 8032 Zurich
Switzerland
Fax: 382-33-09
A training institute in multimodal expressive arts therapy.

Further Reading

Books

Knill, P. J., H. N. Barba, and M. N. Fuchs. *Minstrels of Soul: Intermodal Expressive Therapy.* Toronto: Palmerston Press, 1993.

Levine, S. K. *Poiesis: The Language of Psychology and the Speech of the Soul.* Toronto: Palmerston Press, 1992.

Rogers, N. *The Creative Connection: Expressive Arts as Healing.* Palo Alto, Calif.: Science & Behavior Books, 1993.

Journals

Lusebrink, V. "A Systems-Oriented Approach to the Expressive Therapies: The Expressive Therapies Continuum." *The Arts in Psychotherapy* 5 (1991): 395–403.

Music Therapy

 Music therapy is a profession that believes in the therapeutic potential inherent in music. Qualified music therapists use music and/or musical elements such as sound, rhythm, melody, and harmony with individuals or groups to help people improve, change, or better integrate different aspects of their selves. Listening to, moving to, and creating music are used to help resolve emotional, social, familial, cognitive, physiological, and developmental problems. While recognition of the therapeutic powers of music is ancient and widespread, it formally became a type of therapy in the 1950s.

The Basic Elements of Music

The fundamental elements of music—sound, rhythm, hearing, and movement—and people's prenatal and primary experience with these elements are paramount to music therapists. They consider music's basic elements essential in the development of human beings and deeply rooted in the very beginning of a human life. Research shows that the human fetus can hear after four months in the womb. A developing fetus hears voices, noises, and the sounds of its own and its mother's heartbeats and digestive systems. After birth, a baby continues experiencing rhythm and beat in the sound of its mother's heartbeat and breathing, and in its mother's rocking motions. In fact, music therapists view a baby's very first sign of life, crying, as a combination of the primary elements of music—rhythm, movement, and sound—in the service of self-expression and communication with other people.

Music's Therapeutic Nature

One can find references to the therapeutic powers of music in philosophy, art, and literature throughout the ages. In the Bible, young David, known for his musical talents, is brought to play the lyre before King Saul in the hope that this would alleviate the king's ill humor. Greek mythology ascribed a divine origin to music. In the mythological world, music had magical powers; people believed it could heal sickness and purify the body and the mind. Among the Greeks, music was thought to be an activity related to the pursuit of truth and beauty.

The therapeutic power of music plays an important role in the healing ceremonies of early cultures throughout the world. Healers and shamans use chants, incantations, rhythmic playing of drums and rattles, clapping, and stomping to induce hypnotic or ecstatic states. When in this altered state of consciousness they communicate with the spirit world, which helps them exorcise bad spirits, cure illnesses, and soothe and relax patients.

Everyday experience also points to the psychological effect that music can have on us. Most would agree that even given varying musical tastes, certain types of music create specific moods. A wedding march creates a different mood than does a funeral dirge. Scary movies use ominous music to create suspense. Bands play lively music at sporting events to excite the crowd. A doctor may play quiet, easy-listening or classical music in his waiting room to help soothe patients. Mothers sing to and rock their babies in times of distress.

History

Music therapy was established as a profession in the United States in the 1950s. Professionals from various disciplines, such as music, education, medicine, and psychology, had been using music while working with various populations. Through their clinical experience, they found that music yielded remarkable therapeutic results. Individuals suffering from severe impairments, be they sensory, motor, mental, or emotional, seemed to show startling improvement when working with music. By 1950 the National Association for Music Therapy (NAMT) was created, and training programs for music therapists were initiated in several colleges and universities. Around this time, methodical research expanded, as well as the formulation of theories, clinical models, and professional publications. In 1998 the American Association for Music Therapy and NAMT merged into one association, the American Music Therapy Association.

Today music therapy is practiced worldwide. An extremely varied and flexible profession, it is found within such disciplines as special education, rehabilitation, psychiatry, psychotherapy, and geriatrics. It is practiced in hospitals, clinics, rehabilitation centers, schools, and private settings.

Basic Principles

All models of music therapy encourage an individual to find and express his or her uniqueness through music. Because it fo-

cuses on the process of self-discovery and not on the end product, one need not have any musical skills or talent in order to utilize or benefit from music therapy. The music that is produced is not judged as good or bad.

The therapeutic agents of music therapy are dual: on one hand there is music, and on the other, the relationship between client and therapist. Because music is deeply rooted in the early physio-psychological development of an individual, making music touches on the unconscious in a direct, unmediated way. This enables individuals to connect themselves directly to repressed material and forgotten or masked memories, or to enter into regressive emotional states, which allow further exploration of issues central to the self.

In order for music activity to be therapeutic, it must take place within the framework of a reliable relationship with a therapist, a relationship characterized by trust, respect, and a serious commitment to the process. As this relationship becomes more meaningful, so does the musical activity that takes place within its framework.

Practice

Music therapists use varied techniques and models for their work, which they adapt to their clients' needs and ages as well as the setting of each session (individual versus group, for example). Nevertheless, all types of music therapy search for the individuality of the client as expressed through music. This search is carried out with active help and support from the therapist.

Many clinical models in music therapy use instrumental or vocal improvisation. Because of its spontaneous and expressive qualities, musical improvisation is a particularly potent method of shedding light on aspects of the self that are many times obscured or blocked by one's conscious thinking or behavior. Music therapists are trained to understand improvised music as a unique personal language. In music therapy, both client and therapist set out to explore and reveal the form and meaning of this special language.

For an adult client with emotional problems, a session might begin with a verbal discussion of a current issue. Then, client and therapist find a way to investigate issues through sound in various ways. One might choose to play an instrument, sing, or write words to a song. This musical experience occurs in the here and now but later becomes material for discussion and the development of improved self-understanding.

Another type of music therapy uses recorded music as a stimulus for exploring the self. Clients are introduced to a state of relaxation through breathing and suggestive imagery. Music carefully selected by the therapist is played, and the client is invited to explore images, sensations, memories, and visions prompted by the music. Sometimes the client achieves an altered state of consciousness, which is usually extremely positive and relaxing and can lead to self-discovery. After the listening experience, the client is brought out of the relaxed state and is invited to discuss the experience with the therapist. In some models the client is invited to choose preferred selections and listen, move, or paint to that music.

Music is also used in family and group therapy. Special techniques have been developed to utilize music's inherent social character. One outstanding feature of the art of music is the possibility to produce and perceive several sounds simultaneously as with orchestras, ensembles, and choirs. Although something of this sort takes place in all of the performing arts, its effect is most dramatic in music. Members of a family in therapy may be asked to choose a musical instrument and then improvise a performance. The "music of the family" proves to be enormously indicative in showing who is "in harmony" with whom in the family, who gets the role of making "disturbing noises" or "clashing sounds," who picks a very loud instrument that prevents everybody else from being

heard, or who gives up playing her favorite instrument because someone else demanded it. Group or family musical improvisations often reveal hidden agendas, tensions and dilemmas, self-defeating communication patterns, and other problems. These problems are sometimes easier to perceive, express, and deal with when manifested in music.

Benefits

Music therapy is suitable for individuals of all ages, even young babies. It is used to help autistic children acquire communication skills; to improve the skills of individuals with learning disabilities; and to help people deal with emotional, social, and familial problems. Music therapy is utilized in individual, family, and group settings, as well as with couples. Recipients include individuals recovering from cerebrovascular accidents and major surgery.

—ADVA FRANK-SCHWEBEL

Resources

American Music Therapy Association, Inc.
   8455 Colevill Road, Suite 1000
   Silver Spring, MD 20910
   Tel: (301) 589-3300
   Fax: (301) 589-5175
   e-mail: info@musictherapy.org
   Web site: www.musictherapy.org
   Association of professional music therapists that provides registered music therapist (RMT) credentials. It also publishes the *Journal of Music Therapy* and holds conferences.

Further Reading

Books
Bonny, H., and L. Savary. *Music and Your Mind: Listening with a New Consciousness.* New York: Harper and Row, 1973.

Bruscia, K. E. *Improvisational Models of Music Therapy.* Springfield, Ill.: Charles C Thomas, 1987.

Feder, S., R. L. Karmel, and G. H. Pollock, eds. *Psychoanalytic Exploration in Music.* Madison, Conn.: International Universities Press, 1990.

Maranto, Cheryl Dielo, ed. *Perspectives on Music Therapy Education and Training.* Philadelphia, Pa.: Temple University, 1987.

Nordoff, Paul, and Clive Robbins. *Creative Music Therapy.* New York: John Day Co., 1977.

Priestley, Mary. *Music Therapy in Action.* St. Louis, Mo.: MMB Music, 1985.

Sekeles, Chava. *Music, Motion, and Emotion: The Developmental-Integrative Model in Music Therapy.* St. Louis, Mo.: MMB Music, 1996.

Verney, T., and G. Kelly. *The Secret Life of the Unborn Child.* London: Sphere Books, 1981.

Journals

Noy, P. "The Psychodynamic Meaning of Music– Part II." *Journal of Music Therapy,* 4 (1): 7–23.

Poetry Therapy

 Poetry therapy involves reading, writing, reciting, and/or creating poetry as well as other language arts to cope with emotions related to psychological, physical, and social problems. Poetry therapy uses the imaginative and emotional qualities of all types of literature and is therefore not limited to the specific genre of poetry— metaphor, poetry reading, journal writing, song lyrics, storytelling, and prose writing may be used. It should be noted that bibliotherapy, the use of reading to help individuals, has an extensive history and is now considered a part of poetry therapy. For all practical purposes, the terms are now synonymous. Many social workers, psychologists, nurses, physicians, counselors, and special education teachers use poetry therapy in their work. Other professionals have received advanced training in poetry therapy methods and developed it as their primary method of practice.

History

The notion of poetry as therapeutic has ancient roots. For ages poetry has been a method through which people have pondered the human condition and expressed their sorrows, joys, and epiphanies. The ancient Greeks made Apollo the god of both poetry and healing. In the early eighteenth century psychiatrists started using the various expressive arts in order to soothe patients' anguish and as a medium to encourage dialogue and social interaction. The general population has also used poetry and literature as a form of catharsis. One might be cheered by a limerick or comforted by an eloquent expression of grief that a person feels speaks to her own emotions. Robert Haven Schauffler wrote a prescriptive book called *The Poetry Cure: A Pocket Medicine Chest of Verse,* published in 1925. The book contains numerous poems categorized for use with specific life problems.

The formal development of poetry therapy as a discipline begins with Jack J. Leedy, a psychiatrist, who in 1969 founded the Association for Poetry Therapy (APT) in New York. In 1973 Arthur Lerner, a psychologist and poet, founded the Poetry Therapy Institute in California. APT became formally incorporated in 1981 as the National Association for Poetry Therapy (NAPT). NAPT sponsors annual conventions and has helped set standards and procedures for certification and registration of poetry therapists.

Theory

Language and feelings are central to both poetry and therapy. Similar to other arts therapies such as music and dance, poetry therapy concerns itself with symbolism, verbal and nonverbal expression, rhythm, order, and balance. Psychotherapy, for example, often addresses an individual's interpretation of certain past events or fears about the present and future. Poetry has the capacity to capture similar human experiences through symbols and images. Also, the rhythm of certain poems can affect the reader's mood. Some poems might be used for a calming effect, while others might be used to energize clients.

Poetry therapy provides a vehicle for individuals to express what might be difficult to express under ordinary circumstances. By talking about a poem, one can relate personal material. Often an emotional identification can be made with a poem that reflects a person's thoughts or feelings on a particular matter. A poem can also help a person to feel that he is not alone. Writing a poem (or letter, story, or journal entry) can be empowering by providing a sense of order and control to an individual. The act of writing integrates one's thinking, feeling, and behaving. The sharing of reactions to poetry or the sharing of one's own work also has the potential to build interpersonal relationships and communication skills.

Practice

A variety of techniques can be used depending on the professional's education and training. A social worker might use a poem to validate a feeling or promote insight with a depressed individual in a therapy session. In this situation the poetry is part of the therapy. A poet might start a writing program in a runaway shelter. In this case, the purpose might be educational or life enriching rather than therapeutic; however, the therapeutic aspects of writing are recognized. Following are a number of ways in which poetry is used to help people.

- *Introduce an existing poem to an individual, group, or family and invite reactions.* The theme of the poem should relate to the issues of the individual or group. If a person is having a hard time making an important decision, then a poem such as Robert Frost's "The Road Not Taken" could be connected to the struggle of the individual. A discussion of possible "roads" that the person might take could follow.
- *Collaborative poems.* Sometimes communication breaks down in families and conflicts develop. Each member of a family is invited to contribute one or more lines to a family or group poem, thereby valuing each person's view. The task also allows the family to engage in problem solving (constructing the poem) and working together rather than pointing blame at one another.
- *Creative writing.* The writing could be free writing—that is, covering any topic and using any form—or it could consist of structured exercises. For example, an acrostic—where each line of a poem begins with a letter from a particular word, or the use of sentence stems like "If you knew me . . ."—could provide a structure to facilitate self-expression.
- *Journal writing.* Keeping a journal provides another outlet for an individual to express and sort out a variety of thoughts and feelings.
- *Letter writing.* Sometimes it is difficult or impossible to say things to important people in our lives. Writing a letter to a deceased friend or family member can be helpful in working through grief, anger, and frustration. It could also serve as a positive memorial to a loved one.
- *Recommending specific readings for a particular problem.* In the tradition of bibliotherapy, certain fiction and nonfiction could be used for life guidance. Judith Viorst's *The Tenth Good Thing About Barney* might be a good story to read to a child whose pet died.

Poetry Therapy

PROBLEM	POEM
Decision making	"The Road Not Taken" by Robert Frost
Anxiety	"If I Should Cast . . ." by Stephen Crane
Stress	"Can't Do It All" by Natasha Josefowitz
Family	"Nikki Rosa" by Nikki Giovanni
Grief	"Good Night, Willie Lee . . ." by Alice Walker
Anger	"A Just Anger" by Marge Piercy
Despair	"Hope Is a Thing with Feathers" by Emily Dickinson
Alienation	"Alone/December Night" by Victor Cruz
Communication	"Two Friends" by David Ignatow
Identity	"I'm Nobody" by Emily Dickinson

Limitations

Like any therapeutic tool, anything that has the power to heal also has the power to harm. Poetry therapy should be used by professionals with training in psychology and a good understanding of literature. The individual using it must stay within the boundaries of her profession. Care must be given to the selection and timing of a poem. Sharing a poem or song may bring up feelings one is not ready to deal with at the time. If a particular poem or song is not fully discussed, a destructive or unhealthy conclusion could be reached. Therapists should be sure to choose works that while empathizing with the client's problem, ultimately express hope. The therapist should also know the problems and limitations of the clients. The use of poetry may be insulting, especially if there is a literacy problem and the person is asked to read. Sometimes a poem may serve as a distraction for a client. A person might spend a great deal of time intellectualizing rather than dealing with a pressing problem. If a person focuses on journal writing at the exclusion of interpersonal relationships, his fear and isolation could increase, or conclusions could be reached without the benefit of healthy discussion.

Benefits

Poetry therapy can serve as a nonthreatening means for people to express their thoughts, feelings, and behaviors. It is respectful of different cultures and genders by trying to understand the personalized meanings of each person's language and story. Increasingly, research is indicating that writing has a healing effect and can help people gain emotional strength. It has also been shown that in group counseling, the use of poetry therapy increases cohesion.

Across the United States and around the world, poetry therapy is used in a variety of settings, including hospitals, hospice facilities, correctional institutions, homeless shelters, schools, runaway shelters, and mental health centers. In a time of pervasive social problems and rapidly increasing technology, this therapy touches and affirms our humanity.

—NICHOLAS MAZZA, PH.D.

Resources

Journal of Poetry Therapy
   Human Sciences Press
   233 Spring St.
   New York, NY 10013-1578
   The official quarterly journal of the National Association for Poetry Therapy. It offers a wide variety of original articles, brief reports, dissertation abstracts, and poetry.

National Association for Poetry Therapy
   5505 Connecticut Ave. NW # 280
   Washington, DC 20015
   Tel: (202) 966-2536
   An organization open to all persons interested in the healing capacities of the language arts. There are various levels of membership, including professional, regular, student, and retired. NAPT confers professional credentials—certified poetry therapist (CPT) and registered poetry therapist (RPT). It maintains a registry of practitioners and information regarding training.

Further Reading

Hynes, Arleen McCarty, and Mary Hynes-Berry. *Biblio/Poetry Therapy—The Interactive Process: A Handbook.* St. Cloud, Minn.: North Star Press of St. Cloud, Inc., 1994.

Leedy, Jack J., ed. *Poetry as Healer: Mending the Troubled Mind.* New York: Vanguard Press, 1985. [Note: This book is a combination of two previous classics edited by Leedy, *Poetry Therapy* (1969) and *Poetry the Healer* (1973).]

Lerner, Arthur, ed. *Poetry in the Therapeutic Experience.* St. Louis, Mo.: MMB Music, Inc., 1994.

Lerner, Arthur, and Ursula Mahlendorf, eds. *Life Guidance Through Literature.* Chicago: American Library Association, 1992.

Web Sites

Internet Poetry Archive Home Page
   www.sunsite.unc.edu/dykki/poetry/home.html

National Association for Poetry Therapy
   www.poetrytherapy.org

National Coalition of Arts Therapies Associations
   www.membrane.com/ncata

Sandplay Therapy

 Sandplay therapy is a form of psychological treatment that centers on play with a vast collection of miniature figures and two sandboxes, one that contains damp sand, the other one dry. Unlike verbal therapies that deal directly with inner memories, sandplay involves the construction of scenes in which self-expression can be indirect and nonverbal. This therapeutic approach is considered particularly appropriate for children because it provides a safe way to act out troubling feelings that may be at the root of behavioral problems. Furthermore, the scenes themselves are thought to be a sensitive approach to determine the way mind and body come together in the totality of personal development. Sandplay therapy's most widely used theoretical model makes use of symbols and archetypes derived from the theories propounded by Swiss psychotherapist Carl Jung. Though children are the usual clients of sandplay therapy, it is also used effectively with adults on their spiritual path to individuation.

History

Sandplay therapy began with the research of Margaret Lowenfeld, a child psychiatrist active in England during the 1920s and 1930s—decades when the role of objects in child development attracted general interest among analysts who were working with children. The particular focus of Lowenfeld's work was the inner drama revealed in a child's use of his toys. The world technique, devised by Lowenfeld, transposed such play into structures that lent themselves to observation and analysis, yet did not force the child to adapt to adult logic. Lowenfeld asked the child to make pictures in the sandbox using the available miniatures. She found that a child would fashion intricate scenes that Lowenfeld regarded as representations of the child's world. Interpreting the pictures was difficult, in large part because of the ever-present danger of imposing adult norms on childhood experiences. Nonetheless, she believed that the world technique offered a means of gaining privileged access to the world of the child for both diagnostic and therapeutic purposes.

Dora Kalff, a Swiss therapist, brought Lowenfeld's work into the second half of the twentieth century, and she never doubted the healing powers of this technique. Kalff's training at the Jung Institute in Zurich led her to view the miniatures as a counterpart to Jungian archetypes. Influenced by German Jungian analyst Erich Neumann's studies of child development; she was able to correlate her observations of sandplay constructions with Neumann's theories. According to Kalff, the healing powers of sandplay therapy, as she termed her variant of world technique, are explained by its capacity to help traumatized children in their struggle toward internal ego support and full autonomy.

Philosophy

An understanding of Jungian archetypes and the archetypal level of the psyche is what differentiates this approach to sandplay from other theories. Jung's structure of the psyche proposes that the psyche is made up of three levels: the conscious, the personal unconscious, and the collective unconscious, wherein the archetypes are found. An archetype is simply a model or prototype of

an idea, such as the "Great Mother," the "Wise Old Man," the "Hero," the "Anima/ Animus," or the "Ego/Self." Archetypes are two-sided, having both positive and negative aspects. They are believed to be in the psyches of all people in all cultures. Knowledge of the archetypes allows the analyst to transmit her understanding of the client's struggle, most often nonverbally, in the interactive field. For instance, the analyst is aware that a child's mother has died. It is to be assumed that the child in therapy will seek to connect with the lost mother in some way. If the analyst is aware of the archetypal level of the psyche, she will be able to observe, for example, when the Great Mother archetype (in both her positive and negative forms) emerges. This can enhance the analyst's unspoken understanding of this child's struggle and deepen the connection between child and therapist.

As taught by Kalff, sandplay therapy is based on the belief that symbols and myth constitute a world history of, and psychological "guidebook" to, the ways by which human beings come to an understanding of themselves and their culture. By providing ready access to this system of representation, sandplay therapy enables clients to explore and expand their awareness of the dominant issues in their lives. The Kalffian/Jungian therapist approaches the child as a unique, complex being with an innate capacity for symbolic logic as revealed through an archetypal struggle witnessed in sandplay.

Practice

Sandplay therapy employs sandboxes that are shallow, rectangular, and of a size (20 x 28 x 4 inches) that permits rapid, easy assembly of a picture. Two boxes—one with dry sand, the other with wet sand—are made available. The small size of the sandbox gives the client a sense of security and, at the same time, forces him to make choices, since it can accommodate only a portion of the miniatures displayed on shelves around

Despite Dora Kalff's book *Sandplay* and many lectures, training in sandplay therapy has never been widely available. While some advocates remain committed to the Kalff-Jung legacy and offer a pure form of sandplay, a growing number of analysts and educators approach it on a pragmatic basis as a natural form of healing with strong affinities to art and play therapy.

the sandplay room. After suggesting that the client make a picture, the therapist becomes more or less a silent observer, having been taught to withhold interpretations until the therapy has progressed to the point where the ego is solid enough to accept interpretations. Premature interpretations usually impact the therapy quite negatively. In this technique there is strong emphasis on the nonverbal ability of the psyche to seek its own healing, given the proper milieu.

Benefits and Risks

While sandplay therapy poses no unusual risks to clients, it does require the help of a skilled analyst if the full range of benefits is to be attained. One cautionary note: If there is any overt resistance to using sandplay, it is never pushed because the resistance may be serving a protective psychic function and must always be honored.

—LOIS CAREY

Resources

Association for Play Therapy
California School of Professional Psychology
1350 M St.
Fresno, CA 93721
Holds conferences that include presentations on recent work with sandplay therapy.

Center for Sandplay Studies
252 South Blvd.
Upper Grandview, NY 10960
Tel: (914) 358-2318
Offers beginning and advanced courses in sandplay therapy.

Sandplay Therapists of America
P.O. Box 4847
Walnut Creek, CA 94596
Tel: (310) 607-8535
Organization that holds conferences and publishes a journal on sandplay therapy.

Further Reading

Books

Carey, Lois. *Sandplay with Children and Families.* Northvale, N.J.: Jason Aronson, Inc., 1998.

Friedman, Harriet, and R. Mitchell. *Sandplay: Past, Present, and Future.* London: Routledge, 1994.

Jung, C. G. *The Archetypes and the Collective Unconscious.* Princeton, N.J.: Bollingen Paperback, 1980.

Kalff, Dora. *Sandplay: A Psychotherapeutic Approach to the Psyche.* Santa Monica, Calif.: Sigo Press, 1980.

Lowenfeld, Margaret. *The World Technique.* London: George Allen and Unwin Ltd., 1979.

Neumann, Erich. *The Child.* Boston: Shambhala, 1990.

Stevens, Anthony. *Archetypes.* New York: Quill, 1982.

Wilmer, Harry. *Practical Jung.* Wilmette, Ill.: Chiron, 1991.

Journals

Carey, Lois. "Sandplay Therapy with a Troubled Child." *Arts in Psychotherapy* 17, no. 3 (1990): 197–209.

———. "Family Sandplay Therapy." *Arts in Psychotherapy* 18 (1991): 231–39.

———. "A Child-Centered Approach to Family Sandplay Therapy." *Quaternio: Journal of the Brazilian Society of Jungian Psychotherapy* 1, no. 3 (1992): 6–11.

Part 16:

Body-Oriented Psychotherapies

Body-oriented psychotherapies are healing modalities that use the body to help solve emotional problems. The term *body-oriented psychotherapy* traditionally refers only to methods in which physical body postures or types and physical behavior patterns are used to diagnose and treat emotional disorders. This book expands that definition to include many other methods that rely on a variety of physical activities to affect mental and emotional health. Although some people mistrust these unusual methods, others credit a body-oriented psychotherapy as the only way they were able to change painful, limiting mental and emotional patterns and begin living a healthy and fulfilling life.

The Development of Body-Oriented Psychotherapy

Most body-oriented psychotherapies can trace their origins to the groundbreaking work of the Austrian neurologist and founder of psychoanalysis, Sigmund Freud (1856–1939). Through his work as a neurologist, Freud became aware that many of his neurotic patients' symptoms, including paralysis, headaches, fainting spells, and heart palpitations, were caused by something other than the physical working of their muscles, bones, and nerves. Working in tandem with his friend the physiologist Josef Breuer, Freud discovered that releasing repressed memories of childhood experiences or emotional conflicts while in a hypnotic trance alleviated his patients' physical symptoms. By combining clinical experience with deep insight into the nature of human behavior, Freud created a new model of the human mind that changed Western medical discourse forever.

Contrary to the popular belief that human beings are totally rational creatures, always aware of the causes of their actions, Freud saw the human mind as two parts: the conscious mind, which controls aspects of memory, speech, and logical thinking; and the

BIOENERGETICS

BODYNAMIC ANALYSIS

CORE ENERGETICS

CORESOMATICS®

EMOTIONAL-KINESTHETIC PSYCHOTHERAPY

FOCUSING

GESTALT THERAPY

HAKOMI INTEGRATIVE SOMATICS

HOLOTROPIC BREATHWORK™

MEDICAL ORGONE THERAPY

ORGANISMIC BODY PSYCHOTHERAPY

PESSO BOYDEN SYSTEM PSYCHOMOTOR

PROCESS-ORIENTED PSYCHOLOGY

PSYCHODRAMA

PSYCHOSYNTHESIS

RADIX

REBIRTHING

RUBENFELD SYNERGY METHOD™

UNERGI

unconscious mind, which contains the somatic reflexes such as breathing and heart rate, basic biological drives, dream imagery, and many other memories. Freud believed that when a memory or conflict was too painful for an individual to hold in his conscious mind, it would be repressed by a variety of defense mechanisms into the unconscious mind, where it would affect the physical body and many aspects of behavior. Freud believed that many of these anxiety-producing conflicts were inherent to the human condition, especially in Victorian Europe, where one's basic biological drives contradicted the demands of civilized society.

Freud developed techniques to bring repressed memories to consciousness without the aid of hypnosis. This became the basis of psychoanalysis, a particular approach to psychotherapy consisting of many scheduled verbal encounters between a therapist and patient over a long period of time. The therapist guides the patient in dredging up and sorting through the repressed memories, emotions, impulses, or desires.

Although Freud's theories and practices were controversial, he drew many of the brightest doctors in Europe into his circle. However, as Freud became increasingly inflexible in his methods and his theories about human nature increasingly pessimistic, many of his students eventually moved on. Among them was the Austrian Wilhelm Reich (1897–1957), who was the most influential in developing a body orientation to psychotherapy. Reich broke with Freud by asserting the primacy of the body and biological processes in the cause and treatment of physical and emotional symptoms. In his book *The Function of the Orgasm* (1942) Reich presented the idea that a psycho-physical energy exists that, if not released through sexual orgasm, becomes locked in muscular tensions in the body. From this basic premise he developed an entire model of human psychology in which conflicts were stored not only in the subconscious mind but also in the physical body as a complex of muscular tensions he called "muscular armoring" and a complex of behavior patterns he called "character armoring." Reich's model of treatment, known today as medical orgonomy, uses hands-on manipulation of the body and breathing patterns to release the chronically tight muscles and repressed energy. It became the basis of many forms of body-oriented psychotherapies, including bioenergetics, core energetics, hakomi integrative somatics, organismic body psychotherapy, and Radix.

Both Carl Jung (1875–1961) of Switzerland and Roberto Assagioli (1888–1974) of Italy broke with Freud because they believed he placed too much emphasis on the sexual drive in interpreting human behavior. The two approaches to psychotherapy they developed—analytical psychology and psychosynthesis, respectively—extended the range of Freud's model of human personality to include spiritual drives and goals. They introduced the West to the connection between spirituality and psychology, a connection that had dominated non-Western art, religion, and health practices for centuries. Jung and Assagioli's concepts of motivational drives had a huge impact on the development of techniques used in body-oriented psychotherapies, including core energetics, coreSomatics, emotional-kinesthetic psychotherapy, Holotropic Breathwork™, organismic body psychotherapy, and process-oriented psychology.

As the twentieth century unfolded, psychotherapists continued to develop new models of personality and treatment methods. In the 1960s many approaches to psychotherapy, known collectively as humanistic psychology, developed by individuals such as Abraham Maslow and Carl Rogers, were based on observations of healthy people instead of neurotic ones and on the human potential for growth and change. Especially important to the development of body-oriented psychotherapies was gestalt therapy, created by Fritz and Laura Perls. In gestalt therapy many techniques, some borrowed from Jacob Moreno's psychodrama, are used to physically enact painful experiences and difficult relationships. Gestalt therapy, like all humanistic psychology approaches, emphasizes developing a sense of wholeness, authenticity, and self-esteem through the conscious awareness of feelings and bodily expression in the present rather than by dredging up the past.

At the same time, a new wave of spiritual teachers from non-Western religions came to the United States, filling the burgeoning growth centers across the country with the wisdom of ancient teachings regarding the connections among body, mind, and spirit. As a result, new approaches to psychotherapy evolved, including Leonard Orr's rebirthing, Stanislav Grof's Holotropic Breathwork, and Ilana Rubenfeld's Synergy. These psychotherapies offered new methods to discover psychic wholeness by combining physical, mental, emotional, and spiritual aspects of humanness in varying ways. Today literally hundreds of different body-oriented approaches to psychotherapy influenced by science, religion, or the arts offer individuals a choice from a plethora of paths to psychological healing or self-discovery.

Theories and Practices

All body-oriented psychotherapies are based on the belief that the body, mind, and spirit are interdependent aspects of humanness. While Freud observed the mind's influence over the body, these disciplines reverse this relationship and study how the body affects the mind. They claim that creating a healthy, balanced body will help restore mental and emotional harmony. Body-oriented psychotherapists believe that the emotional and mental experiences of life, which in some methods include prenatal (before birth) or after-death experiences, are imprinted in the body as clearly as the words that are printed on this page. To effect a real and lasting change in a human psyche, they believe, one must work through the physical body.

Unlike Freudian psychoanalysis, which relies exclusively on verbal exchange between therapist and patient, body-oriented psychotherapists believe the body to be primary in both reflecting emotional problems and working toward their cure. Therapists direct the patient's attention to the physical sensations of the body and the relationship of these sensations to other aspects of the whole self. The techniques used range from the direct, sometimes violent physical manipulation of Reichian-based methods to the barely physical guided imagery sessions of psychosynthesis. In some methods, such as Holotropic Breathwork, two patients will work together in a therapeutic process without the direct aid of the therapist. In others, such as Pesso Boyden system psychomotor therapy, a group of people is needed to embody the healing process. Despite the differences, all types of body-oriented psychotherapies use the body, rather than another individual, as the monitor of psychological well-being, the gauge of emotional truth.

Benefits and Risks

Body-oriented psychotherapies aim to give greater freedom and integration to the physical, mental, emotional, and spiritual aspects of human life. Most of the methods included in this section are based on a theoretical foundation, which states that an individual's psychic development will ultimately lead to a spiritual unfolding, evidenced by a growing concern for and action toward the good of the entire community. Body-oriented psychotherapies have helped many people break painful physical or emotional addictions. Others report experiencing increased pleasure, optimism, and spontaneity, and a greater sense of participation in the process of living. Still others describe a stronger feeling of connection to other people and a clearer sense of purpose and value in their lives, as well as life in general.

These rewards are not easily gained. Body-oriented psychotherapies generally require a long-term commitment to a process that can require painful physical and emotional work. In addition, because these methods regard each individual as intrinsically whole, they are generally not appropriate for people suffering from psychoses or people whose self-esteem is so severely damaged that it cannot confront the truth of the body.

—NANCY ALLISON, CMA

Resources

The United States Association for Body Psychotherapy
  111 Bonifant St., Suite 201
  Silver Spring, MD 20910
  Tel: (301) 587-4011
  Web site: www.usabp.com
  A professional association, established in 1998, of body psychotherapy professionals and students that holds conferences and publishes professional journals and newsletters that track research and development in the field of body psychotherapy.

Further Reading

Brown, Dennis, and Jonathan Pedder. *An Introduction to Psychotherapy: An Outline of Psychodynamic Principles and Practice.* London and New York: Tavistock/Routledge, 1979.

Bioenergetics

 Bioenergetics is a form of body-oriented psychotherapy developed by American physician Alexander Lowen in the mid–twentieth century. Based on the groundbreaking work of Austrian psychotherapist Wilhelm Reich, bioenergetics views body, mind, and spirit as interdependent and reflective of one another. By combining active bodywork exercises with verbal therapy, bioenergetics therapists aim to liberate both body and mind from restrictive holding patterns, helping people to live freer, more pleasurable, fulfilling lives.

History

Bioenergetics was developed by Alexander Lowen, M.D. (1910–), a student of Wilhelm Reich, (1897–1957). Reich, founder of medical orgonomy and a colleague of the seminal psychoanalyst Sigmund Freud, is generally credited as the first person in modern Western psychotherapy to incorporate working directly with the body in psychotherapeutic treatment. He explored the body's involuntary responses to emotional situations to arrive at his own theoretical construct of human personality.

Reich believed that neuroses, or personality problems, are anchored in the body as chronic muscular tensions. He observed that chronic muscular tensions decreased a person's general energy level and ability to feel all emotions, particularly pleasurable ones. Reich believed that deepening a person's involuntary breathing process was key to releasing chronic muscular tension and opening muscular tissue to the full streaming of psychological and physical energy.

As a young man, Lowen noted that regular physical activity improved his physical and emotional states. He became interested in techniques that developed the body-mind relationship, such as Emile Jacques Dalcroze's eurythmics, Edmund Jacobson's progressive relaxation, and yoga. But it was not until 1940, when he heard Reich lecture at the New School for Social Research in New York, that he felt he found an answer to his own questions about the nature of the relationship between body and mind. Lowen studied with Reich from 1940 to 1952 and underwent therapy with him from 1942 to 1945. During these exciting and inspiring years he finished his premedical studies and trained to become a Reichian therapist. Lowen saw his first patient in 1945. Disappointed by his progress with his early patients, Lowen studied medicine from 1947 to 1951, earning an M.D. from Geneva University in Switzerland.

Although Lowen believed he had made substantial progress in his own therapy with Reich, he felt that many of his own conflicts had not been fully resolved. He perceived that the physical and emotional freedom gained in his work with Reich did not necessarily transfer to real-life situations. After his return from Europe, Lowen spoke with several other former patients of Reich, most notably John Pierrakos, M.D., who felt the same way.

In 1953, working with Pierrakos, Lowen set out to develop the techniques of Reichian therapy to achieve a deeper, more pervasive improvement. He believed a more active physical approach, as well as a deeper analytical approach, was needed. For three years Lowen experimented with Reich's bodywork techniques, using Pierrakos to apply pressure directly on Lowen's chronically tensed muscles. The exercises he developed form the basis of bioenergetics. During this time Lowen and Pierrakos met regularly with another Reichian associate, William Walling, M.D., in clinical seminars that enriched Lowen's theoretical understanding of Reich's approach as well.

Basic Principles

Bioenergetics is based on a model of the human personality as composed of biological impulses and conscious thought or will. According to Lowen, a healthy person follows her biological impulses completely, suppressing them only in response to a personal sense of desire. He believes neuroses develop when biological impulses are suppressed through conscious, willful control in response to fear.

Lowen believes this process begins very early in human development, for example, when a child consciously controls the impulse to cry in response to parental disapproval. According to Lowen, the child stops crying because she perceives her parents' disapproval as a threat to survival. The reflexive, physical act of restricting breathing that stops her crying is spontaneously developed, Lowen believes, as a survival mechanism. The child ceases to cry and parental affection and protection are secured. When a child alters his physical impulses by responding, as in this situation, to fear rather than pleasure, he creates a sense of personal power over his environment based on willful control of biological impulses. Lowen calls this psychological pattern the "neurotic character structure."

Like Reich, Lowen believes the neurotic character structure to be a survival defense, but it is also an imprisonment for the true nature of the human being. The neurotic character structure can be observed in the body, as well as the psyche, as a form of armor. Bioenergetic therapy strives to break down physical and emotional armoring by loosening rigid muscles and promoting the flow of psycho-physical energy, which Lowen calls bioenergy, through the body.

According to Lowen, "in Bioenergetic Therapy the breakdown of the neurotic character structure does not happen as a single event, but as a series of breakthroughs, each of which is experienced as an energetic release and transformation. With each release the patient begins to feel more alive and

more open and has an awareness of an inner strength and force that he or she had not felt before." As the body becomes more alive, the will loosens its grip on feelings that come through more easily as physical sensations that act as catalysts for new responses to and interactions with others.

Throughout this process bioenergetic therapy includes talking about one's history and current life situation, relationships, and dreams. The verbal therapy enables the patient to integrate the new emotions and physical sensations into her whole personality. Without this conscious integration Lowen believes that muscular tension will simply recur because the mind has not incorporated the physical experiences into a new, balanced personality structure.

Practice

Individual bioenergetic therapy, the most common format, may begin with some initial conversation between therapist and client, but will generally proceed quickly to bodywork exercises. In all formats, group or individual, clients work in leotards, bathing suits, or more commonly, their underwear, which allows the bioenergetic therapist to see the body and its changes more easily.

Most of the exercises involve lying, sitting, or standing in positions that actually increase the tension of chronically stressed muscles. It is believed that breathing deeply while in these positions pulls so much bioenergy into the muscles that it forces the client to release his willful hold on them, thereby allowing an involuntary stream of energy and sensation to flow through them. This stream of energy is experienced by the patient as a current, similar to an electrical current passing through a wire, and can be seen by therapist and client alike as actual physical vibrations in the muscle.

One of the most common series of postures used in bioenergetic therapy is called grounding positions. These standing postures were developed by Lowen to help

Wilhelm Reich had his patients lie on a bed and do deep-breathing exercises. He applied pressure to chronically held muscles to help a person feel the pain of holding them tense, and then to help them release the holding. He would direct a person to change the position of their body in some subtle way that allowed the energy and the feeling to flow out in an open channel. Lowen describes his first therapy session with Reich in his book *Bioenergetics* (1975). Lowen lay on a bed in bathing trunks and began to breathe deeply. When he began to relax, Reich asked him to drop his head back and open his eyes wide. As he did this, he screamed involuntarily, thus releasing a feeling he had unconsciously blocked for many years as well as freeing up the energy that had been used to hold it back.

clients who feel out of touch with reality develop a firm sense of the connection between their feet and the ground. Practitioners believe that allowing the breathing process to deepen while standing in the grounding positions helps pull bioenergy downward through the pelvis and legs. It increases a sense of rootedness and the ability to stand on one's own two feet, as well as literally being able to "stand" the increase in the amount of energy and emotion experienced.

Whichever body posture the client maintains, the bioenergetic therapist may use massage, forceful pressure, or gentle touch to encourage the release of contracted muscles. The client will also be advised to release sounds while holding the postures. The use of the voice increases vibration, sending more bioenergy through the system, thereby forcing the patient to surrender his hold on the body more quickly.

The breathing stool is another device designed by Lowen. Its function is to speed the releasing process, which is also called the surrender to the body. It is a padded wooden structure over which the client rests in a backward bending position. Supported by the stool in this position, clients may experience their current shallow breathing process and its connection to their fears. This position also stretches the torso, opening the entire pelvis and thorax to encourage deep involuntary breathing, the catalyst for releasing chronic muscular tension.

As the therapy progresses, expressive exercises will be added to the stationary lying, sitting, or standing poses. Clients perform actions such as kicking the legs alternately up and down while lying on a bed, or hitting a bed with fists or a tennis racket while standing in order to express anger and aggressive feelings. Bioenergetic therapists believe that experiencing aggression allows a patient to feel that she can defend (or stand up for) herself. Releasing these aggressive feelings also means no longer having to keep them under conscious willful control, thereby releasing muscular tissue to experience pleasurable sensations.

Throughout the course of the bodywork therapy, sessions are interspersed with verbal therapy, allowing the patient to integrate the new sensations and emotions into his life with the support of the therapist. Over the course of an individual therapy, clients may also choose to participate in group intensive sessions that may last a weekend or longer. Bioenergetic group therapy sessions utilize many of the same exercises as individual therapy and may involve working with a partner to increase physical resistance in the positions.

Benefits

Bioenergetic therapy is not short-term therapy. It requires a commitment of time and energy to resolve deep conflicts and to free the body and mind from neurotic, unproductive patterns. However, the bodywork seems to allow this deep healing process to proceed faster than it does with only verbal therapy. Bioenergetics seeks to integrate body and mind as it aims to help a person feel more relaxed, connected, spontaneous, and alive.

—NANCY ALLISON, CMA; WITH CONSULTATION FROM NINA ROBINSON, CMA

Resources

International Institute for Bioenergetic Analysis
144 E. 36th St.
New York, NY 10016
Tel: (212) 532-7742
Offers information about the discipline as well as qualified practitioners.

Further Reading

Lowen, Alexander. *Bioenergetics*. New York: Penguin, 1975.

Lowen, Alexander, and Leslie Lowen. *The Way to Vibrant Health: A Manual of Bioenergetic Exercises.* New York: Harper & Row, 1977.

———. *Pleasure: A Creative Approach to Life.* New York: Penguin, 1987.

Bodynamic Analysis

Bodynamic analysis helps people resolve life problems by building new coping skills, also known as resources, in the body and psyche. Bodynamic analysis describes resources as the normal physical and psychological abilities learned during healthy childhood development. Developed principally by Scandinavian physical educator Lisbeth Marcher in the 1970s, bodynamic analysis is based on an intricate theory that links specific muscular actions to psycholog-

ical abilities. Using Marcher's Bodymap™ as a guide, bodynamic analysis strives to help people develop retarded resources, empowering them to have new experiences and make new life choices.

History

Developed by Marcher and her colleagues in Denmark, bodynamic analysis was derived from the rich tradition of body therapy systems that emerged in Scandinavia early in the twentieth century. It has arrived recently in the United States, with the first U.S. program founded in Berkeley, California, in 1990.

Marcher was originally trained in the" relaxation method," an in-depth body education training system well known in Scandinavia. Dissatisfied with the treatment of psychological issues within the relaxation method, she began to study theories of body-mind integration. Influenced by Lillimor Johnsen, a Norwegian physiotherapist, Marcher developed a theory connecting each muscle action to specific psychological issues. She also noticed how motor patterns and psychological abilities seem to develop according to a very specific timetable during childhood. For example, the muscle associated with saying no is the triceps, a muscle that extends the arm out in a pushing-away motion. The triceps first begins its "no" motion very early, before the child can even say no. Later, as the child begins to say no, the action and the word go together. Finally the "no" movement lessens or disappears and the word "no" stays. In this way Marcher believed the timetables for the evolution of motor patterns and psychological and social patterns are intimately linked.

Theory

Bodynamic analysis is based on a fundamental way of thinking about the role the body plays in shaping who people are and how they think, feel, love, play, work, and grow. By observing the unfolding pattern of motor development in children, bodynamic analysts see how the child's motor system is intimately linked to core self-development. By linking a person's spontaneous movements to the underlying psychological expression, bodynamic analysts believe they are able to pinpoint the origins of the difficulties that people experience in their present lives.

Marcher conceived seven overlapping stages of child development that related to the psychological characteristics of each particular stage. They are the existence stage (second trimester–3 months), when the child first develops a sense of secure existence; the need stage (0–18 months), when physical bonding and contact are established and core body rhythms of eating, sleeping, and so forth, are set; the autonomy stage (8–30 months), when the child begins to move directly out into the world through crawling, walking, and grasping; the will stage (2–4 years), when the child learns to manage power and master loving and angry feelings and begins to develop a structuring of the world through planning and role formation; the love/sexuality stage (3–5 years), when loving and sexual feelings emerge more intensely; the opinion stage (5–8 years), when the child learns to express ideas and compare them with the world around her; and finally, the solidarity/performance stage (7–12 years), when the child masters his own abilities within the context of peer group activity. By determining the stage or age at which a person feels stuck, bodynamic analysis is able to help that person resolve past traumas and move him toward gaining new resources.

The thread that runs through all these stages is the child's intense desire and drive toward establishing deep, powerful connections to the outside world. Bodynamic analysts call this drive mutual connection, and believe it informs the basic movement of life energy. What is ultimately most traumatic to the growing child is when the bond between the child and others is disturbed or broken.

Practice

A typical session often begins with an agreement to focus on a specific issue, such as the ability to establish and maintain fulfilling relationships, or with an ongoing developmental issue or stage. Sessions may focus on body sensations, paying attention to any impulses, movements, images, or memories that emerge. The person's posture, movements, and language begin to tell a story. The story is developed by expanding the movements, and through supportive touch, role playing, or working with early historical experiences. Most healing is accomplished through an integration of sensing, experiencing, moving, and thinking, in the context of the supportive relationship with the practitioner.

To return to the earlier example of learning to say no, a person might have had difficulty during the will stage (2–4 years) with expressing her power. Therapy with such a person includes not only a verbal exploration of the experiences that led to this difficulty, but also teaching the body how to express "no." Practitioners help the person by teaching the muscles to express "no" in a new way. In some situations this may be fairly straightforward, but often this teaching needs to engage the person in a deep and subtle, physical and verbal conversation.

Throughout the process the practitioner and recipient explore sensations and experiences located in the body, the fears and beliefs that hold back the expression of the "no." There is a recognition that each person's defense system is unique and deserves respect and understanding before it can change. It is important to engage the person's sensory-motor system and wake up the developmental movements slowly and gently. Practitioner and recipient stay with a movement and the accompanying thoughts

In bodynamic analysis, there is a way to see our body profile in a muscle test called the Bodymap™. This is a process in which each muscle is tested for four degrees of hyperresponse and four degrees of hyporesponse as well as a healthy response. This is then charted visually on a map of the body, which becomes available for detailed interpretation of a person's early history. Therapists then look to see at what ages and in what ego aspects individuals may be most held or blocked, and in what areas they are the most developed and resourced. This information helps clients understand themselves and guides therapy.

and feelings until it has a chance to resolve. A person is then ready to explore a new movement and its accompanying psychological state.

Benefits and Risks

Bodynamic analysis is unique among body-oriented psychotherapies in its ability to work on specific developmental issues. With this specific goal in sharp focus, people seem to achieve a more complete resolution in the body, developing what bodynamic therapists call a "new imprint." People typically report forming deeper, more intimate relationships after experiencing bodynamic analysis.

Because therapist and recipient are able to focus on specific issues, bodynamic analysis often works well as a short-term intensive therapy; however, it is more often seen as a long-term commitment. While bodynamic analysts try to work from people's innate strengths to help them build new resources, therapy can pose a personal challenge as

deeper issues emerge and more profound changes are indicated.

—PETER BERNHARDT

Resources

Bodynamic Institute
P.O. Box 6008
Albany, CA 94706
Tel: (510) 524-8090
Offers information on national and international activities. The Bodynamic Institute provides a foundation training, a two-year practitioner training, and a two-year analytic training program.

Further Reading

Bernhardt, Peter. *Individuation: Mutual Connection and the Body's Resources. An interview with Lisbeth Marcher.* Alberta, Canada: Bodynamic Institute Monograph, 1992.
———. *The Art of Following Structure: An Interview with Lisbeth Marcher Exploring the Roots of the Bodynamic System.* Alberta, Canada: Bodynamic Institute Monograph, 1995.
Bernhardt, Peter, M. Bentzen, and J. Isaacs. *Waking the Body Ego: An Introduction to Lisbeth Marcher's Somatic Developmental Psychology.* Vols. 1 and 2. Alberta, Canada: Bodynamics Institute Monograph, 1995.

Core Energetics

Core energetics is a mode of healing that combines bodywork, psychotherapy, and a spiritual process called the pathwork to activate the greater consciousness dwelling within every human soul to release and strengthen human energy at all levels—physical, emotional, mental, and spiritual. Unlike conventional psychiatric or medical therapies, core energetics views the spiritual dimension of life as an essential component in the process of recovery and growth. In fact, core energetics therapists believe that illness is a block in the life force said to be at the core of every individual. The core is called energy, love, or soul. According to core energetics theory, the unblocking of emotion promotes self-healing and benefits a variety of mental and physical disorders from depression to chronic fatigue syndrome.

History

Sometimes called the core energetic evolutionary process, core energetics was developed by John Pierrakos, a Greek-American doctor who started his career as a follower of the innovative Austrian psychiatrist Wilhelm Reich. Reich had come to America after the Nazis rose to power and soon began to stir controversy in American medical circles because of his unorthodox views on the fundamental nature of the human organism. He maintained that the body is infused with an invisible energy known as orgone, which also infuses all material aspects of the cosmos. What happens in the body affects what happens emotionally and mentally. Therefore, illness is to be understood as a dual body-mind phenomenon—a notion that was alien to a medical profession then organized around the separation of psychological and physical healing. Reich gave Pierrakos the framework for his life's work as a holistic physician committed to the search for effective body-mind treatments.

In the 1950s Pierrakos and another physician, Alexander Lowen, made Reich's teachings the basis for bioenergetics, a body-oriented psychotherapy that uses the body to diagnose and heal emotional illness. Impressed by the parallels between Reich's notion of orgone and ancient Eastern ideas of human energy, Pierrakos began researching the nature of energy and human energy fields. By the early 1970s he had formulated a theory of the human organism, still Reichian in broad outline, but incorporating the conception of chakras, or energy centers. He developed an innovative system that examined the chakras and correlated what he found to be their normal or abnormal functioning to the person's psychological and physical traits. Pierrakos became proficient at viewing the human energy field and chakras. He observed the energy of people in a medical setting and was able to tell what other physicians needed complex laboratory tests to show.

Eva Broch, a spiritual medium who eventually became Pierrakos's wife, helped him complete his synthesis of Western and Eastern medical teachings. Her confidence in the existence of the spiritual, together with clinical observation that spiritual belief enhances patients' recuperative powers, inspired Pierrakos to risk going beyond the boundaries of Western scientific reason in his definition of human energy. It is ultimately spiritual in nature, he concluded, and cannot be fully understood unless its relationship to the human capacity for love is recognized. The spiritual dimension, love, and the life force became synonymous in Pierrakos's thought during the late 1970s. He built core energetics on his work in bioenergetic analysis and on the inspiration he obtained from the spiritual teachings of the pathwork, a spiritual process that consists of learning to activate the greater consciousness dwelling within every human soul.

In 1980 he founded an institute in New York City for study and training in the approach he called core energetics and regarded it as the culmination of his career. Most forms of body psychotherapy and transpersonal work in this country are informed by Pierrakos's work in bioenergetic analysis and core energetics. His work is unique because "the love force" is "the substance and movement of life." During the last decade interest in core energetics has grown rapidly in the United States and abroad. There are now branches of the Institute of Core Energetics in the United States, Canada, Mexico, Brazil, Germany, Switzerland, and Italy.

Theory

Core energetics is based on the belief that the individual has an innate capacity for love and a need to evolve, and that these together constitute a life force of virtually unlimited creative potential. Further, it is believed that health is a dynamic state found only when the individual realizes his creative potential in a process of personal growth and change. Though the movement receives its impetus from the life force, it occurs in the body, the vehicle through which emotion, thought, and spirit are expressed.

Pierrakos is the first modern Western physician to connect the ancient knowledge of energy and spirituality to the science of new physics and to the current medical practice of psychiatry. He has created a holistic approach by combining work with all five levels of human existence in the human entity. These five levels are the physical body, feelings and emotions, mind and thought, will, and spirit.

Core energetics therapists believe that we are made up of layers of energy. At our center is the pulsing, moving energy of life that Pierrakos calls the core. This is our life force, which, following the laws of physics, seeks to expand and grow. When people are in touch with their life force, they feel love for themselves and their fellow creatures. The next layer is the lower self, which contains our wounded child and the dark side, or shadow part, of our nature. Core energetics theory contends that we block our life force when we are not allowed to express our emotional pain or negative emotions. This energy becomes stagnant and will produce a layer of defense, which becomes physical armoring. Next we put on a social mask designed to protect ourselves. This mask, or

false self, dampens the vibrancy and buoyancy of the life center—the core.

The process of this evolutionary work, therefore, is to unblock our defenses, move the stuck energy to create healthy flow, and transform the negative, distorted emotions back to the core self. This is done by first penetrating the mask, which uncovers the false self; second, by working with the physical body, the body armoring; third, by transforming the negative emotions of the dark side and allowing the primal wounds to be expressed; and fourth, by supporting the core to be experienced as loving, joyful, and connected to all life. Finally, this work organically leads to a deep understanding of a person's task and purpose in life.

According to core energetics theory, it is of primary importance to teach people to use their positive will, the will of the heart, to live in the present, and to be aware that people have the choice in each moment to create their own lives.

Practice

A typical session lasts approximately an hour. The receiver may wear a leotard or bathing suit so that the therapist can easily assess and treat the defenses built into the body. Initial work often involves breathing exercises to charge the system, bring awareness to the receiver, and start the process of release and transformation. There is always intensive work with bodily movement and exercise and emotional expression that unblocks the flow of the life force. The therapist may use hands-on touch to help the receiver mobilize and direct energy through the body. All levels of the human entity—physical, emotional, mental, and spiritual—are addressed as appropriate for the individual.

Treatment will be adjusted to the particular needs of the receiver and be different at each stage of therapy, but is always approached as an evolutionary process that leads from unmasking of the shadow self to expression, and toward the transformation of pain to understanding, and the acceptance that opening the heart and feeling love is the healing agent. Transformation occurs when the client unmasks and expresses the energy of the wounded and lower self, which then allows connection to the core/spirit.

Benefits

Core energetics should not be confused with conventional psychotherapy. It teaches receivers about their capacity for self-healing and launches them on a process of transformation that is ultimately spiritual in nature. Proponents of core energetics credit it with providing a sense of well-being at all levels of human existence. It is also regarded as helpful with weight problems, panic attacks, unresolved anger, posttraumatic stress, sexual dysfunction, repairing troubled marital and familial relationships, making major personal and professional changes, and expanding spiritual awareness.

—PAMELA L. CHUBBUCK, PH.D.

Resources

Institute of Core Energetics International
115 E. 23rd St., 12th Floor
New York, NY 10010
Tel: (212) 982-9637
Fax: (212) 673-5939
Web site: www.core-energetics.org
A training and treatment center that organizes workshops and lectures, publishes a newsletter, and gives referrals to therapists trained in core energetics.

Institute of Core Energetics South
8733 Lake Drive
Lithonia, GA 30058
Tel: (770) 388-0086
Fax: (770) 388-0806
A training and treatment center for core energetics that organizes workshops and lectures and publishes a newsletter.

Training in core energetics requires four years of coursework and extensive personal therapy at an Institute of Core Energetics. Generally, prior involvement in another form of therapy such as chiropractic or osteopathy is required for admission. The curriculum features courses on anatomy, physiology, human energy theory, Reichian theory, bioenergetics, and pathwork spirituality. One year of postgraduate study is required for those who wish to become trainers.

Institute of Core Energetics West
P.O. Box 806
Mendocino, CA 95160
Tel: (707) 937-1825
Fax: (707) 937-3052
e-mail: lisycee@mcn.org
Offers treatment and training in core energetics.

Further Reading

Books
Pierrakos, Eva. *The Pathwork of Self-Transformation.* New York: Bantam, 1990.
Pierrakos, John. *Core Energetics: Developing the Capacity to Love and Heal.* Mendocino, Calif.: Life Rhythm, 1990.
———. *Eros, Love, and Sexuality.* Mendocino, Calif.: Life Rhythm, 1997.

Journals
Energy and Consciousness: International Journal of Core Energetics. Jacqueline Carlton, Ph.D., editor.

Videotapes
Chubbuck, Pamela. *Say Yes to Life: Grounding and Loving Your Body.* Lithonia, Ga.: The Institute of Core Energetics South, n.d.
———. *Say Yes to Life: Expressing Your Emotions and Opening to Your Core.* Lithonia, Ga.: The Institute of Core Energetics South, n.d.

coreSomatics®

 coreSomatics® is a discipline designed to increase awareness of the ways our childhood, emotions, and experiences influence the posture and alignment of our bodies. In coreSomatics, the habitual use of the body is seen as a mirror, reflecting all personal experience, creating a dynamic interdependence between the body and the mind. In the nonjudgmental environment of coreSomatics, individuals identify and change limiting habitual physical behaviors, leading to an improved state of mind and self-image. The discipline combines the Feldenkrais Method® and the Alexander technique with gestalt therapy, Jungian psychology, and the expressive arts therapies.

History

coreSomatics was developed in the 1970s by Kay Miller, who created countless theater games and sound and movement exercises for the improvisational theater company she founded in 1974. The exercises gained recognition for their success with at-risk young adults. Miller began to combine theater exercises with the physical process therapies of the Feldenkrais Method and the Alexander technique. Integrating these with Jungian psychology and gestalt therapy, she created coreSomatics. In 1983 the Somatic Institute, Pittsburgh, was founded as a not-for-profit organization to provide research and education in coreSomatics.

Philosophy

coreSomatics is founded on the premise that what the individual seeks, in order to bring about personal improvement and change, already exists in the unconscious. Negative aspects such as insecurity, self-doubt, fear, rigidity, and tension are believed to be a result of early trauma. These early traumatizing experiences negatively impact an individual's nervous system, shaping the actions and postures used in adult life. Thus, a seemingly ineffectual or poor use of the body may actually be a highly complex reaction to childhood experience or a limited muscular memory that, once brought into awareness, can be released.

Practice

The first objective of the coreSomatics practitioner is to provide a safe environment in which the client is free to express past and current experiences. Having established trust, the practitioner employs touch, uses verbal expression and movement exercises, and works with breathing patterns and existing posture. Body tensions and pain are explored through imagery, sound, humor, and intuition.

In the process of the hands-on physical interventions and verbal expressions, individuals discover that their physical habits are connected to emotional and psychological memories, which are experienced as muscular armor, rigidity, tension, and pain. Through the physical and emotional releases of this process, individuals find more effective ways to manage their lives and experience the exuberance of having reclaimed their fluidity, flexibility, and spontaneity.

Benefits

coreSomatics has been used to reduce stress, relieve tension, and allow individuals to experience their lives more fully. People have experienced significant improvements in intelligence, sensory acuity, memory, and concentration. Improvements in mood, interpersonal relationships, productivity, and general health and wellness follow naturally.

—KAY MILLER

Resources

Somatic Institute, Pittsburgh
    8600 W. Barkhurst Drive
    Pittsburgh, PA 15237
    Tel: (412) 366-5580
    Fax: (412) 367-1026
    Offers coreSomatics training through a two-year certification program, a mastery-level program, an associates program, and a variety of postgraduate internships. Sponsors research and education in coreSomatics and publishes a variety of materials, including the journal *Touch*®.

Emotional-Kinesthetic Psychotherapy

 Emotional-kinesthetic psychotherapy (EKP) is a discipline that incorporates the body in psychotherapy, seeking to help clients integrate the physical, emotional, and spiritual aspects of their selves. It incorporates a variety of techniques, including touch, to facilitate this integrative process. Therapists attempt to create an environment of emotional safety and respect to allow clients to access and reveal their minds, bodies, hearts, and souls.

History

Linda Marks developed EKP from her experience as a trauma survivor, which led her to study approaches to psychotherapy that study the body. EKP draws extensively from Ron Kurtz's hakomi integrative somatics and incorporates aspects of Roberto Assagioli's psychosynthesis and Eugene Gendlin's focusing. EKP responds to clients' particular needs by using character typology, the model of human personality conceived by psychiatrist Wilhelm Reich and developed by Alexander Lowen and John Pierrakos in bioenergetics. Marks founded the Institute for Emotional-Kinesthetic Psychotherapy in 1990, but the principles of EKP had been applied in her private therapy practice and personal growth workshops since 1985.

Theory

EKP believes that there exist three levels of human intelligence: cognitive (consisting of knowledge), emotional, and somatic (consisting of body sensations). According to EKP, the heart is the place where somatic and emotional intelligence meet. Any life difficulty or body sensation can be accessed and explored by asking, "What's happening in your heart?" at a moment in time. Emotional and somatic sensations contain information and experience that inform a person's thought process, and without which a person often cannot move forward in her life.

Practice

An EKP therapist's goal is to help clients achieve a sense of integration that allows them to live meaningful and productive lives. The work aims to allow clients to heal their most wounded parts, meet their simplest unmet needs, and reclaim the deepest part of their selves. A typical session may include the following:

1. Leading the client through a guided meditation, which EKP calls a heart meditation. In this process the client explores the emotional and physical sensations he experiences in his heart in relation to what is happening in important parts of his life, such as work, personal relationships, and self-esteem. A heart meditation begins each EKP session to help the client center himself and

create a safe, spiritually inclusive environment in which to do therapy.

2. Sharing aspects of the client's life to create a context for an ongoing therapy.

3. Calling attention to what is happening in the heart and body in the present moment, to help the client follow emotional and somatic processes.

4. Touching, when appropriate and with permission, to facilitate emotional processes.

5. Guiding a client toward perception of sensations, such as jitteriness, numbness, or tightness. These sensations, referred to as the emotional-kinesthetic charge, are considered the embodiment of the client's inner state. The EKP therapist helps the client follow the emotional-kinesthetic charge to its source, which may be a traumatic experience or unmet needs. This guiding is known as EKP process work.

6. Closing a session by calling attention to the emotions and somatic experiences that have emerged. This is often done with closed eyes so that the client can assimilate his inner experiences of the session. Finally, the client returns to an outer, open-eyed state of consciousness.

Benefits

EKP has many benefits, the most immediate of which can include stress reduction, developing a stronger sense of self, and alleviating pain. At a deeper level, EKP offers a healing context for trauma and neglect, allowing clients to bridge the split between body and mind that often follows traumatic experience. EKP can be used to help one find her voice, develop appropriate work and personal relationships from the core of one's being, and connect with a sense of spiritual purpose. For borderline clients and others in the midst of a serious psychotic crisis, other therapeutic approaches would be indicated.

—*LINDA MARKS*

Resources

Institute for Emotional-Kinesthetic Psychotherapy
3 Central Ave.
Newton, MA 02160
Tel: (617) 965-7846
Fax and Office Line: (617) 332-7262
Provides numerous seminars, workshops, and extended group therapeutic programs, in addition to running a three-year training program.

Further Reading

Liedloff, Jean. *The Continuum Concept.* Reading, Mass.: Addison-Wesley, 1977.

Marks, Linda. *Living with Vision: Reclaiming the Power of the Heart.* Skokie, Ill.: Knowledge Systems, Inc., 1989.

———. *The Emotional-Kinesthetic Study Guide.* Newton, Mass.: Institute for EKP, 1991.

Small, Jacquelyn. *Becoming Naturally Therapeutic.* New York: Bantam, 1990.

Focusing

 Focusing is a process that allows and encourages the mind and body to communicate in order to heed the wisdom that comes from our bodies. The focusing process can be used by itself, or in conjunction with all types of psychotherapy and counseling. It facilitates problem solving, creative endeavors, stress reduction, and spirituality. The six steps of focusing invite people to unlock doors and move into dimensions that cannot be entered through intellect alone.

History

Dr. Eugene Gendlin, a professor, philosopher, and psychologist, developed focusing while at the University of Chicago. The concepts evolved from his work in existential philosophy, which he wrote about in *The Creation of Meaning* (1962), and from his research in psychotherapy, which is described in an article entitled "Focusing" in *Psychotherapy: Theory, Research, and Practice* (Vol. 6., no. 1, 1969).

Since 1969, Gendlin has been teaching focusing all over the world and writing about it in numerous articles and three books. Certified focusing trainers are located throughout North America, as well as in South America, Europe, and Asia. Training programs are available worldwide for those who want to become certified focusing trainers in order to teach or to apply it toward other disciplines.

Theory

In his research, Gendlin posed the question, "Why is some psychotherapy successful and some not?" From analyzing a large number of therapy sessions, he and his coworkers discovered that it is not *what* the client talks about, but rather *how* the client talks about an issue that determines whether a person improves in therapy. Successful clients get in touch with what feels like a vague bodily experience, then concentrate on it as it comes into focus. In essence, they attend to what they don't yet fully understand. In the realm of focusing, the "body" means not only the physiological self, but also the storehouse of experience that is carried there. Gendlin called the body's version a "felt sense." By learning to tune in to the bodily "felt sense" of different experiences or difficulties, we can more easily resolve life issues and problems.

Another important assumption is that every problem has within it some wisdom about its next step, and some positive life energy that wants to move forward or be released. When we accurately name how the body is carrying an experience, we get new information and insights, as well as a physical release that feels good.

Currently, efforts are being made to bring focusing into education, the healing and creative arts, medicine, and spirituality. The potential of this simple yet powerful tool continues to unfold. As Gendlin says, "One step in the body is worth a thousand steps in the mind."

Practice

Focusing can be learned from a book, but is best learned from a person who guides one through the process. Many people begin by learning it in a class or workshop or from a focusing teacher, and then continue to practice with a focusing partner. Partners take turns so that each one has a chance to be the guide and the focuser.

The focusing process involves six steps. In the first step, the focuser is invited to "clear a space," which involves taking an inventory of the concerns or issues that the person can locate in her body at that time and placing each "down" or outside the body. After the simple act of putting the problems down, the person often feels a distinct release. Clearing a space often releases stress and creates a safe distance from the issues or feelings that are being carried around.

Next, the focuser is asked to choose a problem that needs attention right now and to ask in a friendly way, "How does this whole issue feel in my body right now?" After a pause, the focuser checks to see if a word, phrase, or perhaps an image comes that feels as though it matches the sensations inside. If there is a match, the focuser usually feels a "yes" inside, followed by a sense of bodily release. She then proceeds to the next step. If there isn't a match, the focuser tries other words or images until a good fit is found. Then the focuser sits with this body sense, just "keeping it company," or asking it open-ended questions such as "What's the crux of this?" "What does this problem need?" or "What's a step in the right direction?" In the pause after each question, the focuser is invited to let a fresh answer arise from the body sense. There is usually some physical relief or "felt shift," as well as new insight.

For example, a focuser might find on a given day that she is aware of three different and distinct unsettled feelings in her body: one from an uncomfortable conversation with her mother, one from an argument with her boyfriend, and one from worry about a test. After setting them all aside on an imaginary bench for a few moments, she chooses to work on the argument with her boyfriend. At first she thinks the word that best describes the tight feeling in her chest is "angry," but that doesn't quite fit. She finds that "hurt" better captures how she feels after their argument. When she says the word "hurt," she heaves a sigh of acknowledgment and says, "Yes, that's how I really felt when I hung up the phone." She then senses into the whole thing about being "hurt," and finds that it has to do with feeling unrecognized and unseen. When she asks what this feeling of "hurt" needs, it becomes clear that the right step is to talk to her boyfriend about her hurt and disappointment, not about the anger, which has by now shifted.

The instructions for a typical focusing session might be as follows:

1. CLEAR A SPACE
   How are you? What's between you and
      feeling fine?
   Don't answer; let what comes in your
      body do the answering.
   Don't go into anything.
   Greet each concern that comes. Put each
      aside for a while, next to you.
   Except for that, are you fine?
2. USE FELT SENSE
   Pick one problem to focus on.
   Don't go into the problem. What do you
      sense in your body when you recall
      the whole of that problem?
   Sense all of that, the sense of the whole
      thing, the murky discomfort or the
      unclear body-sense of it.

3. GET A HANDLE
   What is the quality of the felt sense?
   What one word, phrase, or image comes
      out of this felt sense?
   What quality-word would fit it best?
4. RESONATE
   Go back and forth between word (or
      image) and the felt sense. Is that
      right?
   If they match, have the sensation of
      matching several times.
   If the felt sense changes, follow it with
      your attention.

When you get a perfect match, the words (or images) being just right for this feeling, let yourself feel that for a minute.

5. ASK
   "What is it, about the whole problem,
      that makes me so _____?"
   When stuck, ask questions:
      What is the worst of this feeling?
      What's really so bad about this?
      What does it need?
      What should happen?
   Don't answer; wait for the feeling to stir
      and give you an answer.
   What would it feel like if it was all OK?
      Let the body answer:
      What is in the way of that?
6. RECEIVE
   Welcome what came. Be glad it spoke.
   It is only one step on this problem, not
      the last.
   Now that you know where it is, you can
      leave it and come back to it later.
   Protect it from critical voices that
      interrupt.

Does your body want another round of focusing, or is this a good stopping place?

Benefits

The benefits of focusing include becoming aware that there is a realm of inner knowing that can be found in the body, reducing stress or tension in the body-mind, and increasing one's life energy. Focusing also offers a way to work through blocks, facilitates effective problem solving and decision making, promotes creativity, improves the effectiveness of psychotherapy, and deepens spirituality.

—JOAN KLAGSBRUN, PH.D.

Resources

The Focusing Institute
    34 East Lane
    Spring Valley, NY 10977
    Tel: (914) 362-5222 or 1-800-799-7418
    e-mail: info@focusing.org
    Web site: www.focusing.org
    Provides training tapes, articles, and information about teachers and focusing-oriented psychotherapists around the world. Publishes the journal *Focusing Folio*.

Further Reading

Boukydis, C. F. Z. "Client-Centered/Experiential Practice with Parents and Infants." In *Client-Centered and Experiential Psychotherapy in the Nineties,* edited by G. Lietar et al. Belgium: Leuven University Press, 1990.

Campbell, P., and G. McMahon. *Biospirituality: Focusing as a Way to Grow.* Chicago: Loyola University Press, 1985.

Cornell, A. Weiser. *The Power of Focusing.* San Francisco: New Harbinger, 1996.

Friedman, Neil. *On Focusing: How to Access Your Own and Other People's Direct Experience.* Self-published (259 Massachusetts Ave., Arlington, Mass. 02174).

Gendlin, E. T. "A Theory of Personality Change." In *Personality Change,* edited by Worchel and Byrne. New York: Wiley, 1964.

———. *Focusing.* New York: Bantam, 1981.

———. *Let Your Body Interpret Your Dreams.* Wilmette, Ill.: Chiron Publications, 1986.

———. *Focusing Oriented Psychotherapy: A Manual of the Experiential Method.* New York: Guilford Publications, 1996.

Gestalt Therapy

 Gestalt therapy is a form of humanistic psychology that attempts to help participants develop awareness of their unresolved needs and emotions. Gestalt therapy's notion of the mind is based on psychoanalysis, gestalt psychology, existentialism, and the theories of Austrian psychiatrist Wilhelm Reich. A person is thought to be psychologically healthy when he is aware of his needs and is able to resolve them in an effective way. Gestalt therapists try to identify when their clients are blocking emotions by observing their movements and postures. Instead of investigating the past, gestalt therapists address clients' problems and emotions as they manifest in the present moment, often using techniques that require the client to act out his emotions. By urging people to confront their emotions, gestalt therapy seeks to help them make choices, interact with others, and relieve the physical symptoms of anxiety and stress.

History

The original theories and techniques of gestalt therapy were formed by Laura and Frederick "Fritz" Perls in the scientific and intellectual atmosphere of Germany in the 1920s. After receiving his medical training, Fritz Perls began working with brain-damaged soldiers at Frankfurt-am-Main in 1926. During this time he became interested in new theories of the mind conceived by the existential philosophy of Martin Heidegger and Martin Buber and gestalt psychology, developed by Max Wertheimer and Kurt Koffa. He became a psychoanalyst, studying with people such as Karen Horney and Wilhelm Reich, who were expanding upon Sigmund Freud's methods. In the 1930s Fritz Perls went into therapy with Reich, who led him to believe that the body was a critical aspect of psychological therapy. Laura Perls studied with Buber and Paul Tillich at the University of Frankfurt. Often writing under her husband's name, she incorporated the principles of existential philosophy and theology into a framework of psychological therapy.

In 1934 Fritz and Laura Perls fled Nazi Germany for South Africa, where they established the South African Institute for Psychoanalysis. *Ego, Hunger, and Aggression,* published in 1942, outlined the principles that were to become the foundation of gestalt therapy. In 1946 the couple moved to New York City, where they began conducting gestalt group therapy sessions in their apartment. The Gestalt Therapy Association of New York was established in 1952, followed by the Gestalt Institute of Cleveland in 1954. Through the 1960s gestalt therapy's popularity grew. Fritz and Laura Perls moved to California in 1960 and conducted workshops on the West Coast. In his workshops Fritz Perls established himself as a leader and a guru, and many participants accused him of abusing his power. He continued to promote gestalt therapy until his death in 1970. The variety of techniques developed throughout the history of gestalt therapy have become a resource for therapists in many other disciplines. At least sixty-two gestalt therapy institutes currently exist throughout the world.

Theory

The theory of gestalt therapy was inspired by the insights into human consciousness developed by gestalt psychology. This theory of mind originated in 1920s Berlin in reaction to the prevailing atomistic and analytical approaches to understanding perception. At that time theorists believed a person identifies a perceived object by mentally assembling each part. Gestalt psychology asserted that this model must be reversed. Instead, a person grasps the whole form of the object first. This whole, or gestalt, then determines the way that one recognizes the component parts. Thus, one's experiences are organized according to basic mental patterns, or gestalts. As gestalt psychologists believe that each person possesses a set of gestalt images, gestalt therapists claim that basic needs, drives, and beliefs are also gestalts. These gestalts impart value to the objects or people in a person's environment, affecting her view of a situation and motivating her to make certain choices. Like existential philosophy, this view emphasizes personal responsibility. To feel more in control of and satisfaction with one's choices, one must become aware of one's freedom instead of blaming external influences. The gestalt therapist's role is to help clients identify how their needs and beliefs shape the ways they see themselves and others.

According to this model, a healthy individual is able to manage her needs by acknowledging what she desires and identifying how to obtain it. Unfortunately, human needs are not always met, and gestalt therapy claims that these unfulfilled needs manifest as anxiety, frustration, muscular tension, and other disturbances. A person's needs may not be met because she is unaware of the needs or is unable to express or fulfill them. Adopting the essential framework of psychoanalysis, gestalt therapy seeks to reveal unexplored parts of a client's personality and allow her to resolve unfulfilled desires responsibly. However, gestalt therapy deviates from traditional Freudian psychoanalysis by replacing the therapist's search into a client's past with a dialogue and enactment techniques that reveal the client's feelings and opinions in the present moment. Gestalt therapy emphasizes the here and now to illuminate the ways that a person's current behaviors and attitudes influence the choices she makes. Despite this emphasis on the present, the client's past remains an important aspect of gestalt therapy. Since unresolved needs from the past are thought to persist in a person's mind, affecting her everyday functioning, important aspects of a client's history will directly or indirectly present themselves during the session. With this approach, the course of a session will be different for each person.

Practice

Throughout a gestalt therapy session, a person's attention is always directed to the present. At any moment a client may be asked to describe what he is feeling. The client and therapist must always speak in the first person and describe events in the present tense. For example, instead of telling the therapist "my back is tense" or "my father makes me angry," a client will be urged to describe his current feelings and behavior with a statement such as "I am tensing my back" or "I feel angry at my father." These statements are phrased to emphasize the person's responsibility. Gestalt therapy techniques are designed to force a client to confront and express his needs and emotions during the session. They are often intense emotional experiences. In one common technique, the client is asked to isolate an emotion or a part of his personality and address it as if it were sitting in an empty chair in the room. A client also may conduct an imaginary dialogue with a person from a dream or from his past.

Gestalt therapy is often practiced in groups, usually consisting of ten people, for two hours. The therapist attempts to create an environment in which each person must express what he feels and listen to others. For example, a person who has trouble expressing criticism may be instructed to make a critical statement about each of the other members of the group. Then the therapist may ask each person to describe her emotional reaction to this confrontation. Through this process a person can identify and overcome his barriers to self-expression, and participants investigate how their problems manifest in their interactions with the group. The therapist mediates the group, giving instructions and setting boundaries.

Therapists ask their clients to monitor how they feel during each exercise, helping them to become aware of the different emotions that may surface. They also observe how a client may be blocking emotions. Borrowing concepts from Reich, gestalt therapy claims that the body may be affected by blocked emotions. Thus, a therapist will look for signs of blocked emotion in a person's movement or posture. The therapist seeks to make clients more aware of how their bodies are affected by their blocked emotions. The goal is to equip an individual with the self-awareness to find effective and authentic ways to resolve his needs.

Benefits and Risks

Many individuals choose gestalt therapy to become more emotionally expressive and more confident in their ability to make decisions, and to develop greater self-awareness. An individual may attend a group session to improve the way she relates to others. A group of family members or coworkers may attend together to develop more successful ways of interacting. Gestalt therapy traditionally appeals to people seeking help with anxiety, depression, or stress. It is not designed to treat individuals with more severe psychological conditions, such as psychoses or schizophrenia. Since a typical session will require confronting one's emotions, it is possible that a participant will encounter a severe emotional experience. For this reason, people who are extremely unstable or vulnerable may choose to avoid this type of therapy.

Resources

Gestalt Center for Psychotherapy and Training
510 E. 89th St.
New York, NY 10128
Tel: (212) 879-3669
Offers training and resources for those interested in gestalt therapy.

Gestalt Therapy Institute of Los Angeles
    1460 Seventh St., Suite 301
    Santa Monica, CA 90410
    Tel: (909) 629-9935
    Promotes the study of gestalt therapy.

Further Reading

Kogan, Gerald. *Gestalt Therapy Resources.* Berkeley, Calif.: Transformations Press, 1980.

O'Connell, Vincent, ed. *Gestalt Therapy Primer: Introductory Readings in Gestalt Therapy.* Springfield, Ill.: Charles C Thomas, 1975.

Van de Riet, Vernon. *Gestalt Therapy: An Introduction.* New York: Pergamon Press, 1980.

Hakomi Integrative Somatics

 Hakomi integrative somatics is a form of therapy that combines bodywork with elements of psychological counseling. It grew out of the hakomi method of body-centered psychotherapy founded by Ron Kurtz. Both forms of hakomi view the mind and body as a single integrated organism, in which past traumas, both mental and physical, are "somaticized," that is, manifested in the body as habitual tension and strain. Fixed attitudes and patterns of behavior are similarly formed. Hakomi integrative somatics seeks to teach students to bring these unconscious habits to conscious awareness, understand them, and change them.

History

Ron Kurtz based his original techniques of hakomi psychotherapy on his knowledge of Taoism, Buddhism, and various body-mind disciplines, including Reichian therapy and bioenergetics. His studies in these areas led him to observe that a person's psychological defenses arise from a desire to avoid pain; thus, Kurtz believed, they are more readily overcome when they are gently supported rather than opposed. He developed hakomi into a method of psychotherapy that strives to evoke and process inner experiences through techniques of "mindfulness," an Eastern meditative technique for becoming aware of one's feelings and sensations in the present moment.

In the mid-1970s Pat Ogden, an apprentice to Kurtz and a student of various bodywork therapies, became intrigued with the pervasive pattern in her patients' dissociation of the mind from the body. She also noticed that bodywork therapies and psychotherapy were generally practiced independently of each other. Wanting to forge the two approaches into a tool for treating body-mind dissociation, Ogden began to include bodywork in psychotherapy sessions. As a result, her patients negotiated the healing process in a more integrated way and with more lasting results. In addition, she found that by incorporating the psychological processing of emotional material during a bodywork session, a patient's physical changes were more enduring. Ogden's efforts to join hands-on bodywork and movement work with psychotherapy resulted in the formation of hakomi integrative somatics.

Basic Principles

Hakomi is founded on the premise that human beings are self-organizing: we continually and creatively adapt our perceptions and behaviors in accordance with our environment. Eventually, however, we may form fixed attitudes about ourselves that may become unconscious attitudes, or "core organizers," that in turn can limit us to habitual, automatic styles of being and relating to the world. Further, they can restrict our creativity and capacity for personal fulfillment. Core organizers are held and expressed in belief systems and emotional habits, as well as in body structure and movement patterns. Hakomi recognizes two distinct types of wounds that affect the formation of core organizers: developmental and traumatic. Developmental wounds arise from the unsatisfactory completion of learning tasks. Such tasks include learning to get one's needs met and learning to be autonomous. Traumatic wounds occur in overwhelming situations in which actual survival is threatened, such as abuse, accidents, and surgery. When we suffer from either kind of wound, we may become habitually dissociated from one or more of our core organizers.

In hakomi integrative somatics, a healing relationship between therapist and patient is established, providing a crucial element in the creation of a context in which the cooperation of the patient's unconscious may be gained. Then, by means of exercises combining bodywork with verbalizations by the patient, core organizers are brought to consciousness and new information about them becomes available. In this experiential, rather than cognitive (analytical, thinking-based) process, the patient can explore new options—both physical and psychological—and spontaneously reorganize toward health. The patient also learns ways to deepen his awareness of the connection between the body and the mind. He becomes more attuned to the ever-changing flow of wordless information that is the language of the body. This awareness becomes a powerful healing tool, for it naturally expands the patient's sense of a physical self—an essential step in correcting the dissociation of the mind from the body.

Practice

The practitioner begins a session by talking with the patient to assess her situation and to establish a healing relationship in which the client feels safe and accepted. The client is helped to access a state of consciousness called mindfulness, a self-reflective state cultivated by gently focusing one's attention inward. Through mindfulness the client observes and describes present inner experience—specifically body patterns, emotions, images, memories, or thoughts. These facets of inner experience reflect basic attitudes such as "I'm not good enough" or "I am always alone." Core organizers are accessible through either body or mind; one level easily accesses the other. By means of verbal and physical experiments, a client begins to re-associate with previously dissociated core organizers. For example, a client is asked to attend to what happens as hands-on bodywork is performed on her shoulders. She may notice that a feeling of sadness arises as she is reminded of being alone as a child. The practitioner continues using such exercises to explore the places in the body that contain patterns of core organization—in this case, the one involved with feelings of loneliness. Throughout the process the client actively participates and verbalizes her inner experiences and emotions.

A session also includes supporting a client's inner resources by developing an awareness of the strengths and potentials an individual already possesses. The therapist approaches the client in a manner that acknowledges that client's abilities, rather than adopting a stance that focuses exclusively on problems and supposed deficiencies.

Benefits

Hakomi integrative somatics can enhance physical, psychological, and spiritual well-being. By working simultaneously with the body and the mind, hakomi can often uncover information that remains unconscious in conventional therapies and can effect physical changes that are more lasting. Participants consistently report greater integration of the body and mind. While specific outcomes vary, results can include the reduction of pain and posttraumatic stress symptoms; improved physical alignment, capacity for intimacy, and creativity; and an overall feeling of being more in tune with oneself.

—*PAT OGDEN, M.A.*

Resources

Hakomi Integrative Somatics
    P.O. Box 19438
    Boulder, CO 80308
    Tel: (303) 447-3290
    e-mail: hakomisoma@aol.com
    Offers workshops in hakomi integrative somatics and training of practitioners.

Further Reading

Kurtz, Ron. *Body-Centered Psychotherapy: The Hakomi Method.* Mendocino, Calif.: Life Rhythm, 1986.

Holotropic Breathwork™

 Holotropic Breathwork™ is a recently developed method of self-exploration that combines rapid, deep breathing, evocative music, and focused bodywork. The term *holotropic* is derived from the Greek *holos*, meaning "whole," and *trepin*, meaning "to move in the direction of." Holotropic Breathwork aims to bring the mind and body together in a trance state, which furnishes access to buried memories and aspects of consciousness hidden under ordinary conditions. While Holotropic Breathwork can be an effective treatment for mental and physical disorders, it is more often approached as shamanic activity for recovery of the deep past and entry into the spiritual realm.

History

The founders of Holotropic Breathwork are Stanislav Grof, a Czech psychiatrist trained in Prague during the 1950s, and his wife, Christine. A study of Jung's theories of the collective unconscious convinced Grof that faith in reason had led modern science to espouse a mechanistic model of the mind, incapable of assessing or utilizing its true range of powers. He was particularly interested in determining the scope and nature of experiences such as visions generally relegated to the category of parapsychological phenomena.

A breakthrough in the manufacture of psychedelic drugs gave Grof a way to experiment with altered states of consciousness. By his own account he soon realized there were broad similarities between certain drug-induced states of mind and the experiences attained through meditative, mystic, and shamanic activity.

After emigrating to the United States in the early 1960s, Grof continued his research into altered consciousness and parapsychology at the Maryland Psychiatric Research Center, Johns Hopkins University, and eventually the Esalen Institute in Big Sur, California.

During the 1970s the Grofs emerged as leaders in the New Age healing and spiritual movement but kept strong ties with psychiatric theory and scholarship. Along with Kenneth Wilber, they are regarded as key figures in the formation of transpersonal psychology, a system integrating Jungian theory with contemporary physiological research and multicultural study of religion. Transpersonal psychology is sometimes the true basis for clinical treatment of mental disorders. The Grofs incorporated its principles into Holotropic Breathwork, which they began to offer in workshop and training programs in 1976. Several books, most notably Stanislav Grof's *Realms of the Human Unconscious* (1975) and *The Holotropic Mind* (1992), have contributed to the steady rise of interest in the Holotropic Breathwork technique and transpersonal psychology.

Theory

Holotropic Breathwork is based on the premise that the psyche is a field of commingled personal and cosmic, or transpersonal, energy. Breath is more than a metaphor for the fluid continuum of personal and transpersonal energy. According to the Grofs, breath acts as a conduit for the energy, sustaining the mind as well as the body. In ordinary holotropic consciousness, one is aware of only a limited portion of the vast spectrum of energies being exchanged. The technique of Holotropic Breathwork is designed to accelerate breathing and at the same time greatly expand awareness of the transcendent forces pervading each moment of human life.

Faster and deeper breathing and music are used to bring about a trance state comparable to the state reached in Sufi dancing or Native American sweat-lodge rituals. The Grofs maintain that in this state it is possible to gain access to different kinds of consciousness experiences: sensory, biographical, perinatal (centered around the time of birth), and transpersonal. In the sensory experience, sight and sound become richer and more compelling. In biographical experiences, the individual accesses buried memories and feelings known as coex systems. Coex systems are systems of condensed experience that have been stored up since childhood and are regarded by some alternative health care professionals as the source of many health problems. In perinatal experiences, the individual relives her birth. This is considered the doorway to transpersonal experience, which corresponds to Jung's collective unconscious. Numinous experience floods the individual, boundaries of space and time are crossed, past life experiences reclaimed, myths and symbols may assume enhanced vitality, and visions of the future sometimes appear.

Grof refers to Holotropic Breathwork as "an adventure in self-discovery" rather than as a therapy or mystic rite. Its therapeutic value is thought to issue from the unblocking of conflicts and traumas stored in coex systems and from the enhancement of the individual's sense of inner potential.

Practice

Two-day workshops in Holotropic Breathwork are presented by facilitators certified by the Grofs. Participants are interviewed, then taught the principles and techniques. The sessions, which last from two to four hours, take place in a dimly lit room.

Participants work in pairs, alternating the roles of breather and sitter. As sitters, they watch over the breathers, providing a sense of shelter and support and attending to any needs the breather may have. As breathers, they lie flat on the floor and undergo a process that leads from relaxation exercises to an extended period of accelerated, deep breathing. Music is played at a high volume throughout the session and generally features little-known classical pieces, film scores, New Age music, Gregorian chants, aboriginal drumming, and other types of music associated with ritual and trance experience. If requested or required, the facilitators provide hands-on touch for the breather, applying pressure to areas of resistance and tension in order to aid in their release.

The breathers soon enter a trance in which consciousness is altered, not lost. The effects vary from individual to individual. Some grow still as if in deep meditation. Others see vivid images and become active, rocking, moaning, weeping, crying out in anger, expressing a sensation or feeling. Within a single session there may be a broad range of emotion from ecstatic rapture to abysmal despair. A breather does not necessarily experience all four categories of experience, and the experiences do not always progress in sequence from the sensory to

Certification at the Grof Transpersonal Training center requires 150 hours of general experience in Holotropic Breathwork, 350 hours of training combining theory and practice, and a final two-week seminar. The instruction focuses on breathwork techniques and correlated issues ranging from childhood sexual abuse to paranormal psychology and shamanism. The certification program takes at least two years to complete.

the transpersonal. Each time the role of breather is assumed, a different response is likely to occur. Usually participants breathe and sit two times each during the course of a workshop.

At the end of the session participants and facilitators work together to release unresolved tensions. Mandala drawing, which involves graphic and symbolic figures, concludes the session. The typical workshop in Holotropic Breathwork includes meditation, lectures, and group sharing.

Benefits and Risks

Holotropic Breathwork is a highly charged, sometimes strenuous experience precluded during pregnancy and for anyone with glaucoma, heart disease, or a severe emotional disorder. Participants report that they receive intuitive insights and clarify troublesome areas of their lives. Practitioners believe the technique promotes self-healing through the release of accumulated stress and trauma and greater connection with physical, emotional, and spiritual parts of oneself.

—KYLEA TAYLOR, M.S.

Resources

Association for Holotropic Breathwork International
P.O. Box 7169
Santa Cruz, CA 95061-7169
Web site: www.breathwork.com
Membership group that organizes conferences and publishes a quarterly newsletter, *The Inner Door,* with articles on Holotropic Breathwork research and practice.

East-West Retreats
P.O. Box 12
Philo, CA 95466
Tel: (707) 895-2856
Organizes Buddhist Vipassana/Holotropic Breathwork workshops.

Grof Transpersonal Training
20 Sunnyside, Suite A-253
Mill Valley, CA 94941
Tel: (415) 383-8779
Web site: www.holotropic.com
Trains and certifies practitioners of Holotropic Breathwork, provides referrals to certified practitioners, and publishes the Grofs' lecture and conference schedule.

Further Reading

Grof, Christina. *The Thirst for Wholeness.* San Francisco: HarperCollins Publishers, 1993.

Grof, Stanislav. *The Adventure of Self-Discovery: Dimensions of Consciousness and New Perspectives in Psychotherapy and Inner Exploration.* Stonybrook, N.Y.: SUNY Press, 1988.

———. *Realms of the Human Unconscious.* London: Souvenir Press Ltd., 1975.

Grof, Stanislav, and Hal Bennett. *The Holotropic Mind.* San Francisco: Harper San Francisco, 1992.

Scotton, Bruce, Allan Chinen, and John Battista, eds. *Textbook of Transpersonal Psychiatry and Psychology.* New York: HarperCollins Publishers, 1996.

Taylor, Kylea. *The Breathwork Experience.* Santa Cruz, Calif.: Hanford Mead Publishers, 1994.

———. *The Ethics of Caring.* Santa Cruz, Calif.: Hanford Mead Publishers, 1995.

Wilber, Kenneth. *The Spectrum of Consciousness.* Wheaton, Ill.: Theosophical Publications, 1977.

Medical Orgone Therapy

 Medical orgone therapy is a unique approach to treating emotional and physical illness by reducing or eliminating those barriers that block the natural expression of emotions and healthy sexual feelings. This method of treatment was developed by Austrian psychiatrist and scientist Wilhelm Reich, M.D. (1897–1957). After years of clinical and experimental laboratory research, Reich concluded that emotions, sexual feelings, and all life processes are expressions of a biological energy in the body. This life energy is related to bioelectricity but is fundamentally different. He called this energy "orgone energy." Reich theorized that orgone energy fills the universe and pulsates in all living things. He believed that deep, genuine love and the ability to experience a gratifying orgasm mutually with one's partner are the fullest and deepest expressions of our being and are central to maintaining optimal health.

Reich contended that in almost all individuals, the flow and release of orgone energy are blocked by chronic muscle contractions in various areas of the body and by emotional attitudes adopted early in life. The "good little girl" who never gets angry and the "strong, brave boy" who never shows fear or sadness are but two examples of such attitudes that prevent the full and rational expression of natural emotions. Blocked emotions interfere with pleasure in life and cause sexual feelings to become disconnected from tender emotions of love. Without emotional release, anxiety devel-ops, which further increases physical and emotional contraction. This cycle results in a range of problems such as feelings of emptiness, depression, irrational fears, and self-destructive behavior. Medical orgone therapy combines direct work on the body, especially on spastic muscles, with verbal therapy to bring about a healthy state accompanied by satisfaction in one's work and love life.

History

Wilhelm Reich began his career as a student and colleague of Sigmund Freud (1856–1939), founder of psychoanalysis. During his work as a psychoanalyst, Reich discovered that the individual's deep emotions were bound up in defensive character attitudes, which he called "character armor." To treat these problems, Reich developed a highly effective technique of character analysis, still used today by other psychotherapies, which focuses on the individual's attitudes and present-day concerns and less so on past relationships within the family.

While working with patients, Reich observed that only those who developed a satisfactory, healthy sexual life fully resolved their neurotic symptoms. Satisfaction was not determined by the mere presence of sexual activity. Rather, it required the ability to give in to both deep, tender, love feelings and the intense sexual sensations that are experienced with a total body orgasm. Reich asserted that this all-encompassing experience is possible only with a partner of the opposite sex, and concluded that only such a complete orgasm could regulate the energy metabolism.

Reich observed that defensive emotional attitudes are not just "in the mind" but are held in the body's muscles, and he called this the "muscular armor." He also found that inhibited feelings were accompanied by restrictions in respiration. These realizations led him to the groundbreaking conclusion that the successful treatment of emotional problems requires work on the body combined with verbal therapy.

Reich's theories about the link among sex, emotions, and the body, and his experimental work with orgone energy were very controversial. Legal action was taken against him by the U.S. Food and Drug Administration. He refused to defend his scientific work in a courtroom, believing the proper venue to challenge his research was the laboratory. He was found guilty of failing to obey an injunction and was jailed. He died in prison in 1957.

His ideas about sexuality have often been misunderstood. This was especially true during the sexual revolution of the 1960s and 1970s, when his name and ideas were associated with the notion that one can become "free" by having sex. In fact, Reich clearly stated that loveless sexuality was neurotic and, when harsh or mechanical, was unhealthy.

Elsworth F. Baker, M.D. (1903–1985), Reich's associate, continued Reich's work in the late 1950s, overseeing the training of medical orgonomists and orgone research. He founded the *Journal of Orgonomy* in 1967 and established the American College of Orgonomy in 1968. The college actively continues the development of the science of orgonomy, and its journal publishes clinical and scientific research.

Theory

Medical orgone therapy is based on Reich's theory of armoring and developed from observations on the movement and blockage of energy in the body. Infants and children naturally feel pleasure and reach out to the world. If these impulses are frustrated, the child contracts and develops methods to adapt to the stress. If frustrations continue, these defensive reactions become chronic and extend into adult life even when they are no longer needed. For example, a child may develop a submissive manner to deal with an angry parent and then as an adult react submissively to all authority figures, even when it would be better to be assertive. Other common examples of character armor are found in individuals who present themselves as aloof, superior, "cool," sophisticated, cute, or special. Medical orgonomists consider these character attitudes to be manifested in actual muscular rigidities (muscular armor), which hold back intolerable or unacceptable emotions such as anger, fear, or sadness. Individuals are usually unaware of their muscular armor or that their physical problems, such as headaches, stiff neck, or back pain, are often rooted in repressed emotions.

Armoring forms in infancy and early childhood as a defense against painful feelings, but it is not a satisfactory solution because it later interferes with healthy emotional life and energy discharge. Medical orgone therapy strives to eliminate chronic armor to restore the individual to more natural functioning in all aspects of life.

Practice

The medical orgonomist is trained to understand the patient in all respects and diagnose the patterns of character and physical armor. Because all medical orgone therapists are physicians who also have had specialized training in psychiatry, they are equipped to diagnose physical conditions and work directly on their patients. Treatment includes character analysis and the release of buried emotions facilitated by breathing and direct work on spastic muscles. The therapy does not focus much on psychological causes or delve deeply into past relationships with parents. It is also used to treat infants and children. The removal of early armoring allows the child to develop with a natural energy flow, emotional aliveness, and a sense of well-being. Treatment helps to prevent the development of chronic character and muscular armor in adult life.

It is important to note that the techniques used in this therapy are not the same as those in other methods used to address physical tension, such as acupressure, massage, and deep breathing. Character analysis also has its own specific techniques, which should not be confused with positive affirmations, guided self-examination, and similar therapeutic approaches.

In the *Journal of Orgonomy* (vol. 28, no. 1), Dr. Charles Konia describes a representative course of orgone therapy: "In medical orgone therapy, armor is intentionally dissolved. This invariably brings about anxiety, because the very function of the armor is to prevent the [individual] from experiencing such painful feelings. The medical orgonomist encourages the individual to experience and tolerate anxiety so that the underlying, contained emotions can be felt and then expressed. This brings about the desired, positive, therapeutic effect: anxiety is eliminated and replaced by a sense of pleasurable well-being."

Benefits

Medical orgone therapy is a unique approach to the prevention and treatment of a wide range of mental and physical conditions. Medical orgonomists report successful treatment of the full range of emotional symptoms and relationship problems. Serious conditions such as depression, schizophrenia, panic disorder, and attention deficit hyperactivity disorder can often be treated without resorting to medications. Reich concluded—and present-day physicians who practice medical orgone therapy concur—that the elimination of armoring, in and of itself, restores natural, healthy functioning. Patients regain their natural capacities to enjoy satisfaction in love, work, and the pursuit of knowledge.

—PETER A. CRIST, M.D.; AND RICHARD SCHWARTZMAN, D.O.

Resources

The American College of Orgonomy
P.O. Box 490
Princeton, NJ 08542
Tel: (732) 821-1144
Fax: (732) 821-0174
Web site: www.orgonomy.org
Trains and certifies medical orgonomists. Provides referrals and offers seminars, conferences, and laboratory courses that are open to the general public. Orgonomic Publications, a division of the American College of Orgonomy, sells numerous in-print and out-of-print books on the subject of orgonomy and publishes the biannual *Journal of Orgonomy*.

Further Reading

Books
Baker, Elsworth F. *Man in the Trap*. New York: The Macmillan Co., 1967.

Reich, Wilhelm. *Character Analysis*. Translated by Theodore P. Wolfe. 3rd ed. New York: Noonday Press, 1949.

———. *Children of the Future: On the Prevention of Sexual Pathology*. New York: Farrar, Straus, and Giroux, 1983.

———. *Cosmic Superimposition: Man's Orgonotic Roots in Nature*. Rangeley, Maine: Wilhelm Reich Foundation, 1951.

———. *The Discovery of the Orgone: Vol. 1, The Function of the Orgasm: Sex-Economic Problems of Biological Energy*. Translated by Theodore P. Wolfe. 2nd ed. New York: Orgone Institute Press, 1948.

———. *The Discovery of the Orgone: Vol. 2, The Cancer Biopathy*. Translated by Theodore P. Wolfe. New York: Orgone Institute Press, 1948.

———. *The Emotional Plague of Mankind: Vol. 1, The Murder of Christ*. New York: Orgone Institute Press, 1953.

———. *Reich Speaks of Freud*. New York: Farrar, Straus, and Giroux, 1967.

————. *Selected Writings: An Introduction to Orgonomy*. New York: Farrar, Straus, and Cudahy, 1960.

Sharaf, Myron. *Fury on Earth: A Biography of Wilhelm Reich*. New York: St. Martin's Press/Marek, 1983.

Journals

Konia, Charles. "Anxiety: Curse or Blessing?" *Journal of Orgonomy*, 28, no.1 (1994):1–3.

Numerous clinical and theoretical articles on medical orgone therapy have been published in the *Journal of Orgonomy* from 1967 to the present. A detailed and complete listing of these articles is available from the American College of Orgonomy.

Organismic Body Psychotherapy

 Organismic body psychotherapy was developed by Malcolm and Katherine Brown, based on their belief that the body, mind, and spirit are interconnected and that life-enhancing benefits can be realized using techniques that involve the body as well as the mind. The discipline is termed *neo-Reichian* because it incorporates ideas put forth by psychiatrist Wilhelm Reich, such as the concept of body armoring, but makes significant modifications to Reich's ideas. One of the most important modifications is the belief that releasing body armor does not have to be strong and highly emotional; rather, organismic body psychotherapy theory recognizes the possibility of a gradual, quiet release. Physical exercise, verbal dialogue, and touch are combined to bring about release and eventual physical, emotional, and spiritual well-being.

History

Malcolm Brown is a clinical psychologist who has been strongly influenced by a variety of therapeutic models, including Fritz Perls's and Kurt Goldstein's writings on gestalt therapy, Abraham Maslow's humanistic psychology, Carl Rogers's client-centered therapy, and Jungian psychology as developed by Carl Jung and Erich Neumann. The writings of Alexander Lowen in bioenergetics introduced Brown to the ideas of Wilhelm Reich and other body-oriented psychotherapists. Brown has worked with Alexander Lowen and European neo-Reichian psychotherapists, including Gerda Boyesan and David Boadella, who are known for developing a more subtle approach to Reich's work.

Katherine Brown is a therapist with a background in gestalt therapy, sensory awareness, and massage therapy. In 1972, after attending a lecture given by Malcolm Brown, she became interested in his theories and eventually began collaborating with him. They subsequently married and started working as cotherapists. Having coined the term *organismic body psychotherapy* for their work, they devoted the remainder of their professional pursuits exclusively to training psychotherapists in their methods. The Browns are now semiretired.

Basic Principles

Organismic body psychotherapy is designed to facilitate an increasing self-reliance on the human faculties, such as the abilities to sense, feel, think, and intuit, that lie within a person's body. The internal flowering of these faculties enables a client to become relatively self-trusting and to lead a rich life. To awaken these self-healing resources, organismic body psychotherapy techniques seek to engage the mental, emotional, and spiritual aspects of a client.

A key tenet of organismic body psychotherapy is that the body as well as the mind must be engaged in the therapeutic process because a client's psychological defenses are also manifested at the body level. This physical manifestation of a client's defenses is called armoring and consists of physical tensions that block emotion, feeling, and the ability to satisfy fundamental emotional needs. These needs include the ability to connect with others, the ability to connect to one's inner self, the ability to see the outer world and one's inner self objectively and make meaning of both, and the ability to fulfill personal goals.

There are three stages of growth in the therapeutic process: loosening the armoring, resolving psychological conflicts, and finally, growth combined with self-actualization. Using these stages as a guide, the therapist attempts to identify a client's current state and to adjust the therapeutic modality accordingly. The process begins with more of a therapist-directed style and gradually becomes more patient directed. Because organismic body psychotherapy is based on the idea that each individual is unique, it is believed that the unfolding and duration of each of these stages will be different for each individual.

Practice

Among the techniques used to dissolve the armoring are mobilization exercises and direct touch. Mobilization exercises are done with a client standing or lying on a padded mat. These exercises are designed to release chronic armoring patterns, which consist primarily of tense muscles. Direct touch is given by the therapist in two forms: nurturing and catalytic. Nurturing is a very soft form of touch used to soften armoring by mobilizing energy within the body, causing the release of armoring. Catalytic is a harder, more aggressive form of touch that releases the armoring. While doing the exercises or receiving direct touch, the client may experience expressive emotional releases, such as crying or screaming, which are a result of the loosening of the armoring.

While working with the body is an elemental aspect of organismic body psychotherapy, sessions are not entirely nonverbal. Discussion of emotional releases, dreams, or insight also plays an important role in the organismic body psychotherapy process.

Benefits

When applied properly, direct touch seems to increase a client's awareness of his primary need to feel connected and related that often has been unsatisfied since early childhood. Moreover, direct touch seems to accomplish this without creating overwhelming anxiety or hardening a client's defenses. Once the armoring has been loosened and healing has occurred through the resolution of psychological conflicts, practitioners of organismic body psychotherapy believe that a person's resources and faculties are accessible for development of the soul.

—ELLIOT GREENE

Resources

Washington Institute for Body Psychotherapy
   Elliot Greene and Barbara Goodrich-Dunn, Directors
   8830 Cameron St., Suite 206
   Silver Spring, MD 20910
   Tel: (301) 588-9341
   Offers a four-year training program in body psychotherapy and workshops on subjects related to body psychotherapy.

Further Reading

Brown, Malcolm. *The Healing Touch*. Mendocino, Calif.: Life Rhythm Press.

Pesso Boyden System Psychomotor

 Pesso Boyden system psychomotor (PBSP) therapy uses group therapy to help patients recall, encounter, and ultimately rebuild in a positive way their reactions to past events. The *psycho* in psychomotor refers to the psyche, or the mind. *Motor* refers to bodily sensations and movements, which include actions that may be blocked in the body by trauma. Through group role-playing activities called structures, PBSP patients relive long-past memories and emotions that have saddled them with traumatizing feelings of dissatisfaction. With the guidance of the therapist and the assistance of the group, the patient undergoes emotional "re-education": the truthful recollection of a painful event with a convincing reenactment of a happier conclusion.

History and Basic Principles

PBSP is based on the studies of Albert Pesso and Diane Boyden-Pesso, classically trained dancers and choreographers who, in the late 1950s, developed their own style of expressive dance. Much of their new style focused on the development of emotional and physical tools that could convincingly communicate internal feelings, visions, and ideas to an audience.

This research led Albert Pesso, in the early 1960s, to publish an essay that placed all movement into three categories: reflex, voluntary, and emotional. Reflex movement includes the reflex that keeps our bodies upright. Voluntary movement is oriented to our environment, that is, those movements that we consciously initiate in order to manipulate and move through the world around us. By contrast, emotional movement includes any movement initiated by our reaction to our inner feelings and how we feel about the environment around us.

These three types of movement are inextricably interwoven. We can voluntarily alter or stop many reflex actions for short periods of time. Similarly, strong emotions can have a marked impact on our voluntary and reflex motions.

Albert Pesso and Diane Boyden-Pesso were not the first researchers to envision such a breakdown of the patterns of movement. Their work built on the established system of French acting and singing teacher François Delsarte (1811–1871), who formulated specific principles of aesthetics based on a set of rules coordinating the voice with body gestures. As the couple continued to develop their style of expressive dance, they began to incorporate more and more exercises aimed at sharpening awareness of the three types of movement into their dance training programs. They found that a dance student, once made sensitive to these three types of movement, could eliminate unwanted and unpredictable motions from her performance by giving them their proper and therapeutic expression. Furthermore, students reported that having full mastery of all three types of movement seemed to allow a more open and healthy expression of their needs in their everyday lives.

Pesso and Boyden-Pesso soon theorized that these same exercises could help emotionally troubled people overcome their problems. To them, a person's emotions stored in the body represent the nearest thing to a true self. Most psychological problems, they believe, can be attributed to the absence and repression of the body's interactive needs that had not been met by the participant's parents. These needs and hungers change the way people look at the world. Depending on the nature of the unfulfilled need, the effect from these unconscious hungers can range from occasional depression to total physical and emotional debilitation on the part of the sufferer.

PBSP tracks down clues to these hidden feelings and seeks to bring expression and healing to the damage they have caused. A patient first meets with a psychotherapist for an observation session, during which the therapist formulates some idea of what might be the underlying root cause of the patient's neuroses or problems. Diane Boyden-Pesso explains, "My goal as a therapist is to make sure that the client works in [PBSP] from where he really is, what is really important and real, and not work on something that he or she may have decided in advance intellectually that it would be good to work on. We have to work on what is valid and spontaneous at the moment."

Practice

In a safe, respectful setting, the PBSP therapist supplies the natural, comprehensive, and carefully crafted technology that uses the resources of the body, mind, and soul to help people complete the five crucial life tasks necessary for intellectual, psychological, emotional, and spiritual well-being. Those life tasks are:

1. Satisfy the basic developmental needs for place, nurture, support, protection, limits, and experience needed by our human nature to fully mature and bear fruit.
2. Integrate and unify the polarities of our biological and psychological being—to own all parts of our body and mind.
3. Develop our consciousness—know that and why we are alive.
4. Develop our self-organizing center, or "pilot"—be in command of our own lives.
5. Realize our personal uniqueness and potential—find our calling and become who we truly can be.

The primary tool of PBSP is a group role-playing activity, called structures, comprised of a seamless series of steps (individually known as a structure) within the total structure. Within a carefully controlled group session the therapist encourages the patient to share what is upsetting him in the present.

To this scene, however, two important characters are added: the "truth stater" and the "witness." The truth stater is used to externalize and illustrate the participant's spoken thoughts and beliefs by stating out loud the "truths" by which the participant lives. If the participant says, "I have to take care of myself because there is no one in the world who will do that for me," the truth stater is instructed to announce, "You have to take care of yourself because there is no one in the world who will do that for you."

Meanwhile, the witness is used to track the emotional reactions of the participant as the therapist queries the participant on what he thinks he is feeling. Witnesses also validate the participant's emotional expressions, naming each emotion and the context of the emotion in a compassionate, accepting manner. A typical statement might be, "I see how bitter you feel as you hear that statement."

The input of the two special accommodators induces a participant to recognizing these current feelings as part of a pattern of behavior from his past. Participants can then see these patterns of dysfunction as a result of past life-shaping events. Memories evoked by these structures are powerful and experienced almost as if they were happening in the present. The participant is thus in the dual position of "reliving" a vivid memory while at the same time becoming aware of himself from a therapeutic perspective. Finally, the patient can express the suppressed longings that were left unfulfilled, such as the isolation and self-loathing that can arise from desertion by a parent. Although absorbed with this memory, the participant is nonetheless able to use his newfound awareness of emotions, body sensations, and impulses to express what he is experiencing.

Once the patient feels thoroughly reimmersed in the recollection, he instructs the other members of the group, called accommodators, to positions and roles that reenact the event as it occurred. Accommodators play the antithesis role of whichever person has denied the patient his specific need. They are meant to provide the ideal role or figure in order for participants to meet the needs that were not met by history. In the above example, the ideal figure would play the role of a new, alternative parent who has deserted the patient. In this scenario, however, the new parent offers clear, positive accommodation to the person, such as "If I had been there, I would not have left you."

Although the activity occurs in the group session, the final and most meaningful locus of reconstruction takes place in the inner theater of the mind. Through this emotional re-education, the participant has gotten in contact with his needs, feeling them again, and then has these needs met by this new positive figure in a way that leaves an imprint in the body-mind memory of the participant. The memory can then be recalled at will by the participant to reinforce the positive experience. This is a step toward final maturity. Through this the participant has abandoned the hope of having his needs redressed by the original person. Instead, he has the need satisfied while he is in touch with the right age by someone representing the ideal mother or father, whichever is needed. The participant has taken an important step toward healing.

PBSP is considered a psychoanalytic process, a behavior modification process, a reparenting process, a gestalt process, a body therapy process, a family therapy process (without the family), and more. It contains so much that is fundamental to all forms of psychotherapy that it relates easily to all major techniques used to treat emotional and mental problems.

Benefits

PBSP gives participants a positive lens through which to see and experience the world. Following PBSP therapy, they are less likely to be ruled by habitual, emotional reactions such as displaced anger, anxiety, depression, and emotionally immature desires.

Clients can function more productively in the reality of present-day settings.

Therapists use PBSP, in groups and one-on-one, with a wide variety of populations. It is successfully used in psychiatric settings, drug and alcohol treatment centers, pain clinics, and obesity treatment programs. The therapy is effective with victims of abuse, incest, and adolescents having trouble with their emotions, the law, and drugs. It has significant value in application to marriage and family problems and is now being used to alleviate executive stress and to deal with other organizational problems.

PBSP is a safe procedure that puts a high emphasis on the comfort of its patients. Nevertheless, it involves complex psychological evaluation that is best handled by professionals. Anyone interested in PBSP therapy should consult a trained PBSP psychotherapist or PBSP institution.

—*Albert Pesso*

Resource

Pesso Boyden System Psychomotor
   Strolling Woods
   Lake Shore Drive
   Franklin, NH 03235
   Tel: (603) 934-9809
   Web site: www.pbsp.com
   Provides information on practitioners as well as the discipline.

Further Reading

Books

Napier, Augustus Y. *The Fragile Bond: In Search of an Equal, Intimate, and Enduring Marriage.* New York: HarperCollins, 1990.
Pesso, Albert. *Experience in Action.* New York: New York University Press, 1973.
———. *Movement in Psychotherapy.* New York: New York University Press, 1969.
———. *Moving Psychotherapy.* Cambridge, Mass.: Brookline Books, 1991.

Journals

Foulds, Melvin, and Patricia S. Hannigan. "Effects of Psychomotor Group Therapy on Ratings of Self and Others." *Psychotherapy: Theory, Research, and Practice,* 2, no. 4 (Winter 1974).

———. "Effects of Psychomotor Group Therapy on Locus of Control and Social Desirability," *Humanistic Psychology,* 16, no. 2 (Spring 1975).

Process-Oriented Psychology

 Process-oriented psychology, or simply process work, is a form of psychotherapy used to help a person become aware of and embrace all aspects of her experience, even those that at first seem too disturbing, strange, or socially unacceptable. The disturbing or traumatic experiences that we cannot accept tend to reappear as dreams, physical symptoms, relationship difficulties, or conflicts with society. A process oriented psychologist, believing that all experience is meaningful, helps a client approach the disturbing experience and explore its connection to current physical and emotional problems. Treating a disturbing experience with love and understanding may help one find a solution.

History and Theory

Process-oriented psychology was founded by the American Jungian analyst Arnold Mindell, who developed methods to help couples and families explore disturbing experiences and worked with a wide variety of individuals not usually treated with psychotherapy. These techniques later became a part of Mindell's work with groups and organizations that were troubled by conflict.

He found that groups, when faced with situations and individuals that challenge their purpose and unity, behave much like troubled individuals. By encouraging silent voices to speak and allowing other members to experience what it feels like to occupy unpopular roles, he helped the majority of the group assimilate new points of view, often leading to unique solutions. Mindell developed these methods into *world work,* a body of theory and practice for working with groups in conflict, even when they contain people from different ethnic and racial groups, socioeconomic classes, sexual orientations, and spiritual affiliations.

At the heart of Mindell's work is the belief that a mysterious, often irrational, and nonverbal current of subjective experience, which he calls the dreaming process, flows alongside each person's conscious, objective, intentional activities of everyday life, leading a person to experience things that conflict with their self-image. When a person puts aside such a disturbing experience, the dreaming process continues to express itself as physical symptoms, relationship difficulties, or conflicts with society. Mindell believes the experiences with which a person least identifies consciously have the most power to produce change and restore the flow of the dreaming process. Because these experiences challenge our personal or collective identities, he believes we stop them from completing themselves, fearing the inner or outer conflict they might produce. By focusing awareness on these experiences and encouraging them to unfold, process-oriented psychology aims to help people find solutions to current problems and to tap into a source for continued personal growth.

Practice

Process work is most frequently practiced as a form of individual psychotherapy. A client typically visits her therapist for an hour-long session. A course of therapy may consist of one session or may last for many years. The client may present a dream, a relationship difficulty, a physical symptom, or any other experience she would like to explore. The process worker focuses on the client's subjective experiences of her concerns and problems, observing movement, body posture, and language. To help identify, clarify, and learn from aspects of the client's subjective experience, the process worker employs a wide array of techniques, some of which are drawn from psychodrama, and art and dance therapy. A therapist may also employ bodywork techniques, including massaging or gently vibrating the client's body to help raise awareness of her physical sensations.

While process workers deal with a broad spectrum of human experiences, it is an adjunct, not a substitute, for medical or psychiatric treatment by a qualified physician or psychiatrist.

—DR. JOSEPH GOODBREAD

Resources

Process Work Center of Portland
2049 N.W. Hoyt
Portland, OR 97209
Tel: (503) 223-8188
Fax: (503) 227-7003
e-mail: pwcp@igc.apc.org
Web site: www.processwork.org
Provides information on process work therapy, seminars, and training.

Further Reading

Books

Goodbread, Joseph, *The Dreambody Toolkit: A Practical Introduction to the Philosophy, Goals, and Practice of Process-Oriented Psychology.* Portland, Ore.: Lao Tse Press, 1997.

Mindell, Arnold, and Amy Mindell. *Riding the Horse Backwards: Process Work in Theory and Practice.* London: Penguin Arkana, 1992.

Journals

The Journal of Process Oriented Psychology, published since 1992 by the Lao Tse Press (Web site: www.lao-tse-press.com), keeps the reader up to date on the latest research and developments in process work.

Psychodrama

Psychodrama is a method for exploring problems by improvisationally enacting them as if in a play. In addition to its being a form of psychotherapy—the process of treating patients by psychological means—psychodrama is often applied in role playing, one of psychodrama's derivatives, to deal with a wide range of situations in education, business, or community relations.

History

Psychodrama was developed by psychiatrist Jacob Levi Moreno, M.D. (1889–1974). Moreno saw a need for spontaneity and creativity in social relations and began developing practical methods to address this need. In 1921, as an avocational interest, he formed perhaps the first modern improvisational dramatic troupe, the Theatre of Spontaneity. Through this group Moreno discovered that the process of improvised role playing seemed to help the actors deal with personal problems; this was the beginning of psychodrama. Moreno then emigrated to the United States in 1925, and later, in 1936, established a psychiatric sanitarium about 60 miles north of New York City. For the rest of his life, in addition to developing his method of psychodrama, Moreno was also a major pioneer of group psychotherapy, as well as of social role theory, and "sociometry," a method for applied social psychology.

Theory

All of Moreno's approaches to understanding and helping people are aimed at the goal of furthering people's creativity. Moreno believed many of humanity's social and psychological problems arose out of people's tendencies to rely excessively on what others had previously created instead of themselves taking on the challenge of creating anew. He also declared that a truly holistic learning and experimental process required involvement through action, similar to the training of astronauts through the use of simulators. In his emphasis on dramatic, physical action, he ran counter to those tendencies in psychotherapy that constrain the process to verbal modes of interaction.

One of Moreno's major insights is that creativity emerges most effectively through spontaneity. Spontaneity isn't mere impulsivity, but rather improvisation, whereby one becomes gradually more involved and allows the insights to emerge. It involves some aim at finding a new solution or a fresh approach to problems, and includes a measure of rationality associated with intuition and feeling. Related to this was Moreno's view—based on his observations—that the best way to promote spontaneity and creativity in interpersonal problem solving was through the use of improvised drama. Instead of engaging in the type of theater that requires actors to memorize and rehearse scripts, psychodrama involves the participants improvising scenes based on themes that they themselves feel are relevant to their lives.

At times the term *psychodrama* has been used inaccurately to describe any psychologically laden piece of theater, literature, or news event. But people in those situations generally play out their parts without exploring other alternatives to the situation being enacted. Psychodrama involves consciously and intentionally pausing and reflecting on one's attitudes and behaviors toward situations or people rather than merely plunging ahead without reflection, which could compound the problem. It may be thought of as a kind of laboratory for examining psychological and social issues in depth. The primary goal is to help people become more creative in their lives. Psychodrama achieves this through structured improvisation and by having the person whose problem is being enacted play the role not only of the main character, but also of other characters in the drama or of the director. This allows the person to participate in discovering new understandings and more effective coping strategies.

Psychodrama offers a rich variety of techniques, many of which have been integrated into other forms of therapy. For example, the idea of talking to someone imagined to be sitting in an empty chair has been used in Fritz Perls's gestalt therapy. Family therapy transformed a psychodramatic technique of setting up family members as if they were a diorama representing the emotional relationships into what is known as "family sculpture." Role playing is now commonly used in assertiveness training or social skills classes. Other psychodrama warm-up techniques, such as structured experiences, action techniques, and nonverbal games, have come to be used widely in group psychotherapy, personal-growth programs, and self-help groups.

Practice

Psychodramas involve five elements:

1. The director (who often is also the therapist), who facilitates the process.
2. The protagonist, whose problem is being explored.
3. Auxiliaries, members of the group who play supporting roles in the enactment.
4. The stage, a special area in which the scene is enacted.
5. The audience, composed of the rest of the group.

The procedure begins with a warm-up, a five- to fifteen-minute general discussion in

To become a certified director, a psychodramatist must obtain both professional training as a psychotherapist and subspecialty training involving hundreds of hours of supervised personal involvement. Psychodrama as a subspecialty of psychotherapy should be differentiated from drama therapy. The latter is one of the creative arts therapies and involves the use of theater itself as an aid to healing. However, in the last decade there have been increasing areas of overlap.

which issues are brought into focus and the level of trust in the group is strengthened. Sometimes structured exercises, like theater games, are used to stimulate the imagination, promote self-disclosure, and allow everyone to share an experience.

The protagonist is chosen and the problem is then presented, usually by having the protagonist show instead of explain the situation. The protagonist's underlying assumptions, which in part cause the problem, are brought into more explicit awareness using various dramatic devices, such as doubling, asides, or soliloquies. Also, in order to appreciate the predicament of the other roles in the enactment, the director has the protagonist switch parts and then take on the challenge of responding to the interpersonal tension from that other person's viewpoint. This technique of role reversal is one of the most powerful ways to expand the imagination, cultivate empathy, and reduce tendencies toward egocentricity. The action proceeds often through a series of several scenes, including subscenes, in which the protagonist can step out of role and reflect on his attitudes and behavior. This phase generally requires about twenty to forty-five minutes.

Finally, the session closes with a period of sharing, in which the members of the audience say how the enactment relates to their own lives. Because psychodramas are at times very emotional, the sharing itself often involves an opportunity for the expression of the evoked feelings in the audience, a catharsis that further supports and encourages the protagonist. A group that experiences a series of these psychodramas seems to build a trust that allows more unconscious material to emerge and be processed.

Benefits and Limitations

The benefits of psychodrama are manifold: shifting roles seems to help develop empathy and greater flexibility in thinking. Improvisation appears to foster a trust of the healthy parts of the mind, especially the creative imagery flowing from the subconscious. The physical movement and direct encounter in enactments bypass the mind's language-based avoidances and thus lead to a deep form of insight.

Psychodramatic methods seem to help improve participants' communication and problem-solving skills and enhance self-awareness. Thus, they may be applied in nontherapeutic contexts, such as schools, professional training, business, religious education, community building, and other settings. However, the participants in a psychodrama must have some degree of mental coherency; they cannot be in states of intoxication, delirium, or psychotic confusion. But in modified form, and applied with reasonable judgment, role-playing methods have been used with patients who are mentally retarded or suffering from delusions, and others who might be inaccessible to ordinary "talk" methods of therapy.

—ADAM BLATNER, M.D.

Resources

The American Board of Examiners in
Psychodrama, Sociometry, and Group
   Psychotherapy
   P.O. Box 15572
   Washington, DC 20003-0572
   Tel: (202) 483-0514
   Information about training and names and
   addresses of certified directors may be ob-
   tained upon written request.

The American Society for Group Psychotherapy
and Psychodrama (ASGPP)
   301 N. Harrison St., Suite 508
   Princeton, NJ 08540
   Tel: (609) 452-1339
   Fax: (609) 936-1659
   Information about regional and national conferences, newsletters, and professional journals may be obtained upon written request.

National Coalition of Arts Therapies Associations
   2000 Century Plaza, Suite 108
   Columbia, MD 21044
   Tel: (410) 997-4040
   Fax: (410) 997-4048
   This is an alliance of professional associa-
   tions that promote the therapeutic nature of
   the arts.

Further Reading

Books

Blatner, Adam. *Acting-In: Practical Applications of Psychodramatic Methods.* 3rd ed. New York: Springer, 1996.

————. "Psychodrama." In *Current Psychotherapies*, edited by R. J. Corsini and D. Wedding. 5th ed. Itasca, Ill.: Peacock, 1995.

Blatner, Adam, and Allee Blatner. *The Art of Play: An Adult's Guide to Reclaiming Imagination and Spontaneity.* Bristol, Pa.: Brunner/Mazel, 1997.

————. *Foundations of Psychodrama: History, Theory, and Practice.* New York: Springer, 1988.

Corey, G. "Psychodrama." In *Theory and Practice of Group Counseling.* 4th ed. Pacific Grove, Calif.: Brooks/Cole, 1994.

Fox, J., ed. *The Essential Moreno: Writings on Psychodrama, Group Method, and Spontaneity.* New York: Springer, 1987.

Holmes, P., M. Karp, and M. Watson, eds. *Psychodrama Since Moreno: Innovations in Theory and Practice.* New York: Tavistock/Routledge, 1994.

Moreno, J. L. *Psychodrama.* Beacon, N.Y.: Beacon House, vol. 1, 1946; with Zerka T. Moreno, vol. 2, 1959; and vol. 3, 1969.

Journals

Blatner, A. "Psychodrama: The State of the Art." *The Arts in Psychotherapy* 24, no. 1 (1997): 23–30.

Journal of Group Psychotherapy, Psychodrama and Sociometry. Heldref, 1318 18th St., Washington, DC 20006.

Psychosynthesis

 Psychosynthesis is a theory of mind used to help a person realize his inner wisdom. There exists within each person a "higher self" that is a source of guidance, value, and creativity. It is the basis of a form of therapy that, through various methods, attempts to bring participants to a greater understanding of themselves. They are encouraged to access their higher selves to help solve problems and make decisions.

History

Psychosynthesis was first developed by Roberto Assagioli (1888–1974). A colleague of Sigmund Freud and Carl Jung, Assagioli was the first person to practice psychoanalysis in Italy. In 1910 he left the psychoanalytic movement because he felt its view of human nature was too limited. He objected to the standardization of ideas and techniques, believing there should be an individual method for each person.

He began to develop his own spiritual model of human development and opened an institute in 1927 in Rome. He chose the term *psychosynthesis* to give a name to the impulse in each person to develop, learn, and evolve. His early work ended in 1940, when he was arrested as a pacifist and jailed by Mussolini's fascist government. After his release, he lived under police surveillance. In 1943 he was persecuted by the Nazis and was forced into hiding. His institute was reopened in 1951 at his home in Florence. There he saw patients and trained professionals until his death in 1974. His work is now continued at more than one hundred psychosynthesis institutes around the world.

Theory

Assagioli's theory of the unconscious deviated from that of many of his contemporaries in psychoanalysis. While others saw unconscious motivation as a collection of base, biological needs, Assagioli claimed that the unconscious also encompasses nobler impulses, such as love, ethics, and creativity. He believed that repressing either impulse could be harmful. In his view therapy should help foster these higher instincts.

The hidden source of wisdom and guidance within each person is considered that person's higher self. The higher self, although part of a person's nature, is different from one's personality. While an individual's personality makes him unique, the higher self is concerned with universal values, such as compassion, truth, and life purpose. The higher self may be considered a part of the brain or mind, although it is just as often experienced in the body. The goal of psychosynthesis is to explore and utilize the concealed resources of human thought.

Practice

A person may experience psychosynthesis therapy individually or within a group. At the start of each session, participants are encouraged to talk about their problems with a therapist or with the group. As a person proceeds to express his thoughts or emotions, the therapist may intervene to help him clarify a particular image or memory. According to psychosynthesis, people can overcome conventional ways of viewing their problems when they are able to access the insight within their imaginations. A therapist may draw from a variety of techniques to help a person enter his imagination. The therapist begins by helping the person to relax and withdraw his attention from the outer environment and concentrate inward. A therapist will then use guided imagery techniques to help a client enter his imagination and focus on a particular thought, feeling, or sensation. Finally, the therapist will ask this person to express these images. Depending on what method works best, a therapist may help evoke these images through visual art, movement, music, analysis, personality study, traditional psychotherapeutic techniques, maps of consciousness, and many other methods. In accordance with Assagioli's theory, the techniques used in a session will vary with each therapist.

Benefits

The higher self is a crucial part of psychosynthesis therapy. Therapy is not intended to develop the higher self, because it is thought to already exist in each person. Psychosynthesis therapy is used to acquaint people with the resources of their higher selves and equip them with the ability to approach problems imaginatively and to better understand themselves. The therapist's role is to help a person gain the inner skills to become aware of his higher self.

—RICHARD SCHAUB, PH.D.

Resources

International Association for Managerial and
Organizational Psychosynthesis
  3308 Radcliffe Road
  Thousand Oaks, CA 91360
  Tel: (805) 942-4815
  Disseminates information on
  psychosynthesis.

New York Psychosynthesis Institute
  2 Murray Court
  Huntington, NY 11743
  Tel: (516) 673-0293
  Provides information and promotes the prac-
  tice of psychosynthesis in the New York area.

Synthesis Center for Psychosynthesis
Distributions
  P.O. Box 575
  Amherst, MA 01004
  Tel: (413) 256-0772
  Offers resources and information regarding
  psychosynthesis.

Further Reading

Assagioli, Roberto. *Psychosynthesis: A Manual of
    Principles and Techniques.* New York: The
    Viking Press, 1971.
———. *Transpersonal Development.* New York:
    HarperCollins, 1991.
Ferrucci, Piero. *What We May Be.* Los Angeles:
    Tarcher, 1982.
Schaub, B., and R. Schaub. *Healing Addictions.* Al-
    bany, N.Y.: Delmar, 1997.
Whitmore, Diana. *Psychosynthesis: Counseling in
    Action.* London: Sage Publications, 1991.

Radix

 Radix teaches students to become conscious of an invisible
life force ("radix") and to restore
its natural pulsation in their
bodies. This requires confronting and changing acquired patterns of breathing and muscular tension that block a person's emotions.
By getting in touch with the physical sensations flowing through their bodies and the
emotions linked to those sensations, Radix
students seek to gain better control over their
life forces and physical defenses and to develop greater capacity for choice.

Dr. Charles R. (Chuck) Kelley founded
the Interscience Research Institute in 1960.
He changed its name to the Radix Institute
in 1974 after he coined the term *radix* to describe his unique concept of the life force. He
reserved the capitalized term *Radix* for the
personal growth program that he developed
with the help of his wife, Erica. He and Erica
began their first bodywork programs in 1970
and ran worldwide training and teaching facilities in southern California until 1987,
when Charles Kelley retired and broke from
the Radix Institute. The Kelleys now practice
in Vancouver, Washington, and Charles Kelley offers training tutorials and supervision
by arrangement. Others now use the Radix
name worldwide for their own work and
training. They are not associated with or en-
dorsed by Kelley unless they display a certificate signed by him.

Kelley was influenced by the psychoanalyst and founder of medical orgonomy, Wilhelm Reich, who believed that people
develop physical defenses against emotions
they consider unacceptable. People build defenses early in life by selectively tightening
muscles and holding their breath in different
ways to inhibit the expression of particular
emotions. This gradually forms the patterns
of tension Reich called muscular armor.
Over time these inhibiting behaviors become
anchored in the bodily structure. They block

feelings, interfere with thinking, and may contribute to chronic disease and emotional difficulties. Nevertheless, Kelley believes that the muscular armor is not a negative attribute, because it is the mechanism of voluntary attention and basis of the will. We need it in order to function effectively as human beings. Radix work aims to help people learn how to use their muscular armor without unconsciously becoming its victim.

Radix teachers work with inhibitions to breathing, with the muscular armor, and with the mental attitudes that support them. They use suggestions, direct body contact, and exercises for loosening tensions and freeing feelings. Clients learn to develop a structure of muscular tensions that contains emotions and forms personal boundaries, resulting in a more effective, flexible type of muscular armor. Most sessions include work with the student lying supine on a mat, clad in shorts or bathing suit, with the teacher kneeling alongside. This enables the teacher to observe skin color—an indicator of the degree of radix charge and flow in the body—and to observe breathing and patterns of muscle tension or flaccidity. A student may stand up for "grounding" exercises that are used to develop a sense of the relationship between the feet and the ground. A student may also stand to perform exercises that help release anger. A student may also sit face-to-face with the teacher to discuss a problem or emotional issue.

There are a variety of Radix programs reflecting the style of the teacher and needs of the student. Many students choose a mix of individual and group sessions. Group sessions are usually small and include periods of individual interaction with the teacher. A typical individual program lasts for fifty minutes on a weekly basis, but other arrangements are often made, including concentrated programs of up to ten sessions within five days.

—ERICA KELLEY

Resources

Kelley/Radix
    Chuck and Erica Kelley
    13715 S.E. 36th St.
    Vancouver, WA 98683-7770
    Tel/fax: (360) 896-4004
    e-mail: Kelley6@ix.netcom.com
    Provides information on Radix, as well as promoting the practice.

Further Reading

Bar-Levav, Reuven. *Thinking in the Shadow of Feelings.* New York: Simon & Schuster, 1988.

Branden, Nathaniel. *Taking Responsibility: Self-Reliance and the Accountable Life.* New York: Simon & Schuster, 1996.

Kelley, Charles R. *The Radix, Vol. I: Personal Growth Work,* and *Vol. II: The Science of Radix Processes.* (Compilation of articles from the 1960s to the 1990s. Also published in Spanish.) Vancouver, Wash.: K/R Publications, 1992.

Reich, Wilhelm. "The Expressive Language of Living in Orgone Therapy." In *Character Analysis.* 3rd ed. New York: Orgone Institute Press, 1949. (Reissued by Farrar, Straus, and Giroux.)

Rebirthing

 Rebirthing is a gentle, meditative breathing technique. Advocates of this therapy believe it enables an individual to become more aware of thought and behavior patterns that may prevent her from enjoying life to the fullest. In this way, those who practice rebirthing reduce limiting psychological and emotional conditions, increase the vital transfer of oxygen to the organs and cells, and release deep-seated tensions from the body, thereby increasing physical comfort.

History

Leonard Orr developed the process in California in the 1970s. Submerging himself in a hot tub, he achieved a relaxed mental and physical state that he said stimulated memories of being in the womb, prior to birth. Orr viewed rebirthing as a therapy for releasing the trauma associated with the birth process and our first breaths as infants. He believes coming to terms with that trauma is the first step in resolving buried emotional and psychological issues. After introducing others to rebirthing, Orr observed that the pattern and quality of breathing attained during the sessions, characterized by a continuous cycle of inhalation and exhalation flowing deeply and fluidly through the mouth, remained constant regardless of who participated. By comparison, normal breathing has a pause between one breath and the next. Orr also noted that the same quality of breathing could remain effective for individuals even out of the water. Currently, the most popular version of rebirthing is the "dry" method, which does not require being submerged in water.

Basic Principles

Proper breathing can produce changes in a person's clarity of thinking and physical state. Controlled breathing has been used for centuries—often in conjunction with meditation—to achieve high levels of calmness and peace. Deep, even breathing has the natural tendency to slow the heartbeat as well as the flow of thoughts. Proper breathing also increases the flow of oxygen throughout the body, which is essential to the smooth functioning of cells and organs and the body as a whole. In fact, the body rids itself of 70 percent of its toxins and other body wastes through respiration.

Rebirthing utilizes breathing techniques to achieve maximum physical and emotional health. Rebirthers (rebirthing practitioners) use these techniques to shed tensions and foster a tranquil mental state. This in turn allows the body rest and recuperation, and the mind a period of clear thinking to sort through complex or long-buried emotional issues. Rebirthing also relies on the use of positive affirmation, the planting of new thoughts in a person's consciousness to replace negative thought patterns that affect behavior. Destructive patterns are viewed as stemming from the birth trauma and from later life experiences, all of which can be locked into the tissues and cells of the body and can prove harmful if not released. Rebirthing seeks to release trauma from the body and support increased well-being.

Practice

Individuals are advised to seek the guidance of a rebirther who has enough training and experience to provide safety and support during the first several sessions. A person should ask a prospective rebirther about the extent of his training and the number of his rebirthing experiences. A series of ten sessions with the same rebirther is recommended. The continuity and trust generated by this relationship is believed to accelerate the progress of healing.

The rebirther begins by asking the individual about her life. Together they look for patterns and habits that the client seeks to change or eliminate. They jointly identify positive thoughts that will help begin this change. This period of discussion is followed by a period of physical relaxation and breathing exercises, guided by the rebirther. The individual lies on a mat or pad on the floor. During this stage the breath slows, allowing tension to dissolve from the body. This results in a state of relaxation during which the individual consciously or subconsciously addresses her concerns. Review of traumatic life experiences may result in discomfort when feelings and long-suppressed thoughts resurface. At the end of a session, thoughts and feelings as well as questions can be shared with the rebirther.

The rebirther may also offer some suggestions or affirmations to focus on until the next appointment. The recommended session length is one to two hours.

Benefits

Throughout life people experience stress, frustration, anger, and worry, which, if not dispersed, can affect their physical and emotional health. Advocates of rebirthing say that their therapy allows the body to recuperate by teaching individuals to breathe in a way that promotes physical and emotional well-being. In addition, rebirthers assert that by upgrading the quality of thoughts while in a deep-breathing mode, quality of life also improves, thus producing greater health, improved relationships, self-esteem, and prosperity. Furthermore, by devoting time to the examination of buried emotional and psychological matters while in a relaxed physical and mental state, people are able to address deep-seated issues that affect behavior and thought patterns and make positive changes in their lives.

—MAUREEN MALONE AND TONY LO MASTRO

Resources

Inspiration University
   P.O. Box 1026
   Staunton, VA 24402
   Source of rebirthing books, audiotapes, and videos.

Loving Relationships Training (LRT)
International
   c/o Clarity Productions
   P.O. Box 160
   Manhattan Beach, CA 90267
   Tel: 1-800-468-5578
   Offers rebirthing seminars, training, certification, and books on related subjects.

The New York Rebirthing Center
   205 E. 95th St., Suite 23A
   New York, NY 10128
   Tel/fax: (212) 534-2969
   Coordinates rebirthing seminars, group rebirths, and similar activities and provides a list of rebirthers in the area.

The Philadelphia Rebirthing Center
   1027 69th Ave.
   Philadelphia, PA 19126
   Tel: (215) 424-4444
   e-mail: tlomas@netreach.net
   Web site: www.philadelphiarebirthing.com
   Coordinates rebirthing seminars, group rebirths, and similar activities and provides a list of rebirthers in the area.

Further Reading

Morningstar, Jim. *Breathing in Light and Love.* Milwaukee: Transformations, 1994.

Orr, Leonard, and Sondra Ray. *Rebirthing in the New Age.* Berkeley, Calif.: Celestial Arts, 1977.

Ray, Sondra. *Celebration of Breath.* Berkeley, Calif.: Celestial Arts, 1983.

———. *Loving Relationships.* Berkeley, Calif.: Celestial Arts, 1983.

Sisson, Colin. *Rebirthing Made Easy.* New Zealand: Total Press, 1989.

Rubenfeld Synergy Method™

The Rubenfeld Synergy Method™ is a holistic healing system for the integration of the body, mind, emotions, and spirit. It was developed in the 1960s by Ilana Rubenfeld, a psychotherapist and bodyworker who sought to teach people how to recognize, express, understand, and manage their emotions, feelings, and sensations. By combining gentle touch and verbalization, the Rubenfeld Synergy Method reportedly brings about beneficial changes in self-image, health, personal and family relationships, and spirit.

History

In the 1950s Ilana Rubenfeld was a conducting student at the Juilliard School of Music when she suffered a debilitating back spasm. Seeking help, she contacted Judith Leibowitz, a teacher of the Alexander technique, who taught her how to use her body efficiently to avoid reinjury. During her therapy, Rubenfeld sometimes expressed intense emotional feelings, but Leibowitz, untrained in treating emotions, suggested that she see a psychoanalyst. The analyst talked but wouldn't touch, and Rubenfeld's feelings did not emerge.

Rubenfeld realized that the Alexander technique's specific methods of physical touch helped her access her memories, while verbal processing helped her understand them. She resolved to create a way of simultaneously integrating bodywork with psychotherapy. She became a master teacher of the Alexander technique and trained extensively with Moshe Feldenkrais in the Feldenkrais Method®, a technique for improving both physical and mental functioning through the learning of new body movements. For years, she taught these body-mind modalities but found that they lacked what for her was the most vital element: processing the emotional material that emerged during lessons. She longed to know the emotional history, stresses, and life problems that created physical dysfunctions in the first place.

Rubenfeld's curiosity led her to train and collaborate with psychiatrist Peter Hogan and with Fritz and Laura Perls, cofounders of gestalt therapy, and to further combine body-oriented methods with psychotherapy. The addition of appropriate verbal processing to body-mind disciplines practiced in a safe, trusting, and nonjudgmental environment seemed to make the various modalities function synergistically, and remarkable results occurred in a short time.

In 1977 Rubenfeld launched the first professional Rubenfeld Synergy training program in New York City. This 1,600-hour, four-year program includes lectures, demonstrations, discussion, and a great deal of supervised practice. Trainees learn self-care, maintain high standards of integrity and competency, and seek supervision, therapy, and continued education for themselves. The code of ethics for Rubenfeld Synergists includes demonstrating respect for people, preserving their confidentiality, showing sensitivity to the difference in power between practitioners and help seekers, avoiding personal relationships with help seekers, and maintaining clear boundaries.

Basic Principles

The goals of the Rubenfeld Synergy Method are to enhance people's natural capacity for self-healing and self-regulation, to teach them to recognize and learn from the truths their bodies tell, and to teach them to use their own resources for change, choice, and self-care. Synergists accomplish these goals by teaching people how to become aware of the messages, memories, and emotions locked in their bodies, causing energy blocks and imbalances.

Using a variety of techniques and elements—including verbal dialogue, movement training, imagination exercises, breathing techniques, and nonsexual, caring touch—Synergists assist people in exploring the relationship between posture and emotions; discovering how body metaphors reveal life patterns; healing their "inner child;" exploring somatic (regarding the body) dreams; and developing a sense of humor. Synergists believe the combination of these techniques engages the help seeker in understanding the causes of discomfort, alleviating physical pain, and resolving emotional issues.

The establishment of a therapeutic relationship of safety and trust is essential, so that each person can journey inward, recognize and release traumas and dysfunctional memories, and reclaim his body, mind, and soul.

Practice

A typical session lasts about forty-five minutes and is conducted privately or in a group, with both Synergist and help seeker(s) fully clothed. Help seekers are usually invited to lie on a padded table, but sessions may also be conducted sitting, standing, or moving. Sessions begin in the here and now, then move into the past and future within the context of each person's needs. No diagnoses are made, nor cures promised. Help seekers are in charge of the pace and direction of the sessions, and they may stop at any time. People interested in practicing the method may learn Rubenfeld bodymind exercises, which ease tensions, foster flexibility, develop strength, and teach "inner listening." These can be practiced anywhere. Although Rubenfeld Synergy may bring insights in a short time, weekly sessions for a period of at least several months to several years are advised for fully integrated and lasting benefits.

Benefits

People who experience Rubenfeld Synergy sessions often report greater self-esteem and self-acceptance; a sense of clarity and purpose; increased energy, body awareness, and body image; deep relaxation; and relief from pain. Trainees conduct pilot studies on such topics as body image, posttraumatic stress disorder, recovery from addictive behaviors, incest and abuse, and stress-related illnesses. There are no known contraindications. Synergists are trained to recognize conditions requiring medical supervision and refer clients to appropriate professionals when necessary.

—ILANA RUBENFELD

Resources

Canadian Association of Rubenfeld Synergists
112 Lund St.
Richmond Hill, Ontario L4C 5V9
Canada
Tel: (905) 883-3158
e-mail: aturner@yorku.ca
Supports members' professional growth and promotes high standards of professional ethics. Also seeks to educate the public about the Rubenfeld Synergy Method.

National Association of Rubenfeld Synergists
1000 River Road, Suite 8H
Belmar, NJ 07719
Tel: 1-800-484-3250, code 8516
Provides referrals to certified Rubenfeld Synergists and distributes information about the Synergists' code of ethics.

The Rubenfeld Synergy Center
115 Waverly Place
New York, NY 10011
Tel: 1-800-747-6897
e-mail: rubenfeld@aol.com
Offers an introductory workshop.

Further Reading

Books

Caldwell, Christine. *Getting in Touch: The Guide to New Body-Centered Therapies*. Wheaton Ill.: Quest Books, 1997.

Claire, Thomas. *Bodywork: What Type of Massage to Get—And How to Make the Most of It*. New York: William Morrow and Company, 1995.

———. "Gestalt Therapy and the Bodymind: An Overview of the Rubenfeld Synergy Method." In *Gestalt Therapy: Perspectives and Applications*, edited by Edwin C. Nevis. New York: Gardner Press, 1990.

Journals

Lerkin, Jan Marie. "Sing the Body Electric." *Changes,* June 1995.

Markowitz, Laura. "Therapists Explore Mind-Body Alternatives." *Family Therapy,* 1996.

Rubenfeld, Ilana. "Ushering in a Century of Integration." *Somatics,* Autumn–Winter 1990–91.

———. "Beginner's Hands: Twenty-Five Years of Simple Rubenfeld Synergy—The Birth of a Therapy." *Somatics,* Spring–Summer 1988.

Simon, Richard. "Listening Hands." *Family Therapy Networker,* September–October 1997.

Unergi

 Unergi is a holistic therapy method that aims to help participants integrate body, mind, emotions, spirit, creativity, and the healing forces of nature. It was developed by Ute Arnold by combining healing forms derived from gestalt therapy, the Feldenkrais Method®, the Alexander technique, and the Rubenfeld Synergy Method™.

Theory and Practice

Unergi combines the words *unity* and *energy,* reflecting Arnold's belief that all people originate in a state of unity and can restore their energy and prevent disease through self-care, self-expression, participation in community, and active involvement with the organic rhythms of nature. According to unergi, there exists a vibrational energy, radiating from our natural environment, that is able to heal by restoring one's internal energy. Like all of the healing methods from which it draws, unergi considers physical and emotional problems to be a result of psychological patterns developed in early childhood. These patterns censor various aspects of our inner lives and self-expression. When a person's body and psyche have been denied expression, unergi practitioners believe that person's whole being will start to feel increasingly ill at ease. One may feel this as aches, pains, or numbness, which over time become more acute. Healing is seen as a release of old ways of being and a return to wholeness.

During a unergi session, a client lies, sits, or moves on a bodywork table, fully clothed. The practitioner employs techniques such as body awareness, touch, and movement exercises to balance the energy through the Hindu chakra system, creative expression, visualization, and dreamwork. These techniques invite a dialogue between a client's body and mind to access deeply buried memories and emotions. The goal is to allow greater freedom of movement and create a safe environment for the expression and healing of a person's hidden qualities.

—UTE ARNOLD

Resources

Unergi Training
P.O. Box 335
Point Pleasant, PA 18950
Tel: (215) 297-8006
Offers a three-year certification program in the unergi method. The training is conducted at retreat centers on the East Coast of the United States and in Europe.

Contributors

Acupressure, Process Acupressure

Aminah Raheem, Ph.D. and Diplomate of Process Work, is a transpersonal psychologist, bodyworker, writer, and originator of process acupressure who has worked for many years with the integration of bodywork and consciousness. She was an adjunct faculty member of the Institute for Transpersonal Psychology for ten years.

Acupuncture

Robert J. Abramson, D.D.S, M.D., had a private dental practice for more than a decade before earning his M.D. from the State University of New York and completing a bachelor's course in acupuncture at the College of Traditional Chinese Medicine in England. He is currently an acupuncturist in private practice in New York City.

Aikido

Clio Pavlantos, M.A., CMA, holds a master's degree in dance, a certificate in Laban movement studies, and a black belt in aikido. She has taught all three disciplines at colleges, universities, and private institutions. Dance and Laban movement analysis helped her in learning and teaching aikido, which she finds to have many of the rhythms and expressive qualities of dance.

Marvin Bookman has been involved in the martial arts for twenty years. He is certified as an aikido instructor by the U.S. Aikido Federation. In 1989 he founded Aikido of Greenwich Village. Currently, Bookman gives seminars and classes throughout the United States.

Alexander Technique

Diane Young, NASAT, is a certified teacher and trainer of the Alexander technique. She has a modern dance background, having choreographed and performed in New York City since 1983. She is on the faculty at SUNY, Stony Brook, in the music department and maintains a private practice in New York and Connecticut. She has written various journals on body-mind healing and has received a grant from the New York Cardiac Center to study and report on complementary medicine.

Art Therapy

Cathy Malchiodi, M.A., ATR, LPAT, LPCC, is the director of the Institute for the Arts and Health in Salt Lake City. She is the editor of *Art Therapy: Journal of the American Art Therapy Association* and the author of several books and articles on the topic of art therapy with trauma, child physical abuse, and medical applications. Malchiodi has lectured at many universities, agencies, and institutions throughout the United States, Canada, Europe, and Asia.

Aston-Patterning®

Allison Funk has been working in the fields of bodywork and movement education for twelve years. A licensed physical therapist assistant, she received her certification in 1996 and is currently enrolled in the faculty training program at the Aston-Patterning Center in Lake Tahoe, Nevada. Funk owns a private Aston-Patterning practice in Winter Park, Colorado, where she uses her skills to assist a variety of clients.

Authentic Movement

Daphne Lowell is a professor at Hampshire College and the Five College Dance Department. She is also codirector of the Hampshire College Program in contemplative dance.

Ayurvedic Medicine

Dr. Vasant Lad, BAMS (bachelor of ayurvedic medicine and surgery), MASc (master of ayurvedic science), is founder, director, chairman of the board, and principal instructor of the Ayurvedic Institute in Albuquerque, New Mexico. He practiced and taught ayurveda in Pune, India, before coming to the United States and teaching at the Santa Fe College of Natural Medicine in 1981.

Bartenieff Fundamentals℠

Janet Hamburg, CMA, M.A., is a professor of dance at the University of Kansas, Lawrence. She was a faculty member of the Laban/Bartenieff Institute of Movement Studies Certificate Extension Program in New Mexico. She has taught LMA classes internationally and throughout the United States. Hamburg's work with athletes has been featured on national television, including the program *Science World.*

Behavioral Vision Therapy

Dr. Joseph Shapiro is a behavioral optometrist with twenty-five years of experience. He is director of the Center for Unlimited Vision in New York City. He received his doctor of optometry degree from the Massachusetts College of Optometry and completed his intern and residency program in vision therapy at the University Optometric Center, State College of Optometry, State University of New York. He has taught rehabilitative optometry at six major hospitals in the New York metropolitan area. He is coauthor of *Out of Sight into Vision,* a consumer self-help book presenting new models of seeing and vision therapy.

Bioenergetics

Nina Robinson, ADTR, M.A., CMA, has been a dance/movement therapist since 1973. She has taught in the New York University dance therapy program, from which she received her master's degree. A member of the Academy of Dance Therapists Registered, she has integrated bioenergetics into her dance therapy work throughout her career. She studied with Alexander Lowen, M.D., from 1965 to 1967.

Biofeedback Training

Les Fehmi, Ph.D., organized and chaired the first national meeting of biofeedback researchers in 1968. He received his doctoral degree in physiological psychology from UCLA and has been recognized by the Association for Applied Physiopsychology and Biofeedback for his contributions to the development of applied physiopathology and biofeedback. He directs biofeedback centers in New York City and Princeton, New Jersey.

Body-Mind Centering®

Vera Orlock is an assistant professor of dance at Kansas State University and has taught at

Indiana University, Bloomington, and the University of North Carolina, Charlotte. Her choreography has been recognized by grants from the Ohio Arts Council and the New York State Council on the Arts. She is on the faculty of the School for Body-Mind Centering® and is also a certified practitioner of structural integration, the work of Ida P. Rolf. Orlock is frequently a guest artist/teacher in Europe and the United States.

Bodynamic Analysis

Peter Bernhardt, MFCC, is director of the Clement Street Counseling Center Faculty at California Institute of Integral Studies in Somatics program, San Francisco, and a founding member of the Bodynamic Institute, USA. He has led trainings and workshops throughout the United States and Europe, has twenty years' experience as a body psychotherapist, and is in private practice near Berkeley, California.

Bowen Technique

Oswald H. Rentsch is the principal and founder of the Bowen Therapy Academy of Australia, the official organization of Bowtech®. From 1974 to 1976 he studied under Thomas A. Bowen, who commissioned Rentsch to document and teach his original techniques. He earned a diploma of osteopathy from the South Pacific Council of Natural Therapies, an honorary doctorate of massage therapy from the Australian Registrar of Massage Therapists, and a diploma of homeopathy ionization principles from the Australian Academy of Homeopathy. Rentsch has twenty-two years of experience with the Bowen technique and, together with his wife, Elaine, has spent ten years as a Bowtech teacher.

Brain Gym®

Lark Carroll has been teaching Brain Gym in the San Francisco Bay area since 1986. She completed certification in educational kinesiology, neurolinguistic programming, acupressure massage, and Bowen therapy. Additionally,

she holds training in a variety of modalities, including CranioSacral therapy, Living Vision™, meditation, Chinese five-element theory, and nutritional approaches to health and balance.

Chiropractic

Dr. Trina Marx is a doctor of chiropractic with a degree in clinical nutrition, also specializing in exercise psychology and holistic treatments. In addition to her private practice, she is the chiropractor for the American Tap Dance Orchestra. Her volunteer work includes providing chiropractic services for the Gay Men's Health Crisis and for children born with addictions and HIV. She has also written the books *Body Almanac* and *Tap Dance*.

Connective Tissue Therapy^{SM}

Jackie Hand, M.A., is a certified Laban movement analyst and a registered movement therapist. She is a movement consultant and a dance specialist, performing movement retraining and bodywork. On the faculty at the Laban/Bartenieff Institute of Movement Studies, she integrates her years of dance training with her movement observation skills to educate clients in movement awareness and observation. She studied anatomy with Irene Dowd and Connective Tissue Therapy^{SM} with Theresa Lamb. She has a holistic approach to movement and bodywork and is nationally certified in therapeutic massage and bodywork.

Contact Improvisation

Paul Langland is a dancer, singer, choreographer, and teacher. A longtime practitioner of contact and other improvisational dance forms, he often presents his own work, as well as performing with others. His work has been seen at Dance Theater Workshop, PS 122, Franklin Furnace, and Movement Research. Since 1983, he has been a core faculty member of New York University's Experimental Theater Wing.

Core Energetics

Pamela L. Chubbuck, Ph.D., LPC, is on the senior international teaching faculty of the Core Energetic Institute in New York City, where she is also director of faculty development. Chubbuck is the director of Core Energetics South and has worked personally and extensively with John C. Pierrakos, M.D., for more than twenty-five years. She is the author of *Passages to Womanhood: Stories of Celebration for Young Women* and numerous articles on the core energetics process.

coreSomatics®

Kay Miller is certified in the Rubenfeld Synergy Method™ and the Feldenkrais Method® and received her gestalt training in the three-year postgraduate program at the Gestalt Institute of Cleveland. She has served in various capacities with the Pennsylvania Department of Education, the University of Pittsburgh, Carlow College, the University of West Virginia, Long Island University, the Gestalt Institute of Cleveland, and the Western Psychiatric Institute.

CORE Structural Integrative Therapy

George P. Kousaleos has been a licensed massage therapist specializing in structural integration and myofascial therapy since 1978. A graduate of Harvard University and the Soma Institute of Neuromuscular Integration, he has practiced and taught in Germany and Greece and throughout America. In 1990 he founded the CORE Institute School of Massage Therapy of Tallahassee, Florida, a state-licensed and nationally accredited program. He trains massage therapists in continuing education certification courses in CORE myofascial therapy and CORE structural integrative therapy. Kousaleos also served as the general manager of the British Olympic Sports Massage Therapy Team (1994–1996).

Gary N. Genna, LMT, is founder and owner of the CORE Institute of Tennessee. A graduate of SUNY, Cortland, with a degree in biology and education, Genna has been an advanced instructor for the CORE Institute since 1989. He has presented at various state and international conferences and spent more than three years working as a neuromuscular therapist at St. Anthony's Hospital Sports Medicine and Orthopedic Rehabilitation Center in St. Petersburg, Florida. He has been both a massage therapist and a massage educator for more than twenty-five years, and served as the head coach for the British Olympic Sports Massage Therapy Team in 1995 and 1996.

CranioSacral Therapy

Kenneth I. Frey, PT, is director of the Institute of Physical Therapy, a private practice and clinical resource center in New York City.

Dance Therapy

Anne L. Wennerstrand is a dance/movement therapist, clinical social worker, and dance educator working in mental health and education. Currently, she is coordinator of undergraduate dance education at New York University, where she teaches and advises students. She has presented and written on the arts in education and therapy. Her clinical work focuses on creative mind-body approaches to helping people with eating problems, anxiety, depression, and chronic mental illness. A former professional dancer, she is also on the staff of Career Transition for Dancers, a nonprofit counseling service.

Do-In

John Kozinski has taught do-in, traditional exercises, and healing through food and natural therapies throughout the United States and in Asia and South America. He offers seminars on do-in, traditional exercises, and the macrobiotic approach to health and healing at the Kushi Institute in Massachusetts, as well as in Connecticut and New York. He also has an active health counseling practice in which he recommends specific traditional foods, remedies, and natural lifestyle practices to foster healing and general well-being.

Drama Therapy

Professor Patricia Sternberg, RDT/BCT (registered drama therapist/board certified trainer), is chairperson of the board of examiners of the National Association for Drama Therapy. She is a full professor of the department of theater at Hunter College in New York and heads the developmental drama program there. She is a playwright with more than twenty-five plays produced and/or published and the author of seven books, including *Sociodrama: Who's in Your Shoes?* (with Antonina Garcia), and is currently working on her eighth, *Theater for Conflict Resolution*. A well-known speaker and workshop leader with experience presenting both nationally and internationally, Sternberg is a practicing drama therapist and for the past ten years has worked with a variety of populations in both psychiatric and educational facilities.

Emotional-Kinesthetic Psychotherapy

Linda Marks has practiced body-centered psychotherapy with individuals, couples, and groups for twelve years. She helped found and has served on the board of the Interface Business Association, the Organization Transformation Network, the Massachusetts Association of Body-Oriented Psychotherapy and Counseling Bodyworkers, and the Somatics Community of the Association for Humanistic Psychology. In 1990 she founded the Institute for Emotional-Kinesthetic Psychotherapy. She has written a column on psychology for *Spirit of Change* magazine for the past ten years. She is the author of *Living with Vision: Reclaiming the Power of the Heart*.

Enneagram

Janet Levine is an author, educator, and organizer. She established Learning and the Enneagram, an educational enterprise dedicated to spreading knowledge of the enneagram system and its applications in education and related fields. She has taught at Milton Academy, Massachusetts, for ten years. She is director of the National Educators Institute for Enneagram Studies at Milton Academy. She has presented her work on education and the enneagram at national conferences and many other venues.

Eurythmy

Beth Dunn-Fox was raised and educated in northern California, where she studied and performed ballet, character, and modern dance. A graduate of Eurythmy Spring Valley, she has toured throughout North America and Europe with its professional ensemble for twelve years. In addition to performing, she has handled the finance and development work of Eurythmy Spring Valley over a number of years.

Eye Movement Desensitization and Reprocessing

Barbara A. Parrett, RN, M.S., is a nurse and psychotherapist who brings a holistic approach to her work with individuals and organizations. She has been thoroughly trained in eye movement desensitization and reprocessing and teaches this discipline to other therapists on an international scale, where she is in much demand as a trainer and educator.

Feldenkrais Method®

Alan S. Questel is a founding member of Delman/Questel Associates, Inc., and is a Feldenkrais practitioner.

Feng Shui

Marilyn Saltzman is a feng shui practitioner. She studied feng shui with Nancy SantoPietro, a certified teacher trained by Master Lin Yun. A certified rebirther and hypnotherapist, she has studied Transcendental Meditation and reiki, and has given lectures and workshops on feng shui.

Flower Remedies

Leslie J. Kaslof is an internationally recognized pioneer, researcher, writer, and educator in the field of holistic health, preventive medicine, and natural approaches to stress reduction. He has written numerous articles in professional and popular publications as well as many other works, including *Herb and Ailment Cross-Reference Chart*, the pioneering book *Wholistic Dimensions in Healing*, and *The Traditional Flower Remedies of Dr. Edward Bach: A Self-Help Guide*.

Focusing

Joan Klagsbrun, Ph.D., is a clinical psychologist practicing focusing-oriented psychotherapy in private practice in Boston. A college professor and certified focusing trainer and coordinator, she has been practicing and teaching focusing for twenty years.

Hakomi Integrative Somatics

Pat Ogden, M.A., is a founding member of the Hakomi Institute, serves on its trainers' board, and is the originator and director of hakomi integrative somatics. Trained in a wide variety of somatic approaches, she is a structural integrator (Guild for Structural Integration) and serves on the faculty of the Ergos Institute (founded by Peter Levine, specializing in healing the effects of trauma) and the Naropa Institute.

Halprin Life/Art Process

Daria Halprin-Khalighi, M.A., CET, is cofounder and director of the Tampala Institute. She maintains a private practice in Marin County and is a certified expressive arts therapist. She is the author of *Coming Alive: The Creative Expression Method*.

Hanna Somatic Education®

Eleanor Criswell Hanna, Ed.D., is professor of psychology and former chair of the psychology department at Sonoma State University, in California. In 1975 she cofounded, with Thomas Hanna, the Novato Institute for Somatic Research and Training in Novato, California. She trained in somatic education with Thomas Hanna in his 1981 Australian training program; she has worked closely with him in the development of the field of somatics over the years. She currently serves as president of the Somatics Society and editor of *Somatics*. A licensed psychologist, she maintains a private practice in psychotherapy, biofeedback, and somatic education. She is the author of *Biofeedback and Somatics*.

Herbal Medicine

Mark Blumenthal is founder and executive director of the American Botanical Council, a leading nonprofit research and education organization in Austin, Texas. He also edits the quarterly magazine *HerbalGram*.

Holistic Health

Suzan Walter, MBA, is cofounder and current president of the American Holistic Health Association and past president of the American Holistic Medical Foundation. She is creator and director of the *Global Health Calendar* on the Internet at HealthWorld Online (www.healthy.net). She also facilitates networking for speakers, practitioners, and health care associations within this Web site.

Holotropic Breathwork™

Kylea Taylor, M.S., is a certified Holotropic Breathwork™ practitioner and has been working in the field of addiction recovery since 1970. Since 1984 she has studied with Christine and Stanislav Grof, M.D., Ph.D., and is a member of the teaching staff of Grof Transpersonal Training. She is the author of *The Breathwork Experience: Exploration and Healing in Nonordinary States of Consciousness* and *The Ethics of Caring: Honoring the Web of Life in Our Professional Healing Relationships*. She has served as editor of the *Inner Door*, the newsletter of the Association for Holotropic Breathwork International.

Homeopathy, Osteopathy

Domenick John Masiello, D.O., DHt, CSPOMM, has been a solo, office-based practitioner of traditional osteopathy and classical homeopathy in New York City since 1986. He was certified with special proficiency in osteopathic manipulative medicine and is also certified in homeotherapeutics. He wrote the foreword to *Osteopathy: An Integrated Whole Body Therapy* and has been published in the *Journal of the American Institute of Homeopathy.*

Hydrotherapy

Douglas C. Lewis, ND, is a naturopathic physician in Seattle.

Hypnotherapy

Oscar A. Gillespie, Ph.D., is president of NY-SEPH, the New York Milton H. Erickson Society for Psychology and Hypnosis, and is on the faculty of its training program. He taught psychology at Fordham University and currently is in private practice in New York City.

Ideokinesis

Andre Bernard teaches ideokinesis, drawing upon his background in science and the performing arts. He studied chemical engineering at the University of South Carolina, where he earned a B.S. degree in chemistry and mathematics. Pursuing a professional acting career, he appeared in more than a hundred theatrical productions. He also studied dance and toured extensively with the Charles Weidman Dance Theater. He studied Mabel Elsworth Todd's movement therapy techniques, the foundation of ideokinesis, with Barbara Clark. He has been a member of the faculty at New York University, teaching Todd's work, since 1966.

Infant Massage

Mindy Zlotnick has worked as a teacher with parents and their families since 1975. She holds an M.A. in special education and worked for many years with deaf children, communicating in sign language. She was trained in massage in 1987 and began communicating through touch in her practice with adults. She became a certified infant massage instructor in 1989, combining her love of teaching with her love of massage. Her practice includes teaching parents with healthy babies as well as parents with babies who are medically fragile or have developmental delays.

Integral Yoga

The Reverend Kumari de Sachy, Ed.D., has been a student of Swami Satchidananda since 1980. In 1981 she became an integral yoga instructor and proceeded to teach at institutes, colleges, universities, and prisons. In 1994 she was ordained as an integral yoga minister. For the past ten years, she and her husband have been living and serving as whole-time members at Satchidananda Ashram–Yogaville with the spiritual master Sri Swami Satchidananda. At Yogaville she has taught English and French, in addition to serving as director of the Yogaville Summer Program for Children and Teens. She is also editor at Integral Yoga Publications, which publishes Swami Satchidananda's books and the quarterly magazine *Integral Yoga.*

Interactive Guided Imagery℠

Martin Rossman, M.D., is a 1969 graduate of the University of Michigan Medical School and is board certified in acupuncture. He is founder and director of the Collaborative Medicine Center in Mill Valley, California. As codirector of the Academy for Guided Imagery in Mill Valley, he has taught clinical guided imagery to more than nine thousand health care professionals since 1982. He was a founding member of the Scientific Advisory Board of the Institute for the Advancement of Health. He has written numerous articles and publications and was a recipient of the American Health Book Award in 1987.

Iyengar Yoga

Janet MacLeod teaches yoga full-time, offering ongoing classes in San Francisco and teaching workshops around the country. She is on the faculty of the Iyengar Yoga Institute of San Francisco teacher training program. She is a certified teacher at the intermediate level and continues to study in Pune, India, with the Iyengar family on a regular basis.

Jin Shin Do® Bodymind Acupressure™

Iona Marsaa Teeguarden, M.A., is the originator of Jin Shin Do Bodymind Acupressure. She founded the Jin Shin Do Foundation and began offering Jin Shin Do teacher training programs. She has written several books and articles on the practice of Jin Shin Do.

Jin Shin Jyutsu® Physio-Philosophy

Ian Kraut is a practitioner of Jin Shin Jyutsu and a licensed massage therapist. He is a member of the staff at Jin Shin Jyutsu, Inc., in Scottsdale, Arizona. He has a B.A. in music from SUNY, Binghamton, and has studied Andean music in South America.

Journal Therapy

Kathleen Adams, M.A., LPC, is a licensed psychotherapist and founder/director of the Center for Journal Therapy in Denver, an organization dedicated to teaching the healing art of journal writing to individuals, groups, and mental health professionals. She has specialized in journal therapy since 1985 and is a pioneer in the field. She is the author of three books on the use of journal writing as a therapeutic tool.

Ju Jutsu, Karate

Stefan Nikander is a certified karate and ju jutsu instructor. Having taught soccer to children since the age of fifteen, he became certified as a soccer trainer in 1983. He is also a certified nursery school teacher and has worked professionally at schools and play centers since 1990. He is vice chairman of the children's committee of the Swedish Budo Federation, a martial arts organization. His writing has appeared in various martial arts magazines in several countries, and he has written columns for Scandinavian newspapers on the subject of martial arts as a means to stop violence. He is currently studying to become a personal trainer and massage therapist.

Kendo

Daniel T. Ebihara is the chairman of Ken Zen Institute, Ltd., and a member of the board of directors of the All United States Kendo Federation. He has written several articles about

the martial arts for various periodicals and is an advanced student of karate, kendo, and judo.

Bruce Robertson-Smith is a first-degree black belt in kendo, having studied martial arts in Japan with the Budo master Fushi Sensei. He has trained extensively in bodywork and structural integration and has done shamanic journeywork.

Kestenberg Movement Profile

Susan Loman is director of a master's program in dance/movement therapy at Antioch New England Graduate School in Keene, New Hampshire, and the author of numerous articles on the Kestenberg Movement Profile (KMP). She has given intensive courses on this material in Germany and Italy. She is the coeditor of a textbook on KMP published in 1997.

Janet Kestenberg Amighi is an anthropologist who has done fieldwork in Iran and Bali. She is the author of *Zoroastrians in Iran: Assimilation, Conversion, and Persistence*. She coteaches a course on KMP with Susan Loman and is coeditor of a textbook on KMP.

Kinetic Awareness

Ellen Saltonstall, M.A., MCKA, is a certified master teacher of kinetic awareness, a licensed massage therapist, and a teacher and practitioner of hatha yoga. She has taught at the New School for Social Research, Columbia University, and Bard College, and is currently on the staff of the Mind/Body Medical Institute of St. Peters Hospital in New Brunswick, New Jersey.

J. Robin Powell, Ph.D., CSW, MCKA, is a certified master teacher of kinetic awareness who teaches at New York University and other institutions, as well as privately. She is a founding board member of the Kinetic Awareness Center, Inc., and participates in the teacher training program.

Michelle Berne, M.A., MCKA, introduced the first university course in body-mind therapies while on the faculty of New York University, where she taught for twelve years. As a professional dancer and choreographer in

New York, she presented original work with her own company and performed with others. She is a certified master teacher of kinetic awareness and currently teaches kinetic awareness, neuromuscular reeducation, and alignment in Los Angeles. She is also a celebration artist who choreographs and produces large-scale community art events for cities and nonprofit organizations across the country.

Kung Fu Wu Su

Oswald Rivera is a senior instructor at Alan Lee's Chinese Kung-Fu Wu-Su Association. He has practiced Shaolin style kung fu for twenty-four years. He is also the author of the novel *Fire and Rain* and the cookbook *Puerto Rican Cuisine in America*.

Laban Movement Analysis

Ed Groff, M.F.A., CMA, is currently director of graduate studies in the department of modern dance at the University of Utah. He has served on the faculties of Temple University, Hampshire College, Connecticut College, Tufts University, and Evergreen State College. He has taught in the certification programs in Laban movement analysis at schools and institutions in New York City, Seattle, Salt Lake City, Columbus, Rotterdam, and Berlin. His choreography has been presented in the United States, Europe, and Asia.

Light Therapy

Dr. Brian J. Breiling is a licensed marriage, family, and child counselor and school psychologist. He is coeditor and publisher of *Light Years Ahead: The Illustrated Guide to Full-Spectrum and Colored Light in Mindbody Healing*, to which he contributed three chapters on the professional and self-care applications of light therapy. For the last ten years, he successfully used flashing colored light stimulation through the eyes to aid his clients in uncovering and working through emotional traumas, depression, and pain, as well as to enhance learning and intellectual performance in adults and children.

Magnet Therapy

Dr. John Zimmerman earned a Ph.D. in biological psychology and neurosciences at the University of Colorado at Boulder in 1981. He is a member of the American Sleep Disorders Association and the North American Academy of Magnetic Therapy. Currently, he serves as laboratory director of the Washoe Sleep Disorders Center in Reno. Zimmerman is also founder and president of the nonprofit organization the Bio-Electro-Magnetics Institute, which researches and provides resources on magnet therapy.

Martial Arts

Dr. Michael Maliszewski received a Ph.D. in psychology from the University of Chicago. He has held a number of positions at the University of Chicago and has conducted research and his writing has been published in a variety of areas ranging from medicine to religious studies. He is currently a consultant in psychiatry at Massachusetts General Hospital and lecturer at Harvard Medical School. He has been involved in the study of martial arts and meditative traditions since 1970 and has studied throughout the United States and Asia. Included among his publications is the book *Spiritual Dimensions of the Martial Arts*, as well as articles that have appeared in the *Journal of Asian Martial Arts*, for which he also serves as an associate editor.

Massage

Katie Scoville is a New York State–licensed massage therapist who practices Swedish massage, shiatsu, medical massage, and pregnancy massage. She has a private practice in Manhattan called Studio of Massage Arts (SOMA), and also works with physical therapists. A shiatsu and clinic instructor at the Swedish Institute of Massage Therapy and Allied Health Sciences in New York City, she is also a member of the American Massage Therapy Association. Scoville holds a B.F.A. in dance and brings to her practice more than fifteen years of dance training and professional dance experience.

Medical Orgone Therapy

Dr. Peter Crist received an M.D. from the UCLA School of Medicine in 1977. Crist is a fellow of the American College of Orgonomy (ACO) and has been its president since 1991. As a member of the ACO training faculty, he has been training medical orgonomists since 1982. He has authored clinical and theoretical articles as well as book reviews and is an assistant editor of the *Journal of Orgonomy*. Crist is also assistant clinical professor in the department of psychiatry at UMDNJ–Robert Wood Johnson School of Medicine, New Brunswick, New Jersey. He has a private practice in Belle Mead, New Jersey.

Dr. Richard Schwartzman, D.O., graduated from the Philadelphia College of Osteopathic Medicine in 1966. He is a member of the faculty of Hahnemann University, where he is an assistant clinical professor of psychiatry, and medical director of the Hahnemann University Correctional Mental Health Program. He is a fellow of the ACO, where he conducts the advanced training seminar. An assistant editor and contributing author to the *Journal of Orgonomy*, Schwartzman also maintains a private practice in medical orgone therapy in Philadelphia, Pennsylvania.

Meditation

Eugene Taylor, Ph.D., is a lecturer on psychiatry at Harvard Medical School. He also serves on the executive faculty at Saybrook Institute and is director of the Cambridge Institute of Psychology and Religion.

Marilyn Schlitz, Ph.D., is a social anthropologist and director of research at the Institute of Noetic Sciences in Sausalito, California.

Meir Schneider Self-Healing Method

Carol Gallup works as a member of the staff at the Center for Self-Healing in San Francisco.

Movement Pattern Analysis

Warren Lamb developed movement pattern analysis with Rudolf Laban. In 1950 Lamb joined Paton Lawrence & Co., management consultants, to apply the newly developed as-

sessment method. He has been a professional dancer, a producer of plays, and a lecturer in the United Kingdom and United States. In 1952 he founded his own consulting firm to use movement pattern analysis for top management teams worldwide. His publications include *Posture and Gesture, Management Behavior, Body Code,* and more than one hundred journal articles.

Multimodal Expressive Arts Therapy

Susan Spaniol, Ed.D., ATR-BC, LMHC, is assistant professor in the expressive therapies division of Lesley College in Cambridge, Massachusetts. She received her Ed.D. at Boston University and is a board-certified art therapist and a licensed mental health counselor. She serves as associate editor of *Art Therapy: Journal of the American Art Therapy Association* and is an associate in psychiatry at Harvard Medical School.

Phillip Speiser, Ph.D., REAT, RDT, is director of Arts Across Cultures, Boston. Speiser is a psychodrama, drama, and expressive arts educator/therapist who has been developing and implementing integrated arts programs since 1980. He is an adjunct professor at Lesley College and has taught and lectured extensively at training institutes and colleges throughout Scandinavia, Europe, Israel, and the United States. He is former chairperson of Very Special Arts, Sweden, and the International Expressive Arts Therapy Association.

Mariagnese Cattaneo, Ph.D., ATR, LMHC, is a professor in the expressive therapies division at Lesley College. She is an expressive therapist and has trained expressive therapists for more than twenty-five years. Presently, she is coordinator of art therapy specialization and director of field training.

Muscular Therapy

Ben E. Benjamin holds a Ph.D. in sports medicine and education and is founder and president of the Muscular Therapy Institute in Cambridge, Massachusetts. He is the author of *Are You Tense?—The Benjamin System of Muscular Therapy, Sports Without Pain,* and *Listen to Your*

Pain—Understanding, Identifying, and Treating Pain, all widely used books in the field. He has been a regular contributor to the *Muscular Therapy Journal* since 1986. He has been in private practice for more than thirty-five years and has been leading workshops in muscular therapy internationally since 1973.

Mary Ann diRoberts, LICSW, CMT, is on the faculty of the Muscular Therapy Institute in Cambridge, Massachusetts.

Music Therapy

Adva Frank-Schwebel has been a music therapist for fifteen years. Her work in music therapy has included child psychology, group therapy, and private practice. She studied musicology and anthropology at the Hebrew University of Jerusalem, and classical guitar in Israel and London. She holds a master's degree in musicology from Bar Ilan University and teaches at the Institute for Art Therapy of David Yellin College in Jerusalem and in the department of music therapy of Bar Ilan University.

Myofascial Trigger-Point Therapy

Elliot Shratter has been practicing trigger-point myotherapy since 1987. He is board certified by the National Association of Trigger-Point Myotherapists Certification Board, and the American Academy of Pain Management. He has served as president and journal editor of the National Association of Trigger-Point Myotherapists and chairperson of the Trigger-Point Myotherapists National Certification Board. He is currently in practice in Albuquerque, New Mexico, at Synergy Physical Therapy.

Naturopathic Medicine

Lauri M. Aesoph, ND, a graduate of Bastyr University, is a medical writer, editor, and educator. Over the past ten years, Aesoph's work has appeared in dozens of magazines and numerous books. She makes her home in Sioux Falls, South Dakota, with her husband and two sons.

Network Chiropractic

Donald Epstein, DCA, is a chiropractor and developer of network spinal analysis. He is president of the Association for Network Chiropractic. He is also the author of several articles on the practice of this discipline.

Organismic Body Psychotherapy

Elliot Greene, M.A., is a counselor who has specialized in body psychotherapy for the past twenty-four years. His principal training has been in organismic body psychotherapy with Dr. Malcolm Brown and Katherine Ennis-Brown. He is also trained in bioenergetics, gestalt, and other related body-oriented methods. In addition, he is nationally certified as a massage therapist and served as president of the American Massage Therapy Association from 1990 to 1994. He has a private practice in Silver Spring, Maryland.

Orthomolecular Medicine

California freelance writer Martin Zucker has written for many years about health, nutrition, and preventive medicine. A former Associated Press foreign correspondent, he has written numerous articles, coauthored five books, ghostwritten several others, and scripted many safety and environmental videos for the National Safety Council and other organizations. He has been a contributing editor to *Let's Live*, a leading health magazine, since 1978.

Pesso Boyden System Psychomotor

Albert Pesso cofounded Pesso Boyden system psychomotor (PBSP) psychotherapy with his life partner, Diane Boyden-Pesso, in 1961. He is president of the Psychomotor Institute, Inc., Boston, a nonprofit organization that promotes PBSP internationally. He has been supervisor of psychomotor therapy at the McLean Hospital in Belmont, Massachusetts; consultant in psychiatric research at the Boston Veterans Administration Hospital; and director of psychomotor therapy in the pain unit of the New England Rehabilitation Hospital. Pesso is the author of *Movement in*

Psychotherapy (1969) and *Experience in Action* (1973), and coeditor with John Crandell of *Moving Psychotherapy: Theory and Applications of Pesso Boyden System/Psychomotor Psychology* (1991).

Pilates Method of Body Conditioning®

Leah Chaback, director of the Movement Center, is a certified Pilates instructor and teacher-trainer. She began studying the Pilates Method in 1986 at SUNY, Purchase, New York. Chaback has trained and worked extensively with Romana Kryzanowska, disciple of Joseph Pilates and master teacher of his method for more than fifty years. After teaching the Pilates Method in New York City studios, she opened the Movement Center in 1990.

Poetry Therapy

Nicholas Mazza, Ph.D., is a professor in the School of Social Work at Florida State University. He is also editor of the *Journal of Poetry Therapy*. He has lectured and published extensively on the use of poetry and music in clinical practice.

Polarity Therapy

John Beaulieu, ND, Ph.D., is the author of the *Polarity Therapy Workbook* (1994).

Process Oriented Psychology

Dr. Joseph Goodbread is a longtime student and colleague of Arnold Mindell. He is a co-founder of the Research Society for Process Oriented Psychology in Zurich, of the Process Work Center of Portland, Oregon, and of the Global Process Institute in Portland. He is the author of *The Dreambody Toolkit: A Practical Introduction to the Philosophy, Goals, and Practice of Process-Oriented Psychology* and *Radical Intercourse: How Inevitable Relationships Are Created by Dreaming*, a book on the dynamics of therapeutic relationships. He practices and teaches process work in Portland and throughout the world.

Psychodrama

Adam Blatner, M.D., is the author of several books and articles on the practice of psychodrama.

Psychoneuroimmunology

Leonard A. Wisneski, M.D., is a board-certified physician in internal medicine and in endocrinology and metabolism. He is also certified in acupuncture and homeopathy, which he has incorporated into his practice. Wisneski is a member of the board of directors of the Integral Health Foundation.

Leonard Sherp is a medical writer and reiki practitioner. He is program director of the Integral Health Foundation.

Psychosynthesis

Richard Schaub, Ph.D., cofounded the New York Psychosynthesis Institute with Bonney Gulino Schaub, M.S., RN, CS. The Schaubs have worked in every phase of mental health, alcohol and drug rehabilitation, and health care in careers that span thirty years. They teach internationally in the fields of psychotherapy, recovery, higher self-education, clinical imagery, and contemplation. They have published numerous professional articles, are associate editors of *Alternative Health Practitioner*, and are the authors of *Healing Addictions*.

Qigong

Kenneth S. Cohen, M.A., director of the Qigong Research and Practice Center in Colorado, is an internationally renowned China scholar, qigong master, and health educator. He has been teaching qigong for more than twenty-five years and is helping to build a bridge between qigong and medical science. He was one of nine "exceptional healers" studied in the Menninger Clinic's Copper Wall Project, where he demonstrated unusual physiological control while practicing qigong. Cohen has written more than 150 articles and is the author of *The Way of Qigong*.

Radix

Erica Kelley has shared the growth of Radix since its inception in the late sixties, including its teaching, training, facilities, and administration in the United States and Europe. She maintains a part-time practice in Vancouver and administers Kelley/Radix and K/R Publications.

Rebirthing

Maureen Malone is director of the New York Rebirthing Center.

Tony Lo Mastro is director of the Philadelphia Rebirthing Center.

Reflexology

Laura Norman is a certified reflexologist and New York State–licensed massage practitioner. She is also author of *Feet First: A Guide to Foot Reflexology*. With a B.S. from Boston University and three master's degrees from Adelphi University, she originally embarked on a career in education. She discovered the potency of reflexology when she used it in her early work with hyperactive and emotionally dysfunctional children at Maimonides Institute in Brooklyn. She established the Laura Norman Method Reflexology Training Center in New York, offering a comprehensive training and certification program.

Reiki

Elaine J. Abrams is a reiki master instructor. In private practice in New York City since 1987, she brings her extensive experience with more than eight hundred clients and knowledge as a reiki instructor to her workshops. As founder of the Reiki Group, she provides a continuing support system for her practitioners.

Relaxation Response

Richard Friedman, Ph.D., was a professor of psychiatry at SUNY, Stonybrook.

Herbert Benson, M.D., is the Mind/Body Medical Institute Associate Professor of Medicine at Harvard Medical School; chief of the division of behavioral medicine at the Beth Israel Deaconess Medical Center; and founding president of the Mind/Body Medical Institute. A graduate of Wesleyan University and Harvard Medical School, he is the author or coauthor of more than 150 scientific publications and six books.

Patricia Myers is a research associate at the Mind/Body Medical Institute at the Beth Israel Deaconess Medical Center at Harvard Medical School. Her areas of interest include the economics of behavioral medicine and the use of behavioral interventions in the treatment of pain.

Rolfing®

Allan Davidson was trained by Ida Rolf in Big Sur and San Francisco, California, from 1973 to 1975 and has been lecturing and writing about Rolfing ever since. In the 1980s he cofounded the Chicago School for Advanced Bodywork, a pioneering clinic and forum for new ideas and technologies. He now codirects the Structural Therapy Institute, where he teaches bodywork problem-solving courses to health professionals. He is also trained in the hakomi method of body-centered psychotherapy and in CranioSacral therapy.

ROM Dance

Patricia Yu, M.A., cocreator of the ROM dance, is director of the T'ai-Chi Center in Madison, Wisconsin. She originally learned t'ai chi ch'üan and tao kung meditation in 1970 with Master Liu Pei Ch'ung in the Republic of China. She continues to practice daily.

Rosen Method

Ivy Green is a professor of psychology, a certified Rosen method practitioner, a certified teacher of the Alexander technique, and a licensed massage therapist. Her book on the Rosen method, a psychospiritual bodywork, was published in 1998.

Rubenfeld Synergy Method™

Ilana Rubenfeld, a pioneer in integrating bodywork with psychotherapy, has been an influential healer for the past thirty-five years. She originated the Rubenfeld Synergy Method in the early 1960s and started its professional training program in 1977. Formerly on the faculties of the New York University Graduate School of Social Work and New School for Social Research, she currently teaches at the Omega and Esalen Institutes and the Open Center.

Sandplay Therapy

Lois Carey, MSW, BCDSW, is a practitioner of sandplay therapy.

Sensory Awareness

Mary Alice Roche was cofounder, with Charlotte Selver, of the Sensory Awareness Foundation. She served as managing secretary until she retired in 1988 but continued as bulletin editor and archivist. She has a private practice and is a member of the Sensory Awareness Leaders Guild.

Shamanism

Hal Zina Bennett, Ph.D., is a longtime student of shamanism. He is also the author of twenty-five books on health (such as *The Well Body Book*, with Mike Samuels, M.D.), psychology (*The Holotropic Mind*, with Stan Grof, M.D.), and Native American spirituality (*Zuni Fetishes*). He is an adjunct faculty member at the Institute of Transpersonal Psychology, a private graduate school in Palo Alto, California. Bennett is a frequent contributor to *Shaman's Drum* magazine and *Sacred Hoop*, published in England.

SHEN®

Richard Pavek is director of the SHEN Therapy Institute, which provides information regarding SHEN research, development, and certification procedures.

Shiatsu, Therapeutic Touch

Thomas Claire is a licensed massage therapist and author of the authoritative book *Bodywork: What Type of Massage to Get—and How to Make the Most of It.* A graduate of the Swedish and Ohashi Institutes, he is a reiki master and a practitioner of Swedish massage, shiatsu, CranioSacral therapy, myofascial release, and

therapeutic touch. His work has been featured in numerous publications, and he is a frequent guest on radio and television programs.

Skinner Releasing Technique

Joan Skinner is the originator of the Skinner releasing technique. She earned a B.A. from Bennington College and an M.A. from the University of Illinois. She is Professor Emeritus at the University of Washington and was a member of both the Martha Graham and Merce Cunningham dance companies.

Soma Neuromuscular Integration

Marcia W. Nolte, LMP, has a background in movement studies ranging from performance dance, as a professional ballet and modern dancer and teacher, to a variety of therapeutic modalities of movement. She has been in private practice in soma bodywork since 1979 and continues to explore with her clients the use of movement as medicine.

Karen L. Bolesky, M.A., CMHC, LMP, has been a mental health counselor since 1972 and a soma practitioner since 1985. Karen trained with Elisabeth Kübler-Ross, M.D., and Gregg Furth, Ph.D., in interpretation of spontaneous drawings as an aid to the creative process.

Somatorespiratory Integration

Donald Epstein is a chiropractor and developer of network spinal analysis. He is president of the Association for Network Chiropractic. He is also the author of several articles on the practice of this discipline.

Sounding

Don Campbell is an internationally renowned expert in music, sound, health, and learning. In 1988 he founded the Institute for Music, Health, and Education in Boulder, Colorado, and served as executive director until 1995. He has written several books on the relationship among music, health, and education, and he travels extensively, teaching musicians, teachers, physicians, therapists, and trainers. Presently, Campbell directs year-long study programs on the therapeutic and transformational uses of sound and music.

Spatial Dynamics℠

Jaimen McMillan is the originator of Spatial Dynamics. He has trained hundreds of students as movement specialists and has worked with a broad spectrum of clients ranging from Olympic athletes to severely handicapped children. He is director of the Spatial Studies Institute, Inc., as well as the Spatial Dynamics Institute.

Swedish Massage

Janie McGee is a licensed massage therapist who has been in private practice in New York City for fifteen years. She is also a licensed staff physical therapist in a geriatric facility. She studied physical therapy at Long Island University and was enrolled in premedical studies at Hunter College.

Taekwondo

Mark V. Wiley, an internationally renowned martial arts master and scholar, has been involved in the martial arts for twenty years. He has written the best-selling books *Filipino Martial Arts: Cabales Serrada Escrima* and *Filipino Martial Culture* and is the author of more than fifty articles that have appeared in leading martial arts magazines and journals. He currently serves as martial arts editor of the Charles E. Tuttle Publishing Company and associate editor of the *Journal of Asian Martial Arts*. He is cofounder of talahib-marga, a contemporary, cross-cultural, martial-meditative discipline.

T'ai Chi Ch'üan

Sophia Delza was the first Western female master of t'ai chi ch'üan and was also a dancer, lecturer, and writer. She is credited as being the first Westerner to bring t'ai chi to the United States. She was the 1996 recipient of the Chinese Martial Arts Association's Lifetime Achievement Award. She died on June 27, 1996.

Tomatis Method

Dr. Billie Thompson, founder and director of Sound Listening & Learning Centers in Phoenix, Arizona, and Pasadena, California, received a Ph.D. from Arizona State University in 1979. Thompson was one of the pioneers who brought the Tomatis method to the United States. She edited the English translations of Tomatis's autobiography, *The Conscious Ear*, and his first book, *The Ear and Language*. She established the Phoenix center in 1987 to provide both corrective and accelerated learning opportunities for individuals, corporations, and other organizations.

Traditional Chinese Medicine

Cindy Banker is a certified instructor and practitioner of Oriental bodywork therapy. She began her shiatsu training with Shizuko Yamamoto in 1976 and now uses both five-element shiatsu and Chinese herbal medicine in her private practice. Banker is currently the national director of education for the American Oriental Bodywork Therapy Association. She is an active member of the National Certification Commission for Acupuncture and Oriental Medicine's task force, which is developing the first national certification exam for oriental bodywork therapy. Since 1983 she has been teaching shiatsu in complete training programs and currently owns and teaches at the New England Center for Oriental Bodywork in Brookline, Massachusetts.

Trager Psychophysical Integration

Deane Juhan has been on staff at the Esalen Institute since 1973 and a Trager practitioner there since 1978. He lectures on anatomy and physiology for bodyworkers and has recently published a major work on that subject, *Job's Body: A Handbook for Bodywork*. Deane is also an instructor at the Trager Institute.

Transcendental Meditation

Robert Roth is the author of the popular book *Transcendental Meditation*, which has been translated into ten languages. Roth has lectured and taught TM for more than twenty-five years to tens of thousands of people in the United States and Canada and throughout Europe. He is a senior adviser to the Maharishi Corporate Development Program, the nonprofit organization that teaches the TM program in business and industry, as well as a founder of the Institute for Fitness and Athletic Excellence, which teaches the technique to amateur and professional athletes.

Tui Na

Gina Martin is a licensed massage therapist and chair of the Eastern studies department of the Swedish Institute School of Massage Therapy. She was chair of the New York State Board of Massage Therapy from 1994 to 1998 and is a current board member. Martin is recognized by the American Oriental Bodywork Therapy Association as a certified instructor in five-element style shiatsu. She has been featured in the magazine *First for Women* and is a contributing author to the *Reader's Digest Family Guide to Natural Medicine*. Her book, *The Shiatsu Workbook*, is an Eastern anatomy coloring book published by the Swedish Institute. She maintains a private practice in Eastern bodywork, specializing in shiatsu, tui na, and nuad bo ran.

Unergi

Ute Arnold is an artist and therapist in private practice and is the director of the Unergi Center. She is a certified Rubenfeld Synergy practitioner and trainer and holds degrees in art and design from Schaeffer School of Design, San Francisco, and Chelsea School of Art, London. She has been leading workshops and trainings since 1978 in Scandinavia, France, Canada, and the United States.

Wellness

Brian Luke Seaward, Ph.D., is a faculty member of the University of Colorado. He is recognized internationally as a leading expert in the fields of stress management, mind-body-spirit healing, and human spirituality. Seaward is the author of the critically acclaimed collegiate textbook *Managing Stress: Principles and Strategies for Health and Well-Being,* and the popular best-seller *Stand Like Mountain, Flow Like Water: Reflections on Stress and Human Spirituality.*

Yoga

Lillo (Leela) Way is certified by the Integral Yoga Institute to teach hatha yoga asanas (poses), prenatal yoga, pranayama (breathing practices), deep relaxation, chanting, and meditation. She is an actor and dancer and has been director of her own dance company. Way taught at New York University for seven years. She also taught at Hunter College and was a visiting professor at Princeton University. In addition to her private practice, she is currently on the faculty of the Integral Yoga Institute and the Soho Sanctuary in New York.

Zero Balancing®

The originator of Zero Balancing, Fritz Smith has taught body energy work to hundreds of health care practitioners since 1973. He is an osteopathic M.D., acupuncturist, and teacher. Smith is a pioneer in the blending of Eastern energy systems with Western science and bodywork. He is the author of *Inner Bridges: A Guide to Energy Movement and Body Structure.*

Index

A

action profiling, 302
acupoints, 162, 163, 168
acupressure, 129-30, 160, 162-73
  basic principles, 163
  benefits and risks, 163
  history, 162–63
  practice, 163
  self-, 163
  styles of, 162–63
acupuncture, 23, 74, 98, 130, 160, 164–67
  applications, 160
  body, mind, and spirit and, 164, 166
  history, 164–65
  philosophy, 165
  practice, 166
  uses, 165
  Western theories of, 166
acu-yoga, 163
Adams, Kathleen, 324
Adler, Janet, 313, 315
affirmation, 379
Africa, 205, 244–46, 249–50
aikido, 245, 247–48
  basic principles, 247
  benefits, 247
  history, 247
  practice, 247–48
Akiyama, 251
Alexander, Frederick M., 142, 179–80, 183–84
Alexander technique, 142, 180, 183–85, 350, 381
  benefits, 184

history, 183
practice, 184
theory, 183–84
Alexander the Great, 130
allopathic health care model, 1, 8
  cost and side effects, 1
  dissatisfaction with, 1, 2
  goal of, 3
  institutionalization of, 2
alternative health care models, 1–27
  defined, 1
  goal of, 3
  healing crisis and, 3
  historical survey, 1–2
American Dance Therapy Association, 317
American Medical Association, 2, 42
American Music Therapy Association, 329
American Polarity Therapy Association, 116, 117
archetypes, 311, 334, 335
Aristotle, 2, 60, 130
armoring
  increasing flexibility of, 378
  releasing, 168, 363–65, 366, 367, 377–78
Arnold, Ute, 383
aromatherapy, 80, 81–83
  benefits and risks, 82
  defined, 81
  history, 81
  limbic system and, 81, 82
  practice, 82
  precautions, 82
  theoretical basis, 81–82

arts. *See also* expressive and creative arts
     therapies
   changing role of, 306–7
art therapy, 311–13
   benefits, 312
   history, 311–12
   practice, 312
   theory, 312
Asian bodywork, 159–77
Asian meditative techniques, 282
Assagioli, Roberto, 172, 338, 351, 375–76
Aston, Judith, 185, 197
Aston-Patterning, 185–87, 197
   benefits, 186
   practice, 186
aura, human, 42
authentic movement, 313–15
   basic principles, 313–14
   benefits, 315
   history, 313
   practice, 314–15
ayurvedic medicine, 2, 4–6
   benefits and risks, 5
   diet and, 47–48
   history, 4
   lifestyle management and, 4, 5
   philosophy, 4–5
   polarity therapy and, 116
   practice of, 5

B

babies
   massage of, 139–41
   music and, 328
Bach, Edward, 78, 90–91
ba-gua, 111, 112
Baldwin, Christina, 323
Barnes, John F., 143
Bartenieff, Irmgard, 187–88, 299
Bartenieff Fundamentals, 187–89
   benefits, 189
   history, 187–88
   practice, 189
   theory, 188–89
Bates, William, 83
Bates method, 83–85, 204
   benefits and risks, 84
   history, 83–84

practice, 84
   theoretical foundation, 84
behavioral model of health, and Bates
     method, 84
behavioral vision therapy, 85–88
   conditions helped by, 87
   history, 85
   practice, 86–87
   theoretical foundation, 86
Benjamin, Ben, 142–43
Benson, Herbert, 283, 284, 286–87
Bernheim, Hyppolyte, 68
bhakti yoga, 272
bibliotherapy, 331
bioenergetics, 341–44
   basic principles, 342
   benefits, 343–44
   practice, 342–43
biofeedback training, 63–65, 74
   Bates method and, 83
   benefits, 64–65
   history, 63
   practice, 64
   theory of, 63–64
   uses of, 65
   visual, 86–87
biofield, 125
Bleuler, Eugen, 311, 316
Bodymap, 346
body-memory, 152
Body-Mind Centering, 190–92
   basic principles, 190–91
   benefits, 191
   history, 190
   practice, 191
body/mind medicine. *See* mind/body
     medicine
bodynamic analysis, 344–46
   benefits and risks, 346
   history, 344
   practice, 345–46
   theory, 344–45
body-oriented psychotherapies, 337–83
   benefits and risks, 340
   history and development, 337–39
   theories and practices, 339
bodywork. *See also* Asian bodywork
   defined, 105, 159

bodywork therapy
    Chinese, 23
    defined, 29
Bothmer gymnastics exercises, 238
Bowen, Thomas A., 135
Bowen technique, 135–36
    history, 135
Boyden-Pesso, Diane, 368, 369
Braid, James, 68
brain
    creative arts and, 307–8
    EMDR and, 88–89
    flower remedies and, 90
    guided imagery and, 66
    light and, 96–97
    limbic system, 80, 81, 82
Brain Gym, 218–20
    benefits, 219
    history, 218
    practice, 219
    theory, 218–19
Brazil, 248
breathing
    bioenergetics and, 342, 343
    continuum and, 224
    Holotropic Breathwork, 360–63
    rebirthing techniques, 378–80
Bresler, David E., 71–72
Breuer, Josef, 337
brief strobic phototherapy (BSP), 97–98
bright-light therapy, 98
Broch, Eva, 347
Brown, Katherine, 366
Brown, Malcolm, 366
Buber, Martin, 355, 356
Buddhism, 121, 283
Burmeister, Mary, 167, 170–71

C
Campbell, Don, 100, 101
cancer, and massage therapy, 133
capoeira, 244, 245, 248–51
    basic principles, 249–50
    benefits, 250
    history, 248–49
    practice, 250
Cartesian principle, 25
certified movement analyst (CMA), 188–89

Chace, Marian, 316
chakras, 116–17, 172, 347, 383
Charcot, Jean-Martin, 316
chi, 106, 116–17, 162, 164, 165, 253.
        See also qi
    defined, 159
    feng shui and, 110–13
    manipulating, 159–60
child development stages, 345
China, 6, 20–22, 107, 111, 116, 118–20, 162,
        215, 216, 243–44, 306
    kung fu wu su, 262–63
    massage techniques, 129–30, 160, 175–77
    t'ai chi in, 239–40
Chinese medicine, traditional.
        See traditional Chinese medicine
        (TCM)
chiropractic, 29, 30, 31, 33–35
    defined, 33
    education for, 34
    history, 33–34
    network chiropractic, 38–40
    practice, 34–35
chiropractors, 30, 31–32
Choi Hong Hi, 266
Church, Hudson, 220
Clark, Barbara, 200
Cleveland Homeopathic College, 12
Cohen, Bonnie Bainbridge, 190
colonic irrigation, 94
colorpuncture, 98–99
complementary therapies. See alternative
        health care model
connective tissue, 149
Connective Tissue Therapy, 132, 136–38
    benefits, 137
    history, 136
    practice, 137
    theoretical basis, 136–37
    theory, 136–37
Conrad-Da'oud, Emilie, 216, 222, 223–24
constitutional types
    ayurvedic medicine and, 4, 5
contact improvisation, 220–22
    basic principles, 221
    benefits and risks, 222
    history, 220–21
    practice, 221–22
continuum, 222–24

history and theory, 223–24
practice and benefits, 224
core energetics, 346–49
    benefits, 349
    history, 347–38
    practice, 348–49
    theory, 348
CORE myofascial therapy, 138
coreSomatics, 350–51
CORE structural integrative therapy,
        138–39
    benefits, 138
    practice, 138
costs of health care, 1, 2, 56
Coué, Emile, 68
Cousins, Norman, 73–74
craniosacral system, 36–37
CranioSacral therapy, 31, 35–38
    basic principles, 36–37
    benefits, 37
    defined, 35
    history, 36
    practice, 37
    practitioners, 36–37
creative arts therapies. See expressive and
        creative arts therapies
creativity, 373
Cullen, William, 9
Cyriax, James, 142

D

dance
    African, 249
    authentic movement, 313–15
    contact improvisation, 220–22
    dance therapy, 315–18
    Gurdjieff movements, 226–29
    Halprin life/art process, 322
    Skinner releasing techniques and, 235
dance therapist registered (DTR), 318
dance therapy
    basic principles, 317
    benefits, 318
    history, 315–17
    practice, 317–18
decision-making, 302, 303
de Hartmann, Thomas, 228–29
Dennison, Gail, 216, 218

Dennison, Paul E., 216, 218
Desai, Amrit, 278
de Salzmann, Jeanne, 227
Descartes, René, 25, 60, 66
Dicke, Elizabeth, 136
diet. See nutritional and dietary practices
disease
    ayurvedic medicine on, 5
    germ concept of, 6
do-in, 108–109
    benefits, 109
    history, 108
    practice, 109
    theoretical basis, 108
doshas (life energies), 4, 5
Downing, John, 97
drama therapists, 320–21
drama therapy, 318–21, 374. See also
        psychodrama
    basic principles, 319
    history, 319
    practice, 320–21
drugs, pharmaceutical, 48, 78–79
    herbs and, 52, 53
Durham, Else Henscke, 207

E

ear lavage, 94
Edson, Susan, 12
Egypt, ancient, 81, 93, 130, 306
Ehrenfried, Lily, 207
Einstein, Albert, 272
electronic measuring instruments, 63–64
Eliade, Mircea, 270, 271
EMDR. See eye movement desensitization
        and reprocessing
emotional-kinesthetic psychotherapy,
        351–52
    history and theory, 351
    practice and benefits, 351–52
emotions
    flower remedies and, 90, 91, 92
    immune system and, 73, 74
    mind/body medicine and, 61
    SHEN and, 124–26
empathy, 317, 374
endorphins, 166
energy forces. See also subtle energy
        practices

ayurvedic philosophy of, 4–5
Chinese holistic system and, 163
core energetics and, 347, 348
orgone energy, 363–64
Pressure Acupuncture and, 172
theories of, 1–2
traditional Chinese medicine and, 22–23
vibrational, unergy and, 383
Zero Balancing and, 44–45
enkephalins, 166
enneagram, 291, 293–95
    basic principles, 294
    benefits and risks, 295
    history, 293–94
    practice, 294–95
environment, and feng shui, 110–13
Epstein, Donald, 38
Erickson, Milton H., 68–69
Esalen Institute, 307, 360
essential oils, 81–82
European health care models, 2
eurythmy, 224–26
    basic principles, 225
    benefits, 226
    history, 224–25
    philosophy, 225
    practice, 225
expressive and creative arts therapies,
        305–36
    benefits, 309
    brain and, 307–8
    exploring, 309
    social and emotional skills and, 308
    theoretical orientation and, 308
eye care. See Bates method; behavioral
        vision therapy
eye movement desensitization and
        reprocessing (EMDR), 88–90
    benefits and risks, 89–90
    history, 88
    practice, 89
    theoretical foundation, 88–89

F

fascia, 143–44, 198
    Connective Tissue Massage and, 136–37
    Hellerwork and, 198
    myofascial release and, 143–44
    soma and, 208

feet. See reflexology
Feldenkrais, Moshe, 180, 192, 194, 195, 381
Feldenkrais Method, 192–94, 350, 381
    benefits, 192, 193–94
    history, 192
    modalities of learning, 193
    practice, 192–93
felt sense, 353–54
feng shui, 105, 110–13
    basic principles, 110–12
    benefits, 113
    practice, 112–13
Fenichel, Clare, 207
Field, Tiffany, 140
flower remedies, 78, 80, 90–92
    benefits, 92
    defined, 90
    practice, 91–92
focusing, 352–55
    history and theory, 352–53
    practice, six steps in, 353–54
Freud, Sigmund, 60, 66, 68, 106, 306–7, 308,
        311, 337–38, 339, 355, 363, 375
Fromm, Erich, 207
Fuller, Betty, 212
Funakoshi, Gichin, 256–57

G

Gach, Michael Reed, 163
Gendlin, Eugene, 351, 352–53
gestalt therapy, 255–58
    benefits and risks, 357
    history, 355–56
    practice, 357
    theory, 356–57
Gindler, Elsa, 151, 180, 201, 206, 207
Goldstein, Kurt, 366
Graham, Sylvester, 48
Greece, ancient, 6 0, 48, 65, 81, 93, 106, 130,
        215, 243, 293, 306, 326
Greeks, ancient, 2, 78, 331
Green, Elmer and Alyce, 61, 63
Grof, Christine, 360, 361
Grof, Stanislav, 339, 360, 361
group psychotherapy, 368–69, 372
Guest, Anne Hutchinson, 299
guided imagery, 60, 62, 65–67
    benefits, 67
    defined, 65

history, 65–66
Interactive Guided Imagery, 66, 71–72
practice, 66–67
theory of, 66
Gurdjieff, George I., 216, 226–28, 293
Gurdjieff movements, 226–29
history, 227–28
practice, 228–29

H

Hahnemann, Samuel, 2, 9–10, 11, 106
hakomi integrative somatics, 358–60
basic principles, 358–59
benefits, 359–60
practice, 359
Hall, Edward T., 237
Halprin, Anna, 322
Halprin, Daria, 322
Halprin life/art process, 321–23
history, 322
theory and practice, 322
Hanna, Thomas, 195, 196, 215
Hanna Somatic Education, 194–97
benefits and precautions, 196
history, 195
practice, 196
Harlowe, Diane, 216
hatha yoga, 269, 271–72. See also yoga
Hayashi, Chijuro, 122
Head, Henry, 136
healing. See also self-healing abilities
holistic approach to, 8
healing crisis, defined, 3
heart meditation, 351–52
Heller, Joseph, 180, 197, 198
Hellerwork, 197–99
basic principles, 197–98
benefits and risks, 198–99
herbs/herbal medicine, 52–55, 53, 54
basic principles, 53
benefits and risks, 54–55
Chinese, 166
drugs and, 52, 53
history, 52
practice, 53–54
preparation of, 53–54
traditional Chinese, 23
uses of, 54

Hewitt, James, 270
Heyer, Lucy, 151
Hippocrates, 30, 33, 48, 56, 65, 78, 106, 130
history of alternative health models, 1–2.
See also history under specific types of
therapy
Hoffer, Abram, 56, 57
Hogan, Peter, 381
holism
osteopathy and, 43
Still and, 41
wellness programs and, 25
holistic health care methods, 6–9
allopathic model and, 2
basic principles, 7, 8
benefits, 8
goal of, 6
history, 6–7
naturopathy and, 14
Holotropic Breathwork, 360–63
benefits and risks, 362
history, 360–63
practice, 361–62
theory, 361
home, feng shui and, 110–13
homeopathy, 9–13, 106
ayurveda and, 4
basic principles, 11–12
benefits of, 12–13
defined, 9
history of, 9–11
as holistic, 11
practice of, 12
in United States, 10–11
Hull, Clark, 68
humanistic psychology, 338–39, 355
Hunt, Valerie, 223
Hute, Evan and Wilfrid, 56
Huxley, Aldous, 83, 282
hydrotherapy, 78, 92–95
benefits and risks, 94
defined, 92
history, 93
theoretical basis, 93–94
hypnosis
benefits, 70
self-, 66
hypnotherapists, 70
hypnotherapy, 60, 68–71

defined, 68
history, 68–69
practice, 69–70
self-, 70
theory of, 69

I

Ichazo, Oscar, 293
Ideokinesis, 199–201
    benefits, 201
    history, 200
    practice, 200–201
    theory, 200
imagery
    in Bartenieff Fundamentals, 189
    symbolic, 311
    unconscious, 311
immune system
    journal writing and, 324
    nervous system and, 73, 74
    reiki and, 123
    stress and, 73, 74
India, 4, 6, 216, 243, 270, 272, 283, 288,
        289, 306
infant massage, 139–41
    history, 139
    theory, 139–40
Ingham, Eunice, 147
integral yoga, 276–77
    history and principles, 276
Interactive Guided Imagery, 66, 71–72
    benefits and risks, 72
    defined, 71
    history, 71–72
    practice, 72
interdependency, and holistic health, 6, 7
International Association for Infant
        Massage, 139
International Somatic Movement and
        Education Therapy Association,
        180, 181
Iyengar, B. K. S., 277
Iyengar yoga, 277–78
    history and philosophy, 277

J

Jacoby, Heinrich, 180, 206–7
Japan

aikido, 247–48
    judo, 254
    ju jutsu, 251
    karate, 256–57
    kendo, 259–60, 262
    shiatsu, 173–75
Javal, Emile, 78, 85
jhana yoga, 272
Jigoro, Kano, 192, 254–55
Jin Shin Do Bodymind Acupressure, 162,
        167–69
    basic principles, 168
    benefits and risks, 169
    history, 167–68
    practice, 168–69
Jin Shin Jyutsu Physio-Philosophy, 167,
        169–71
    basic principles, 170–71
    history, 169–70
    practice, 171
Johnsen, Lillimor, 344
journal therapy, 323–25
    benefits, 324, 325
    history, 323
    philosophy, 323–24
    practice, 324
journal writing, 331, 332, 333
Joy, Brugh, 197
judo, 192, 254–56
    basic principles, 255
    benefits, 255
    history, 254–55
    practice, 255
ju jutsu, 251–53
    history, 251–52
    philosophy and benefits, 253
    training and techniques, 252–53
Jung, Carl, 116, 151, 172, 306, 308, 311, 313,
        334, 335, 336, 338, 360, 366, 375

K

Kabat-Zinn, Jon, 283
Kagan, Alfred, 142
Kalff, Dora, 335, 336
Kamiya, Joe, 63
Kanemon, Terada, 254
Kano Jigoro. *See* Jigoro, Kano
kapha, 4, 5

karate, 256–58
   history, 256–57
   philosophy and practice, 257
   styles, 257
   training, 258
karma yoga, 273
Kelley, Charles R. (Chuck), 377–78
Kelley, Erica, 377
Kellogg, John Harvey, 93
kendo, 259–62
   basic principles, 260
   benefits, 261–62
   history, 259–60
   practice, 260–61
Kenkichi, Sakakibara, 259
Kestenberg, Judith S., 296, 297, 299
Kestenberg movement profile, 291, 296–98
   applications, 297–98
   basic principles, 297
   history, 296–97
ki. See chi; qi
kinetic awareness, 201–3
   basic principles, 201–2
   benefits, 203
   history, 201
   practice, 202–3
Klenner, Fred, 56
Kneipp, Sebastian, 2, 14, 78, 93
Knill, Paolo, 326
Konia, Charles, 365
Korea
   taekwondo, 265, 266
Kousaleos, George P., 138
Kraeplin, Emil, 311
Kramer, Edith, 311–12
Krieger, Dolores, 127
kripalu yoga, 278–79
   practice and benefits, 278–79
Kripalvananda, 278
Kübler-Ross, Elisabeth, 27
kundalini yoga, 272
kung fu wu su, 262–65
   benefits, 265
   history, 262–63
   practice, 264
   styles, 263–64
Kunz, Dora, 127
Kurtz, Ron, 351, 358
Kushi, Michio, 48, 108

L

Laban, Rudolf, 187, 188, 291, 296, 299, 301–2
Laban movement analysis, 188, 291, 298–301
   history, 299
   philosophy, 299–300
   practice, 300
Lamb, Warren, 296–97, 299, 302
Lao-tzu, 165
Lawrence, F. C., 301–2
Leedy, Jack J., 331
Leibowitz, Judith, 381
Lewis, Penny, 296
Liberman, Jacob, 97
Liebault, Auguste Ambroise, 68
life cycle, Kübler-Ross on, 27
life force, 105–6. *See also* chi; qi
lifestyle
   holistic health, 6, 7
   wellness and, 7
light therapy, 80, 95–100
   basic principles, 96–97
   benefits and risks, 99
   defined, 95
   forms of, 97–99
   history, 95–96
   medical applications, 99
   practice, 97–99
limbic system, 80
   aromatherapy and, 81, 82
Ling, Per Henrik, 131, 155
Loman, Susan, 296
love force, 347–48
Lowen, Alexander, 341, 342, 343, 347, 366
Lowenfeld, Margaret, 334–35
Lust, Benedict, 14, 78
lymph drainage, 132

M

Machado, Manoel dos Reis, 249
McClure, Vimala, 139, 140
McMillan, Jaimen, 216, 236–37
macrobiotics, 48, 108
magnet therapy (magnetotherapy), 33, 113–15
   benefits, 115
   history, 113–14
   philosophy, 114

practice, 114
management teams, movement pattern
    analysis of, 302, 303
mantra yoga, 272
Marcher, Lisbeth, 344–45
Marks, Linda, 351
martial arts, 243–68, 244
    basic principles, 244–45
    benefits and risks, 245
    choosing, 245
    country of origin, 246
    external, 244
    internal, 244–45
    learning, 245
    theories of development, 243–44
Maslow, Abraham, 339, 366
massage therapy, 129–57
    basic approaches, 132
    benefits and risks, 133
    history, 129–31
    licensure, 132
    precautions, 133
Maudsley, Henry, 316
Maury, Marguerite, 81
mechanistic paradigm, 25
medical orgone therapy, 363–66
    benefits, 363
    history, 363–64
    practice, 364–65
    theory, 364
medical orgonomy, 338
meditation, 281–90. See also relaxation
        response; Transcendental Meditation
    benefits, 284
    in EKP, 351–52
    history in West, 281–82
    mindfulness, 358, 359
    practice, 283
    role in health, 284, 287
    understanding, 282–83
megavitamin therapy. See orthomolecular
        therapy
Meir Schneider self-healing method, 203–6
    benefits, 205
    philosophy, 204
    practice, 205
Melzack, Ronald, 166
mentastics, 213
meridians, 163, 165, 168, 172

Mesmer, Anton, 68
Mesmerism, 33
miasms, 10
Miller, Kay, 350
mind/body medicine, 59–75
    ancient disciplines and, 60
    basic beliefs, 61–62
    defined, 59
    development in West, 60–61
    in future, 62
    uses of, 59
Mindell, Arnold, 172, 371
mindfulness meditation, 283, 358, 359
mirroring movement, in dance therapy,
        316, 317
Montague, Ashley, 139
Moreno, Jacob, 339
Moreno, Jacob Levi, 372–73
motivation, personal, and healing, 61–62
movement, symbolic, 317
movement pattern analysis, 292, 301–3
    history, 301–2
    practice, 302–3
    theory, 302
movement patterns
    movement therapies and, 181
    psychophysical evaluation frameworks
        for, 291–303
movement therapists, 180–82
movement therapy methods, 179–214
    versus bodywork methods, 179
    educational process, 181
    pioneers in, 179–80
    unifying principles of, 181–82
Mowrer, Hobart G., 63
multimodal expressive arts therapy, 325–28
    benefits, 327
    history, 325–26
    theory and practice, 326–27
Murai, Jiro, 162, 167, 168, 170
muscular therapy, 142–43
    history, 142
    practice, 142
music
    babies and, 328
    Holotropic Breathing and, 361
    psychological effects, 328–29
music therapists, 328, 329
music therapy, 328–31

basic principles, 329
benefits, 330
history, 329
practice, 329—30
types, 329–30
myofascial release, 132, 143–144
benefits, 144
history, 143
practice, 144
theoretical basis, 143–44
myofascial trigger-point therapy, 132, 145–46
benefits, 146
history, 145
practice, 146
theoretical basis, 145–46

N

Naranjo, Claudio, 293
National Association for Drama Therapy, 319, 321
National Association for Poetry Therapy, 331
naturopathic medicine, 13–16
basic principles, 14
benefits of, 15
defined, 13
doctors of, 13–15
history and development, 14
practice of, 14–15
naturopathic physicians, 13–15
Naumburg, Margaret, 311
network chiropractic, 38–40
benefits and risks, 39–40
history, 38
philosophy, 39
practice, 39
Neumann, Erich, 335
neurosensory development, 97
Nugent, John J., 33–34
nutritional and dietary practices, 47–58
history, 47–49
practitioners, 49
theoretical foundation of, 49

O

Ogden, Pat, 358
Ohashiastsu, 174
Okinawa, 256–57

Omega Institute, 307
Optometric Extension Program, 85
optometrists
Bates method and, 84
behavioral, 85, 87
organismic body psychotherapy, 366–67
basic principles, 366–67
history, 366
practice and benefits, 367
Organon of Rational Medicine (Hahnemann), 9–10
orgone therapy. See medical orgone therapy
Oriental bodywork. See Asian bodywork
Orr, Leonard, 339, 379
orthomolecular medicine, 48, 55–58
basic principles, 56–57
benefits and risks, 57, 58
goal of, 55
history, 55–56
practice, 57–58
precautions, 57
orthomolecular physicians, 57–58
Osmond, Humphrey, 56
osteopaths, 30, 31–32, 42
osteopathy, 29, 30, 31, 40–44. See also CranioSacral therapy
cranial, 36
defined, 40
history, 40–42
philosophy, 42–43
practice, 43
Ouspensky, P. D., 227

P

pain
magnet therapy and, 113–14
myofascial release and, 143–44
myofascial trigger-point therapy and, 145–46
St. John method and, 154–55
Palmer, Bartlett Joshua, 33, 34
Palmer, Daniel David, 30, 33, 34
Pastinha, Vincente Ferreira, 249
Patanjali, 269
Pauling, Linus, 48, 55–56
Pavek, Richard R., 124–25, 126
Paxton, Steve, 216, 220
Pennebaker, James, 324

Perls, Fritz, 207, 339, 355–56, 366, 381
Perls, Laura, 339, 355, 356, 381
personality
   enneagram system and, 293–95
   movement and, 315
Pesso, Albert, 368
Pesso Boyden system psychomotor, 368–71
   benefits, 370
   history and theory, 368
   practice, 369–70
physicians, and holistic principles, 8
phytomedicines, 53
Pierrakos, John, 341, 347–48
Pilates, Joseph, 216
Pilates, Joseph H., 229–30
Pilates Method of Body Conditioning, 216,
      229–32
   basic principles, 230
   benefits, 231
   history, 229–30
   philosophy, 230
   practice, 230–31
pitta, 4, 5
Plato, 306
PNI. See psychoneuroimmunology
poetry therapy, 324, 331–34
   benefits and risks, 333
   history, 331
   practice, 332
   theory, 331–32
polarity therapy, 115–18, 132
   ayurveda and, 4
   benefits, 118
   history, 115–16
   practice, 117–18
posttraumatic stress disorder (PTSD), and
      EMDR, 88
preventative medicine, 14
Priessnitz, Vincent, 78, 93
Process Acupuncture, 171–73
   basic principles, 172
   history, 171–72
   practice, 172
process-oriented psychology, 371–72
   history and theory, 371
   practice, 371–72
Progoff, Ira, 323
Prudden, Bonnie, 145

psychodrama, 372–75. See also drama
      therapy
   benefits and limitations, 374
   history, 372–73
   practice, 373–74
psychoneuroimmunology, 25, 73–75
   applications, 74
   defined, 73
   history, 73–74
psychophysical evaluation frameworks,
      291–303
   concepts in common, 291–92
   defined, 291
   using, 292
psychosynthesis, 375–77
   history and theory, 375–76
   practice and benefits, 376

Q

qi, 22, 106, 118–19, 125, 164, 173, 175.
      See also chi
qigong, 108, 118–21
   applications, 118, 119
   basic principles, 119–20
   benefits, 120
   defined, 118
   history, 119

R

Radix, 377–78
Raheem, Aminah, 163, 171–73
Rainer, Tristine, 323
raja yoga, 271
rebirthing, 378–80
   history and principles, 379
   practice and benefits, 379–80
reflexology, 146–48
   basic principles, 147
   benefits and risks, 148
   history, 147
   practice, 147–48
Registered Movement Therapist, 180
Reich, Wilhelm, 106, 142, 168, 338, 341, 342,
      347, 355–56, 357, 363–64, 366, 377
reiki, 121–24, 132
   benefits, 123
   philosophy and methods, 122

practice, 122–23
training, 123
relaxation response, 283, 286–87
history, 286
practice and benefits, 287
theory, 286–87
Rentsch, Oswald and Elaine, 135
Robertson-Smith, Bruce, 261
Rogers, Carl, 339, 366
role playing, 318–20
PBSP, 368, 369–70
psychodrama, 372–74
Rolf, Ida P., 149, 180, 185, 197
Rolfing, 132, 149–51, 197
basic principles, 149, 150
benefits and risks, 150
practice, 149–50
ROM dance, 232–33
basic principles, 232–33
benefits and risks, 233
history, 232
practice, 233
Rosen, Marion, 151–52
Rosen method, 151–53
basic principles, 152
benefits and risks, 153
practice, 152–53
Rosenthal, Norman, 96
Rossman, Martin L., 71–72
Rubenfeld, Ilana, 339, 381
Rubenfeld Synergy Method, 380–82
basic principles, 381–82
history, 381
practice and benefits, 382

S

SAD. *See* seasonal affective disorder
St. John, Paul, 154
St. John method of neuromuscular therapy,
154–55
benefits, 155
practice, 155
samadhi, 271, 274
sandplay therapy, 334–36
benefits and risks, 336
philosophy, 335
practice, 335–36
Sands Point Movement Study Group, 296

Satchidananda, 276
Scafidi, F. A., 140
Scandinavia, 344
Schauffler, Robert Haven, 331
Schneider, Meir, 203–5
seasonal affective disorder (SAD), 96, 98
self-healing abilities, 3
CranioSacral therapy and, 37
motivation and, 61–62
movement therapy methods and, 181
network chiropractic and, 38, 40
osteopathy and, 40
Selver, Charlotte, 207
Selye, Hans, 61
sensory awareness, 206–8
benefits, 208
history, 206–7
practice, 207
sensory-motor amnesia, 196
sensory recruitment, 67
sensory therapies, 77–104
history, 77–78
revival for, 79
in Western medicine, 78, 79–80
shamanism, 1, 16–20, 60, 74
benefits of, 19
defined, 16
history and philosophy, 17
practices, 18–19
resources and reading suggestions,
19–20
shamans, 16–20
Shapiro, Francine, 88, 89
SHEN, 106, 124–26
benefits, 125–26
history, 124–25
practice, 125
shiatsu, 132, 133, 160, 162, 173–75
benefits and risks, 174–75
history, 173
practice, 174
Siegel, Bernard, 66
Simons, David, 145
Simonton, Carl, 66
Skeffington, A. M., 85
skeletal manipulation methods, 29–51
history, 29–32
inborn healing potential and, 30–31
practitioners, 30, 31

Skinner, Joan, 216, 234
Skinner releasing technique, 234–36
    basic principles, 235
    benefits, 235
    history, 234
    practice, 234–35
sleep, 108
    REM, 89
Smith, Fritz F., 44–45
Smith, William, 41
Smuts, Jan Christiaan, 6
Socrates, 6
soma neuromuscular integration, 208–10
    basic principles, 209
    benefits, 209
    history, 208–9
    practice, 210
somatic practices, 215–41
    defined, 215
    experiencing, 217
    theoretical foundations, 216–17
somatorespiratory integration, 210–11
    history and practice, 210–11
Sossin, Mark, 96
sound
    eurythmy and, 224–25
    mantra yoga and, 272
sounding, 100–102
    benefits, 101–2
    history, 100
    practice, 101
sound therapy. See sounding; Tomatis
    method
Spatial Dynamics, 216, 236–38
    benefits, 138
    philosophy, 237–38
    practice, 238
Speads, Carola, 201, 207
Spencer, Herbert, 42
spinal adjustments, chiropractic, 33–35
spirit world, 1
Spitler, Harry, 79, 96, 97
spontaneity, 373
Steiner, Rudolf, 216, 224–25, 238
Still, Andrew Taylor, 30, 36, 40–41, 42
Stone, Randolph, 115–16
stress, 204, 218–19
    meditation and, 283
    rebirthing and, 380

structural integration, 149. See also Rolfing
subluxation of vertebrae, 34
subtle energy
    locating and alleviating blockages,
        106–7
    research on, 107
subtle energy practices, 105–28
    defined, 105
Summers, Elaine, 201–2
Sutherland, William, 35–36
Suzuki, Daisetz Teitaro, 282
Swedish massage, 131, 133, 155–57
    basic techniques, 156
    benefits and risks, 156–57
    history, 155–56
    practice, 156
Sweigard, Lulu, 200
symptoms, alternative model view of, 3, 8

T

taekwondo, 265–68
    basic principles, 266
    benefits, 267
    history, 265–66
    practice, 266–67
t'ai chi ch'üan, 215, 216, 232, 239–41, 245
    benefits, 240–41
    history, 239
    philosophy, 239–40
    practice, 240
Takata, Hawayo, 122
tantric yoga, 273
Taoism, 110–11, 165, 176, 215
Tappan, Francis M., 129
Taylor, Charles Fayette, 131
Taylor, George Henry, 131
Teeguarden, Iona Marsaa, 162, 167–69
therapeutic touch (TT), 126–28
    benefits, 128
    history, 127
    practice, 127–28
    theoretical basis, 127
Tillich, Paul, 356
Todd, Mabel Elsworth, 180, 200
Tomatis, Alfred, 79, 102–3
Tomatis method, 79, 102–4
    benefits, 104
    history, 102–3

touch, 105, 106, 117, 133, 367
    infant massage and, 139–40
    therapeutic touch (TT), 126–28
traditional Chinese medicine (TCM),
        2, 20–25, 60, 159, 160, 162, 164–65, 166,
        173, 175, 176. *See also* acupressure;
        acupuncture
    basic principles, 22–23
    benefits and risks, 24
    diet and, 47–48
    finding practitioners of, 24
    herbology, 23
    history, 20–22, 173
    practice, 23–24
Trager, Milton, 180, 212
Trager psychophysical integration, 211–14
    basic principles, 212–13
    benefits and risks, 213
    history, 212
    practice, 213
trance states, 68, 69
Transcendental Meditation, 272, 283,
        288–90
    basic principles, 288–89
    history, 288
    practice and benefits, 289–90
transpersonal psychology, 361–62
Travell, Janet, 145
tui na, 162, 175–77
    basic principles, 176
    benefits and risks, 177
    history, 175
    practice, 176–77

U

Ueshiba, Morehei (O Sensei), 247
unconscious mind, 338, 376
unergy, 383
    theory and practice, 383
Upledger, John E., 36, 37
Usui, Mikao, 121–22, 123

V

Valnet, Jean, 81
vata, 4, 5
Vazquez, Steven, 97
vision, 86. *See also* Bates method;
        behavioral vision therapy;

Meir Schneider self-healing method
        development of, 97
visualization, 66, 272, 383. *See also*
        guided imagery
    shamanism and, 17
    yantra yoga and, 272
vitamins. *See* orthomolecular medicine
voice, 100–101, 179, 225, 307

W

Waldorf School, 225, 226, 238
Walling, William, 341
water. *See* hydrotherapy
Watts, Alan, 207, 282
well-being, physical, mental, emotional
        and spiritual, 26–27
wellness/wellness programs, 25–27
    ayurveda and, 4
    basic principles, 25–26
    benefits, 27
    body, mind, and spirit and, 25–26
    concept of, 25
    history, 25
    holistic health view, 7, 8
    lifestyle and, 7
    origination of concept, 41
    paradigm, 25–26
    practice, 27
    services, 26
Wells, David, 85
Wertheimer, Max, 355
Western thought
    Aristotle and, 2
Whitehouse, Mary, 313, 316
Wilber, Kenneth, 360
Williams, Bill, 180, 208–9
Williams, Ellen Gregory, 180, 208–9
Williams, Roger, 57
Winternitz, William, 93
women
    homeopathic physicians, 12
    in osteopathy, 41
writing. *See* journal therapy; poetry
        therapy

Y

yantra yoga, 272
yin and yang energy, 22, 110–11, 165

yoga, 61, 269–79
    benefits, 274
    hatha yoga, 60
    history, 269–70
    integral, 276–77
    practice in West, 273–74
    spiritual goal of, 271
    systems of, 271–73
yoga therapy, 274

Z

Zen Buddhism, 256
zen meditation, 282
Zen sitting, 283
Zero Balancing, 31, 44–46, 132
    benefits, 45–46
    defined, 44
    history, 44
zone therapy, 147